Controlled Release Polymeric Formulations

Controlled Release Polymeric Formulations

D. R. Paul, EDITOR
University of Texas

F. W. Harris, EDITOR
Wright State University

A symposium jointly sponsored by

the Division of Organic Coatings and

Plastics Chemistry and the Division of

Polymer Chemistry at the 171st Meeting

of the American Chemical Society,

New York, N.Y., April 7–9, 1976.

ACS SYMPOSIUM SERIES **33**

AMERICAN CHEMICAL SOCIETY

WASHINGTON, D. C. 1976

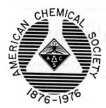

Library of Congress CIP Data

Controlled Release Polymeric Formulations.

(ACS symposium series; 33, ISSN 0097-6156)

Includes bibliographical references and index.

1. Polymers and polymerization—Congresses. 2. De-layed-action preparations—Congresses.

I. Paul, Donald R., 1939–   . II. Harris, Frank W., 1942–   . III. American Chemical Society. Division of Organic Coatings and Plastics Chemistry. IV. American Chemical Society. Division of Polymer Chemistry. V. Series: American Chemical Society. ACS symposium series; 33.

QD381.8.C66   661'.8   76-29016
ISBN 0-8412-0341-5   ACSMC8 33 1–317   (1976)

ACS Symposium Series

Robert F. Gould, *Editor*

FOREWORD

The ACS SYMPOSIUM SERIES was founded in 1974 to provide a medium for publishing symposia quickly in book form. The format of the SERIES parallels that of the continuing ADVANCES IN CHEMISTRY SERIES except that in order to save time the papers are not typeset but are reproduced as they are submitted by the authors in camera-ready form. As a further means of saving time, the papers are not edited or reviewed except by the symposium chairman, who becomes editor of the book. Papers published in the ACS SYMPOSIUM SERIES are original contributions not published elsewhere in whole or major part and include reports of research as well as reviews since symposia may embrace both types of presentation.

CONTENTS

PREFACE

The "controlled release" concept has made significant advances in the last decade because of substantial research efforts by private companies, institutions, and governmental agencies directed towards solving some specific problems by this method. While there are many recognized uses of controlled release, most of the above-mentioned programs have been concerned with either the prolonged delivery of drugs at optimal rates or control of a wide range of pests with minimal pollution of the environment. Previous symposia have focused on these application areas. A number of common techniques or concepts applicable to the different areas of application have emerged, each of which employs polymeric materials as a vital part of the controlled release mechanism. Therefore, controlled release technology has become a new area in which to apply or develop interesting concepts of polymer chemistry and engineering.

It was timely to organize a symposium on controlled release within the two divisions of the American Chemical Society most concerned with polymer chemistry and engineering for the purpose of focusing on the polymer-related aspects of this subject. The contents of this book are based on 25 of the 28 papers presented at this symposium. An attempt was made to include papers that traversed the spectrum from fundamentals to commercial products while also covering a wide range of applications and techniques. The individual papers deal with the role of the polymer to varying levels of detail, but the overall objective is served by the total collection of papers.

The manuscripts for this book were collected several weeks after the symposium so that the authors could incorporate their most recent results and take cognizance of the discussions that took place at the symposium. An introductory chapter, not presented at the symposium, is included here primarily as background and perspective for the reader who is new to this field and wishes to use this book as a beginning point to learn the state of the art in controlled release technology.

University of Texas   D. R. PAUL
Austin, Texas 78712
May 10, 1976

Polymers in Controlled Release Technology

D. R. PAUL

Department of Chemical Engineering, University of Texas, Austin, Texas 78712

Controlled release technology emerged actively from the 1960's with promises to solve a diversity of problems that have in common the application of some active agent to a system with the objective of accomplishing a specific purpose while avoiding certain other possible responses this agent might cause. A number of techniques for effecting controlled release have been identified and analyzed, and most of these have been considered for or embodied in commercial devices or formulations which already are or soon will be on the market. Most of these concepts have been described in the literature (patents, journals, books, etc.) The proceedings of previous symposia (1-3) and recent reviews (4-16) provide a rapid way to learn the present state of the art of this technology. One of the common features of many of these techniques or formulations is the judicious selection of a polymeric material to act as a rate controlling device, container, or carrier for the agent to be released. The contents of this book are the results of an American Chemical Society Symposium organized primarily to emphasize the role of the polymer and its selection as opposed to focusing on a particular application or methodology although aspects of the latter are included by necessity. The polymer choices in some cases are the result of sophisticated considerations while in others evolution from historical successes had dictated this selection. Both extremes illustrate the considerable opportunity for tailoring polymers to meet the demands of this developing technology.

The purposes of this introductory chapter are to make this book somewhat more autonomous and, therefore,

hopefully of more value to the reader by placing
its contents in perspective by reviewing briefly
previous developments in concepts, techniques, principles, areas of application, and commercial products.
This purpose is largely fulfilled by including in
the bibliography a compendium of symposium proceedings, review articles, books, and other references
which have been selected to provide the reader with a
quick introduction to the literature of this field.
From these references and the comments that follow,
the reader will see that the present papers deal with
only some of the concepts which have developed in
this area although a broad and important sampling is
represented.

Rationale for Controlled Release

Conventionally, active agents are administered
to a system by non-specific, periodic application.
For example, in medicine drugs are introduced at
periodic intervals by ingestion of pills, liquids,
etc. or by injection and then distributed throughout
much of the body rather than directed to a specific
target. Similarly in agricultural practice, fertilizers, pesticides and the like are distributed to
crops at periodic intervals by broadcasting, spraying, etc. Immediately following these application
pulses the concentration of the active agent rises
to high levels system-wide. In some cases, these
initially high concentrations may produce undesired
side effects either to the target area of the system
and/or the environment around the target. As time
passes after this spike of active agent, its concentration begins to fall because of natural processes
such as elimination from the system, consumption, or
deterioration. Before the next application, the
concentration of the active agent may fall below the
necessary level for the desired response. Thus
periodic applications are frustrated by concentrations of active agent which may be alternately too
high or too low within the same cycle when the time
between doses is long while on the other hand more
frequent application of smaller doses results in
more inconvenience and expense of application. In
addition, a cyclic regime is usually rather ineffi-
cient in that a considerable fraction of the active
agent never gets to perform the intended function
either because of deterioration or loss to the system

environment. In many cases the latter may be quite
serious, and in all cases both factors inflate the
cost of the treatment. Certainly a more desirable
regime would be to release the active agent at a controlled rate that maintains its concentration in the
system within optimum limits, and it would be even
better to release this agent directly to the target
area of the system if one exists or can be identified.
The latter are the objectives of controlled release
technology in general whether the active agent is a
drug, pesticide, or sex attractant or whether the
purpose is to control the growth of weeds or to prevent barnacles from forming.

Areas of Application

Controlled release technology has been considered
for a wide variety of applications of which a large
fraction are either medically related or for pest
control. Some of the papers incorporated in this
book are general in scope and the formulations or
principles discussed might be applicable to a number
of different areas; however, most deal with particular objectives. It is of interest, therefore, to
summarize these objectives here and to mention examples of other specific problems of active interest
which are not dealt with in this book.
In the medical area, contraception or fertility
control has historically been one of the most publi-
cized applications, and this is reflected in the
papers which follow. However, also covered here more
briefly, are formulations to deliver narcotic antagonists, fluoride for dental purposes and drugs to com-
bat cancer and cardiac arrhythmia and a drug to induce hypertension for experimental studies. Many of
these papers deal with techniques of general applicability as drug delivery systems. An example of a
medical area not covered here is the recently commercialized device for control of glaucoma (8).
A number of the following papers deal with the
control of pests such as snails, weeds, marine fouling organisms, roaches, flys through the release of
toxicants or pheromones. None of the present papers
deal in detail with the release of fertilizers,
pesticides, or growth regulators for agricultural
purposes but activities in these areas are summarized
by one of the authors.

Techniques and Release Kinetics

One of the central problems in controlled release formulations is to combine the active agent with its carrier in an economical manner yet achieve a release profile that best fits the situation. These two desires are often in opposition of one another so compromises must be made. Frequently the desired release profile is a constant rate of delivery of the active agent which in analogy with chemical kinetics has become known as a "zero order" process since it does not depend on how much of the agent has been delivered or remains. Many of the formulations used in controlled release technology do not meet this objective. At this point it will be useful background to categorize as generally as possible the techniques of formulation that are employed in the subsequent papers and to discuss their inherent release kinetic characteristics. Following this, some other techniques not employed here will be mentioned.

The classification scheme preferred here divides the devices of interest into the following basic types which in some cases may be combined in various ways:

I. Erodible Devices that Disappear

In this category the active agent is released as the carrier is eroded away by the environment through physical processes such as dissolutioning or by chemical processes such as hydrolysis of the polymer backbone or crosslinks. The kinetics of release cannot be simply stated since they depend on the details of the erosion mechanism and geometry. The central distinction is the complete disappearance of the device in time which has obvious advantages providing the erosion products are of no health or environmental concern.

II. Membrane Encapsulated Reservoir Devices

In this category a rate controlling membrane completely encloses a cavity which contains the active agent appropriately dispersed. These systems have also been referred to as depot devices (8). The membrane may be porous or non-porous, and in the case of the latter the environmental fluids may or may not appreciably swell the membrane. The most useful situation is when the reservoir contains a suspension of the active agent in a fluid since this will maintain a

constant activity of the agent in the reservoir until
the excess has been removed. This situation creates
a constant steady-state release rate by diffusion
across the membrane as illustrated below for an idealized situation:

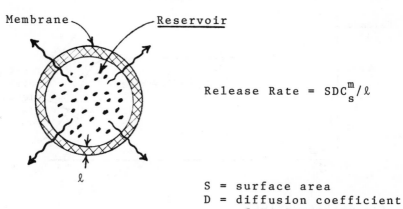

Release Rate = SDC_s^m/ℓ

S = surface area
D = diffusion coefficient
of active agent in
membrane

C_s^m = solubility of active
agent in membrane

If the active agent is totally dissolved in the
reservoir fluid, then its activity will change and the
release rate will decay more or less exponentially
with time as expected for "first order" kinetics.
These devices may be rather large (macroencapsu-
lation) or very small in which case <u>microencapsulation</u>
is the usual terminology (10-16).
In general the release profile for encapsulated
systems has the form shown by the graph at the top of
the next page. The duration and rate for each of the
three stages shown can usually be engineered within
certain limits by the design of the device.
A special case of encapsulated devices depends on
rupture of the membrane by some mechanical action to
release the active agent (13).

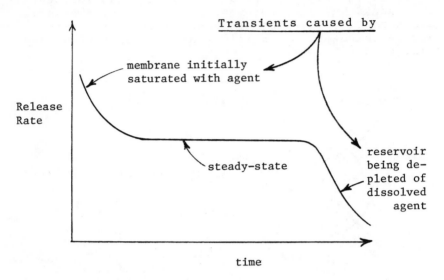

III.   Matrix Devices

In this type of system there is no membrane per
se but rather the active agent is dispersed in a
carrier - usually a polymer - from which it is ultimately extracted.   These have also been referred to as
monoliths (8) and have obvious advantages of fabrication, but generally they do not yield "zero order"
release kinetics.   Matrix devices may be divided into
two categories depending on the mechanism by which the
agent is released:

A.   Release Caused by Simple Diffusion of Agent.
In this case the active agent always has some mobility
within the carrier and its release depends on the jux-
taposition of a suitable exterior sink.   We can
further divide this category depending on whether the
initial loading per unit volume of the agent within
the matrix, A, exceeds the agent's solubility in the
matrix, C_s, or not

1. $A < C_s$

For this situation all of the agent at equil-
brium is dissolved in the matrix and release involves
its diffusion from the device following simple notions
similar to desorption as treated in most classical
works on diffusion (17-19, 22).   The total amount

released in time t, M_t, follows the usual $\sqrt{t}$ relation
as shown below until about 60% has been removed and
then the rate falls off more rapidly.

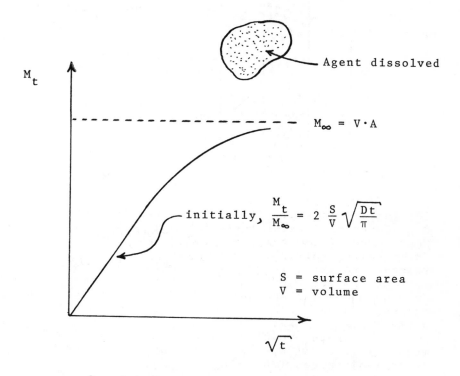

Agent dissolved

$M_\infty = V \cdot A$

initially, $\dfrac{M_t}{M_\infty} = 2 \dfrac{S}{V} \sqrt{\dfrac{Dt}{\pi}}$

S = surface area
V = volume

$\sqrt{t}$

2. $A > C_s$

    In this case, the excess agent above that which
is dissolved at equilibrium is dispersed in the matrix
as small particles. The details of the extraction may
be very complicated; however, for the usual case when
diffusion is rate limiting rather than other processes
such as dissolutioning, Higuchi (25,26) has shown that
a very simple but extremely clever pseudosteady-state
analysis describes the release rather accurately (30).
The figure at the top of the next page shows the physical picture envisioned. The mathematical result
Higuchi obtained for the release rate from planar
geometrics is

$$\text{Release rate} = S \sqrt{\dfrac{DC_s(A - 1/2\ C_s)}{2t}}$$

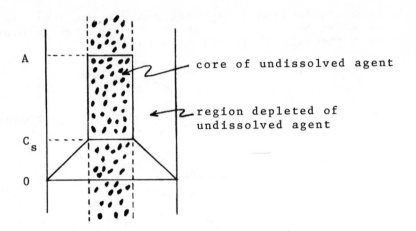

core of undissolved agent

region depleted of
undissolved agent

The release in this situation follows the same $\sqrt{t}$
dependence that exists when A < C_s; however, the
dependence of the rate on loading, A, is not the same.
While neither situation gives true "zero order"
release profiles, it is generally felt that the rate
characteristics can be made adequate for some purposes
by proper design, and this drawback must be weighed
against the ease and economy of fabricating such
devices.
    The Higuchi model has been extended to other geo-
metrical shapes (26, 27) and to include boundary
layer resistances (28, 30).

    B. Release Triggered by Ingression of Environ-
mental Agent.   In this case the agent may be dispersed within the matrix either physically or chemically bound to it, but in either case it is initially
not mobile - for physical dispersions this may be
owing to very small diffusion rates. Its release may
be triggered by the penetration of some environmental
agent, e.g. water, into the matrix. This event could
lead to a chemical reaction to unbind the agent, e.g.
hydrolysis, or simply to plasticize the matrix to
allow physically bound molecules to diffuse. The release rate may be controlled by the penetration of
the environmental agent or the reaction it produces
or some combination thereof and then the exact form
of the rate depends on the details of the particular
system. This class of devices differs from erodible
systems in that the matrix remains physically intact.

IV. Reservoir Devices Without a Membrane

This final category of devices covered in this book confines the active agent in a reservoir but does not employ any membrane to control its release. A simple example is hollow fibers which hold the agent in their bore and release it by diffusion through the air layer above the agent in the bore. A somewhat more complex example is porous networks in which the agent is physically imbibed into the pores and released by diffusion through the fluid which fills these pores. Strictly speaking this configuration might also be thought of as a matrix device. Both of these examples ordinarily may be expected to follow a $\sqrt{t}$ type release pattern although external factors may moderate the diffusion and change the release profile. This is true for all of the other devices described earlier, and it is not uncommon for the external resistances to make systems composed of devices with an intrinsic $\sqrt{t}$ release profile approach "zero order" kinetics.

The above concepts are discussed in one form or another in the papers which follow. There are concepts which have been or could be used that are not included in this book and "osmotic pumps" (8,29) are an important example.

Role of the Polymer

As mentioned earlier, one of the objectives of this book is to focus on the function and selection of the polymer used in the controlled release formulation. The requirements of the polymer are obvious in some cases but it is useful to summarize here what a few of the considerations in its selection might be:

1. Diffusion and solubility characteristics with the active or environmental agents to provide the desired release control (see e.g. 19,20,21,23,24,31).

2. Compatibility with the environment (e.g. not toxic or antagonistic in medical applications).

3. Stability in the environment (should not degrade or change undesirably).

4. Compatibility with the active agent (no

undesirable reactions or physical interactions).

5.   Mechanical properties.

6.   Ease of fabrication.

7.   Cost.

Testing: Laboratory Versus Field

In developing controlled release formulations it
is inevitably cheaper to do initial testing in a
laboratory under controlled conditions that match
closely the application situation (in vitro in
medical terminology), but ultimately field testing
under actual circumstances (in vivo in medical
terminology) is necessary. In medical applications
in vivo use may involve placing the device in the
body by insertion through a body orifice, ingestion,
implantation, injection, or by application to the
skin. The papers that follow deal with various
stages of testing and in some cases direct comparisons between them are made. It is useful to summarize here a few of the factors that could contribute
to different performance in the field than the
laboratory:

1.   External hydrodynamic boundary layers. In
     the lab these can be extremely well con-
     trolled compared to the field. Frequently
     in the lab these are made small intentional-
     ly in order to study the intrinsic charac-
     teristics of the device. In the field these
     effects may be different than in the lab and
     in fact may be variable in time. The conse-
     quences may be dramatic. For example, a
     matrix device may show a $\sqrt{t}$ release pattern
     in the lab where the external boundary layer
     effect is small, but in the field a "zero
     order" release rate could be observed (28)
     because this effect is large - and this
     could be advantageous!

2.   Environmental factors not considered in the
     lab: wind, sun (e.g. UV degradation),
     temperature fluctuations, interference by
     environmental chemicals and organisms, etc.

3. Fabrication Variability. Generally formu-
    lations for laboratory testing are made by
    hand or by proto-type processes whereas
    field testing requires scale-up of the pro-
    cess to commercial or near-commercial con-
    ditions. This may produce differences or
    variabilities not anticipated.

Commercial Products

In spite of the relatively short life of controlled release technology, a number of commercial
products have already been introduced. The following
Table I summarizes a sampling of these products. It
is still too early to know much about what the fate
of this technology will be in the market place, but
the next few years should be interesting. Several of
the papers included here deal with devices which are
already commercial or soon will be. As a consequence,
some do not delve deeply into the more interesting
technical details owing to understandable proprietary
restraints.

Literature Cited
Proceedings of Major Symposia on Controlled Release

1. Tanquary, A.C. and Lacey, R.E., Editors, Con-
    trolled Release of Biologically Active Agents,
    Vol. 47 of Advances in Experimental Medicine and
    Biology, Plenum Press, N.Y., 1974.
2. Cardarelli, N. F., Editor, Controlled Release
    Pesticide Symposium, The University of Akron, 1974.
3. Harris, F. W., Editor, Proceedings 1975 Inter-
    national Controlled Release Pesticide Symposium,
    Wright State University, Dayton, Ohio, 1975.

Books and Reviews on Controlled Release

4. Williams, A., Sustained Release Pharmaceuticals,
    Noyes Development Corp., Park Ridge, N.J., 1969.
5. Allan, G. G., Chopra, C. S., Friedhoff, J. F.,
    Gara, R. I., Maggi, M. W., Neogi, A. N., Roberts,
    S. C., and Wilkens, R. M., "Pesticides, Pollution,
    and Polymers", CHEMTECH (1973), 3, 171-178.
6. Colbert, J. C., Controlled Action Drug Forms,
    Noyes Data Corp., Park Ridge, N.J., 1974.
7. Cardarelli, N. F., "Concepts in Controlled Re-
    lease - Emerging Pest Control Technology",
    CHEMTECH (1975), 5, 482-485.

Table I

Some Commercial Controlled Release Products

Trade Name	Company	Comments
NOFOUL	B. F. Goodrich	Antifouling rubber coating. Matrix device (some versions employ a membrane in addition)
NO-PEST STRIP	Shell	A matrix device for release of insecticide
HERCON DISPENSER	Health-Chem	A laminated membrane device for release of pesticide and other agents
PRECISE	3M	Microencapsulated fertilizer
OSMOCOAT	Sierra	Microencapsulated fertilizer
PENNCAP-M	Pennwalt	Microencapsulated methyl parathion insecticide
OCCUSERT	Alza	Laminated membrane device for release of pilocarpine in the eye for glaucoma control
PROGESTASERT	Alza	A membrane reservoir device for release of progesterone in the uterus for birth control
BioMET SRM	M&T	A matrix device for release of a molluscicide
INCRACIDE E-51	International Copper Research Association	A matrix device for release of a molluscicide

⋆ 8. Baker, R. W. and Lonsdale, H. K., "Controlled
      Delivery - An Emerging Use for Membranes",
      CHEMTECH, (1975), 5, 668-674.
  9. Cardarelli, N. F., Controlled Release Pesticides
      Formulations, CRC Press, Cleveland, Ohio, 1976.

       Books and Reviews on Microencapsulation

 10. Chang, T. M. S., Artificial Cells, C. C. Thomas,
      Springfield, Ill., 1972.
 11. Gutcho, M., Capsule Technology and Microencapsu-
      lation, Noyes Data Corp., Park Ridge, N. J., 1972.
 12. Vandegaer, J. E., Editor, Microencapsulation-
      Processes and Applications, Plenum Press, New
      York, 1974.
 13. Fanger, G. O., "What Good Are Microcapsules",
      CHEMTECH, (1974), 4, 397-405.
 14. Goodwin, J. T. and Somerville, G. R., "Microen-
      capsulation by Physical Methods", CHEMTECH,
      (1974), 4, 623-626.
 15. Chang, T. M. S., "Artificial Cells", CHEMTECH,
      (1975), 5, 80-85.
 16. Thies, C., "Physicochemical Aspects of Microen-
      capsulation", Polymer-Plast. Technol. Eng., (1975),
      5(1), 1-22.

       Selected Books and Reviews on Diffusion

 17. Barrer, R. M., Diffusion In and Through Solids,
      Cambridge Univ. Press, London, 1941.
 18. Jost, W., Diffusion in Solids, Liquids, and Gases,
      Academic Press, N. Y., 1960.
 19. Crank, J. and Park, G. S., Editors, Diffusion in
      Polymers, Academic Press, N. Y., 1968.
 20. Flynn, G. L., Yalkowsky, S. H., and Roseman,
      T. J., "Mass Transport Phenomena and Models:
      Theoretical Concepts", J. Pharmaceutical Sci.,
      (1974), 63, 479-510.
 21. Hopfenberg, H. B., Editor, Permeability of
      Plastic Films and Coatings to Gases, Vapors, and
      Liquids, Vol. 6 of Polymer Science and Technology
      Plenum Press, N. Y., 1974.
 22. Crank, J., The Mathematics of Diffusion, 2nd Ed.,
      Clarendon Press, Oxford, 1975.

Specific References

23. Chemburkar, P. B., "Evaluation, Control, and Prediction of Drug Diffusion Through Polymeric Membranes", Ph.D. Dissertation, Univ. of Fla., 1967.
24. Neogi, S. A. N., "Polymer Selection for Controlled Release Pesticides", Ph.D. Dissertation, Univ. of Washington, 1970.
25. Higuchi, T., J. Pharm. Sci., (1961), 50, 874.
26. Higuchi, T., J. Pharm. Sci., (1963), 52, 1145.
27. Roseman, T. J., and Higuchi, W. I., J. Pharm. Sci., (1970), 59, 353.
28. Chien, Y. W., Lambert, H. J. and Grant, D. E., J. Pharm. Sci., (1974), 63, 365 and 515.
29. Theeuwes, F., J. Pharm. Sci., (1975), 64, 1987.
30. Paul, D. R. and McSpadden, S. K., J. Membrane Sci., (1976), 1, 33.
31. Michaels, A. S., Wong, P. S. L., Prather, R., and Gale, R. M., A.I.Ch.E. J., (1975), 21, 1073.

Structural Factors Governing Controlled Release

C. E. ROGERS

Department of Macromolecular Science, Case Western Reserve University,
Cleveland, Ohio 44106

Polymer membranes have been used extensively over the years as protective permeation barriers such as coatings or packaging films. More recently, polymer membranes have been developed to serve as specific media for the separation of penetrant mixtures by reverse osmosis desalination, hyperfiltration, dialysis, ion exchange, etc. A realm of applications which now is achieving both credence and feasibility is the use of polymer materials, usually in membrane form, as media for controlled dispensing of active chemical or biological agents. The range of present and potential applications in industrial, biomedical, agricultural, and other fields is very impressive.

The concept and practice of controlled release from membrane systems encompasses many types and mechanisms of release kinetics and application specifications. The slow release technique, whereby a dissolved or dispersed agent is desorbed from a suitable matrix over a prolonged period of time, has been used for many applications over the years. Sustained release systems, in which a nearly constant desorption rate is maintained over prescribed time periods, have been developed over the past few years with some commercial products now on the market. Examples, variations, and combinations of these, as well as other, often quite novel systems, have been well documented in the literature (1-3, and references therein).

Major factors affecting controlled release systems are well recognized. The often overriding effects of boundary layer phenomena and/or membrane fouling are serious problems. The mathematical representation and analysis of transport and solution behavior have proceeded on many levels of sophistication with consequent cycles of confusion and enlightenment. The development of viable systems has been perplexed by considerations of environmental compatibility, dependable quality control, and economics. There obviously is much work yet to be done.

The underlying basis of the behavior of all membrane systems - be they for barrier, permselective, or controlled release applications - is common insofar as the solution, transport,

and other properties of the materials are governed by the
physiochemical composition and structure of the components under
given environmental conditions. The phenomena of controlled release are similar (often identical) to those involved in plasticizer technology, environmental resistance of polymers, and related areas of polymer technology. The extensive investigations
in those areas, and in the science and technology of membrane
transport, per se, serve as both theoretical and practical guides
for an elucidation of controlled release systems (4-6).

The objective of certain of our past and present studies in
this area (6-13) has been to obtain a better understanding of the
interplay between solution and transport penetrants in terms of
variations in polymer composition, structure, and morphology.
These variations can be the result of changes in the original
nature of the polymer, or as a result of subsequent specific
chemical or physical modifications, or as a result of the
presence of the agent or other penetrant and/or other temporal or
spatial effects of the environment on the system during the
period of use. These studies have endeavored to utilize information from all of the areas mentioned as well as advances in our
knowledge of synthesis, characterization, and property analysis
of polymers. Most recently, we have been concerned primarily
with advantages and disadvantages of using multicomponent polymers for applications which can be related to controlled release.
The versatility of this wide class of materials gives an enhanced
degree of design flexibility for obtaining useful, perhaps
unique, systems.

With these concepts and objectives in mind, we will discuss
aspects of the general dependence of diffusion and solution
processes on various structural factors. We want to emphasize
certain underlying principles and phenomena common to many types
of application while, at the same time, calling attention to a
few otherwise neglected or misunderstood points. The feasibility
and benefits of controlled modifications in polymer structure is
a topic of particular interest. It is suggested that the onset,
time-dependence, or release rate of suitable systems can be
altered by use of polymers which undergo various transitions in
response to changes in temperature, relative humidity, or other
environmental factors. The development of viable controlled release systems can be based on these and related structural
factors with due consideration given to the effects of boundary
layer phenomena and environmental compatibility.

Factors Affecting Membrane Permeability

The general dependence of transport properties of homogeneous polymers on external experimental conditions (e.g., pressure
and temperature) and on internal structure and thermal history of
the polymer are fairly well established and predictable. On the
other hand, transport behavior of heterogeneous polymer membranes

(e.g., graded composition "asymmetric" membranes, ion-exchange
membranes, and chemical or structural composities or blends) is
much more complex and not as easily predictable. At the same
time, these membranes show the most promise for unique permeation/
release processes.

In all cases, the diffusion flow or flux, J, of a substance
in a mixture with other substances can be defined as the amount
passing during unit time through a surface of unit area normal to
the direction of flow, independent of the state of aggregation of
the mixture. In many cases of interest for release applications,
it is necessary to realize that the total flux may be a combination of a pure diffusive flux and a convective mass flow related
to the swelling of the polymeric matrix. Suitable corrections to
account for the frame of reference for such systems have been
discussed (4-6). These corrections seldom have been made in
practice so that the interpretation of most published data is subject to reappraisal in terms of inferences which are made on the
basis of concepts and theories for diffusive mechanisms of
transport.

For corrected pure diffusive flux, it can be shown (6) that
the flux in the steady-state (or pseudo-steady-state over relatively short time periods) can be expressed as:

$$J = -D^* \frac{d\ln a}{d\ln \bar{c}} \frac{d\bar{c}}{dc} \frac{dc}{dx} = -DK \frac{dc}{dx} \tag{1}$$

The diffusion coefficient D^* is a measure of the average mobility
of penetrant molecules within the diffusion medium. The apparent
Fick's Law diffusion coefficient is the product of the non-
negative mobility factor and a thermodynamic factor related to
the ideality of the penetrant-polymer mixture:

$$D = D^* \frac{d\ln a}{d\ln \bar{c}} \tag{2}$$

where a is the activity and $\bar{c}$ is the concentration of penetrant
in solution in the polymer phase.

When the mixture is a thermodynamically ideal solution,
$d\ln a/d\ln \bar{c}$ is unity. However, most mixtures exhibit deviations
from ideal behavior of a magnitude proportional to the concentration. The concentration dependence of D thus arises from two
sources: the concentration dependence of the mobility, which is
usually the dominant factor, and a concentration dependence
attributed to the nonideal nature of the system.

It is well to note that the thermodynamic term also can be
expressed as:

$$1 + \frac{d\ln \gamma}{d\ln \bar{c}} \tag{3}$$

where γ is the activity coefficient. If, for any reason, these thermodynamic terms become negative in sign, diffusion may occur against the concentration gradient. The presence of unstable phase regions within the diffusion medium, due, for example, to sudden local changes in temperature, composition, morphology or applied stress, will lead to this so-called "uphill" diffusion behavior which is phenomonologically similar to "activated" transport in the biological sense.

The distribution factor (solubility coefficient)

$$K = \frac{d\bar{c}}{dc} \qquad\qquad (4)$$

is a measure of the partitioning of penetrant between a polymer solution phase, $\bar{c}$, and an ambient penetrant phase, c. The latter phase may be the external phase to the membrane or the enclosed reservoir for desorption release. This Nernst-type distribution function is a parameter characterizing the penetrant-polymer system which may be a function of pressure or concentration as well as temperature.

The product of the mobility and distribution parameters can be defined as the permeability $\underline{P} \equiv DK$. It is to be emphasized that these expressions do not impose any restrictions as to the functional dependence of the parameter on experimental conditions. Interpretation of the significance of the parameters must be made in light of refined and realistic theories which take into consideration the nature of the system as regards dominant transport mechanism, frame of reference, boundary-layer effects, etc. At the very least, the parameters serve as phenomenological coefficients which describe the system under given conditions.

The actual migration of a penetrant molecule through a medium can be visualized as a sequence of unit steps or jumps under the influence of a concentration (chemical potential) gradient by a cooperative action of the surrounding complex of molecules during which the molecule passes over a potential barrier separating one position from the next. The precise details of the relative motions which occur during diffusion, as well as the molecular configurations of the resultant mixtures, are uncertain.

It is apparent that the physical and chemical properties of the components as well as the experimental conditions will govern the equilibrium site or hole concentration, its size distribution, and the height of potential barriers between successive sites. The ease of hole formation depends on the relative mobilities of penetrant molecules and polymeric chain segments as they are affected by changes in size, shape, concentration, and interaction between components. The other major factor affecting transport is the number, size, and distribution of defect structures, such as voids, capillaries, and domain boundaries, within the polymer matrix. The inherent morphological nature of the polymer, coupled with the particular fabrication and processing conditions, determine the detailed defect structure.

In relatively homogeneous polymers the dependence of permeability on the anticipated controlling factors can be stated quite generally. For example, the temperature dependence of permeability over reasonable temperature ranges can be represented by the Arhennius-type equation

$$\underline{P} = \underline{P}_0 \, \exp(-Ep/RT) \tag{5}$$

where Ep is the activation energy for permeation equal to the sum of the apparent activation energy for diffusion and the heat of solution. Consequently, any factor which acts to reduce the ease of hole formation for diffusion can be expected to decrease the overall rate of permeation. These effects are quite noticeable in studies of diffusion of a series of penetrants of increasing molecular size and shape since the overall transport process is extremely sensitive to the magnitude and size distribution of "holes" available per unit time and volume for diffusive jumps as determined by the inherent or modified polymer chain segmental mobilities.

The local segmental mobility or chain stiffness may be affected by chain interactions arising from hydrogen bonding, polar group interactions, or simple van der Waal's attractions. As the number of these groupings per unit chain segment length increases, the degree of interaction increases, the segmental mobility decreases, and therefore the permeation rate also decreases. These effects are especially pronounced for the case of symmetrical substitution of polar groups since the packing of adjacent chain segments is somewhat facilitated leading to more efficient interactions.

Other modifications (5-7) which serve to decrease chain segmental mobility, and therefore decrease permeation, are sufficiently high degrees of crosslinking, the presence of solid additives (fillers) onto which the polymer is strongly adsorbed, and the occurrence of crystalline domains within the polymer itself (5, 6). An increase in density and crystalline content results mainly in a corresponding decrease in solubility since crystalline regions are not generally accessible for sorption. However, the concurrent permeability decrease is substantially greater, indicating that the diffusion coefficient also is decreased, presumably because of the restraining effects of crystalline regions on local chain segmental motion in adjoining non-crystalline regions and a more tortuous path through the mixture of amorphous and crystalline domains.

The local chain segmental mobility of a polymer is enhanced by the presence of an added plasticizer, resulting in a lowering of the glass transition temperature of the polymer. The permeation of solvents in a polymer is similar in that the sorbed and diffusing solvent acts to "plasticize" the polymeric system. The

net result of the much higher sorbed concentrations of good
solvents in a polymer (a high K value) times the attendent plasti-
cizing action which increases the corresponding diffusion
coefficient is a marked increase in the overall permeation rate.

Typically, for low concentrations (up to about 10 percent by
weight) of a sorbed penetrant, where Henry's Law is reasonably
valid, the diffusion coefficient varies with concentration as:

$$D = D(c=o)\exp(\alpha c) \qquad\qquad (6)$$

where $D(c=o)$ is the extrapolated value of D at zero concentration
and α is a characteristic parameter which can be related, for
example, to the Flory-Huggins interaction parameter (5, 6). For
wider ranges of sorbed concentrations, better representations are
obtained in terms of solvent activity, a:

$$D = D(c=o)\exp(\alpha' a) \qquad\qquad (7)$$

This includes the regions of sorbed concentrations where Henry's
Law is no longer obeyed, but rather the sorption follows the
Flory-Huggins equation or the related expression (6, 7):

$$K = K(c=o)\exp(\sigma c) \qquad\qquad (8)$$

Combination of Equations 7 and 8 for the case when σ approaches
zero leads to Equation 6. Detailed theories have been proposed
to rationalize the observed concentration dependence of diffusion,
mainly in terms of free volume concepts (5 - 7), and to account
for the phenomena of penetrant cluster formation within the
polymeric matrix (5 - 8).

In most investigations of diffusion and solution in
polymers, the tacit assumption has been made that the accessible
regions are structurally homogeneous so that diffusion can be
considered to occur by a single activated mechanism within the
continuum. Recently, however, evidence has been presented for
the presence of a microporous structure in certain amorphous
polymers below or near their glass temperature, and in semi-
crystalline polymers above their glass temperature.

The distribution of void size and shape, dependent on the
manner of membrane preparation and fabrication, may range from
submicrovoids of the order of unit-cell dimensions to porosities
and cleavages of much greater dimensions with non-random configurations. These voids are to be distinguished from the free
volume associated with liquids or amorphous solids and their
magnitude is not a thermodynamic quantity. In glassy amorphous
polymers as the temperature is lowered below the glass temperature, the actual total volume occupied by a polymer becomes progressively greater than the equilibrium volume of an equivalent
liquid. Since segmental mobility is low, this volume difference
must result in the formation of different density regions on the

microscale. The less densely packed regions then correspond in
effect to voids within the surroundings more densely packed
matrix. This phenomenon may be even more pronounced for cellu-
losic polymers which exhibit very low rates of conformational rearrangement due to their inherent low segmental chain mobility.

The conditions of processing, such as casting temperature,
solution composition, and subsequent annealing treatments, will
have a marked effect on the microstructure of the membrane. In
many cases, the resultant structural heterogeneities can be considered as voids within the terms of the above discussion. The
void content will be characterized by a magnitude and size distribution which will then change with time as the membrane is
subjected to more extreme environmental conditions during its use.
The void distribution is directly related to the polymer chain
conformation statistics.

The effect of a microporous structure on the solubility and
transport properties depends on the continuity of path afforded
by the distribution of microvoids and on the nature of the penetrant contained within such voids. The presence of interconnected
micropores, small channels, cracks, or other flaws in polymer
structure permits convection of penetrant to occur through the
medium in addition to activated diffusion. Such capillary flow
does not show very pronounced differences for various penetrants
unless the diffusing molecule is of a dimension comparable with
that of the capillary.

For the case of a homogeneous distribution of non-inter-
connected microvoids the overall rate of transport would be
expected to increase somewhat owing to the smaller structural
packing density afforded by the presence of the lower density
void regions. However, when the cohesive forces between penetrant molecules are greater than the attractive forces between
penetrant and polymer, the incoming penetrant tends to cluster
within the polymer. With reference to the overall diffusion
flux, a molecule within a cluster generally will be less mobile
than an isolated free molecule owing to the additional energy required to break free from the cluster. A detailed discussion of
the dependence of the diffusion flux on cluster formation as it
varies with penetrant concentration, void content, time, and
other factors has been presented (6, 7).

A more fundamental and comprehensive approach to the general
problem of diffusion in multicomponent systems is afforded by the
theory of irreversible thermodynamics. The rate of flow of a
substance in such a system is dependent not only on its own
gradient of chemical potential (i.e., concentration gradient) but
also on the gradients of chemical potential of the other components as well as external force gradients (stress, electric
fields, temperature, etc.) For systems not far removed from
equilibrium, this interdependence may be assumed to be linear.
The resultant cross terms have been neglected or considered
negligible in almost all past investigations of diffusion.

However, these terms certainly are significant in many cases, such
as in so-called "active" biological transport, and therefore
should be included to obtain a more complete understanding of
diffusion phenomena.

Modification of Polymer Structure and Properties

An aspect of particular interest, and some promise of uniqueness
and utility, is the change of polymer composition, structure, and
morphology as a function of time under, or following, a change of
environmental conditions. If and when these changes can be prescribed by initial selection and fabrication procedures it could
allow a further element of control over the desired transport release properties.

The modification of polymer structure, where the term
structure is used in its widest context, can be achieved by a
number of methods and procedures. Three general considerations,
with some overlap in definition, are composition, morphology, and
geometry. This is especially evident for the case of multicomponent materials where one can alter chemical compositions, propor-
tions, and spatial arrangements of the components. This includes
polymer blends, fillers and other additives, and copolymers.
Particularly attractive classes of materials are graft and block
copolymer systems which allow the possibility of making nearly
independent changes in polymer composition and morphology (12).

The solution and diffusion properties of certain membrane
materials can be drastically altered by careful graft copolymerization procedures. It is possible to prepare series barriers,
permselective control layers, internal blocking, or enhanced
sorption volumes by the control of the grafting process. The
synthesis of spatially asymmetric composition membranes gives
materials with useful directional swelling and transport
properties (10).

The dependence of polymer membrane permeation properties on
the nature of grafted polymer chain length, conformation, and
domain formation have been elucidated using several membrane
materials subjected to controlled graft copolymerization procedures. (11) Improved permeation barrier characteristics of
poly(isoprene-g-methylmethacrylate) to inert gas penetrants were
found for short chain or densified graft domains as compared with
long chain or extended domains. In another study (13), it was
found that the presence of short graft chains acts as relatively
inert filler, or excluded volume by chain packing effect, more
effectively than does longer graft chains. The short chains are
considered to be distributed along the backbone chain allowing a
more efficient packing and structural densification than do the
relatively isolated compacted long chain domains even though
those local domains may be more impermeable, per se. The detailed dependence of solubility and diffusion coefficients on the
nature of the graft copolymerization process and the related

variations in polymer structure and composition shed further
light on the mechanism of transport and property-structure
relationships.

A comparison of the effects of graft content on diffusion
and solution processes suggests that the dominant effect of grafting, in the system under study, is to impede the migration of
penetrant rather than cause much variation in the equilibrium
amount or distribution of penetrant molecules within the polymer.
Effectively the same number of sorption sites exist but these
sites are less readily accessible. The minor change in sorption
level further suggests that sorption is probably taking place in
an environment quite similar to that in the original elastomer
sample. The effects of excluded sorption site volume or overall
change in site energies, related to chemical composition and
interaction variations, are not apparent. These considerations
lead to the proposition that the graft polymer exists within
domains in the more readily accessible regions of the original
polymer. Their presence in those regions would be expected to
reduce the subsequent rates of penetrant transport without substantial changes in the eventual sorbed penetrant content.

Polymer blends, graft and block copolymer, filled or other
composite polymer systems offer definite advantages for formation
of controlled release systems. The discrete domain structure
characterizing these multicomponent, usually multiphase, systems
can be used as suitable solution/diffusion media or controlled
porosity media in which the system composition and morphology can
be altered to obtain favorable solubility and diffusivity behavior (12) suitable for enhanced release characteristics. A
dispersed, molecularly bonded domain structure within a continuous matrix corresponds to selective penetrant reservoirs within a
diffusion-controlling matrix. The inherent viscoelastic and
other mechanical properties of such systems contribute to the
overall solution/release behavior in contrast to many gross dispersed multiphase reservoir systems.

Control of the diffusion characteristics of the matrix, or
of a component domain parallel or normal to the release diffusion
axis, can be achieved by a number of techniques. Selective
chemical reactions such as direct substitution or surface laminate formation (surface grafting or plasma polymerization)
directly affect segmental mobility, density, interactions, etc.
Crosslinking, crystallinity, or the addition of reinforcing
fillers have similar effects. Orientation of surface structure,
for example, by controlled casting procedures, can have a profound effect on release characteristics (9).

Porosity in a polymer system can be achieved by variations
in fabrication procedures, selective leaching of soluble components (polymer blends or volatile diluent/plasticizers), or careful microdeformation of certain crystalline or glassy polymers.
The swelling of polymers under application environmental conditions in effect increases the porosity, hence the release rate.

This type of behavior is of considerable significance both for understanding the course of existing release systems and for the development of new systems with enhanced performance characteristics.

Temporal and Spatial Controlled Release Systems

It is considered advantageous if controlled release systems can be developed which will respond to given stimuli-triggers, so to speak. The use of glassy or semi-crystalline polymers which undergo transitions at fairly well defined temperatures is an example in point. The incorporation of suitable agents within such matrices can be achieved by normal methods. The release characteristics undergo sharp increases when the application temperature exceeds the transition temperature, especially in the case of the semi-crystalline polymer. Specimen continuity and geometry are easily preserved by moderate degrees of crosslinking which otherwise do not significantly affect either the transition behavior or solution/diffusion characteristics.

Another class of materials with this category of properties are those which undergo progressive swelling over prolonged time periods. Certain block copolymer systems, especially those with ionic domains connected to non-anionic domains, swell with gradual destruction of domain continuity under the influence of the (osmotic) swelling stress (12). The gradual, predictable, and controllable swelling can serve to increase the rate of desorption of contained materials as the concentration of materials decreases.

A final class of materials includes those subject to chemical, physical, or biological attack by environmental agents. Several systems have been developed or suggested with these characteristics including biodegradable, UV degradable, erodible, etc. One can speculate on the development of more sophisticated systems sensitive to trace stimuli-agents such as enzymes or changes in pH.

Conclusion

Examples of many of the above aspects of release characteristics by control of polymer composition, structure, morphology, and system geometry can be given. Modifications of these system variables can be achieved by careful selection, fabrication, and post-fabrication chemical and/or physical treatments. The use of multicomponent polymer media offers advantages for enhanced solution reservoir characteristics coupled with controlled diffusion release kinetics by changes in segmental mobilities, swelling and defect composition and distribution (porosity). The development of such composite membrane systems offers tangible benefits for various controlled release applications.

Literature Cited

1. Tanquary, A. C. and Lacey, R. E., eds., "Controlled Release of Biologically Active Agents," Vol. 47, Advances in Experimental Medicine and Biology, Plenum Press, New York, 1974.
2. Flynn, G. L., Yalkowsky, S. H., and Roseman, T. J., J. Pharm. Sci., (1974), 63, 479.
3. Proceedings of 1975 International Controlled Release Pesticide Symposium, Wright State University, 1975.
4. Crank, J., "Mathematics of Diffusion," Oxford, New York, 1956.
5. Crank, J. and Park, G. S., eds., "Diffusion in Polymers, Academic Press, New York, 1968.
6. Rogers, C. E., in "Physics and Chemistry of the Organic Solid State," D. Fox, M. Labes, and A. Weissberger, eds., Vol. 11, Wiley-Interscience, New York, 1965, Chap. 6.
7. Rogers, C. E. and Machin, D., CRC Critical Reviews of Macromolecular Science, (1972), 1, 245.
8. Machin, D. and Rogers, C. E., J. Polym. Sci. A2, (1972), 10, 887; (1973), 11, 1535; (1973), 11, 1555.
9. Sudduth, R. D. and Rogers, C. E., J. Polym Sci., Phys. Ed., (1974), 12, 1667.
10. Sternberg, S. and Rogers, C. E., J. Appl. Polym. Sci., (1968), 12, 1017.
11. Ostler, M. I. and Rogers, C. E., J. Appl. Polym. Sci., (1974), 18, 1359.
12. Ostler, M. I., Covitch, M., Chung, H. Y. and Rogers, C. E., to be published.
13. Rogers, C. E., Yamada, S., and Ostler, M. I., Polym. Sci. Tech., (1974), 6, 155.

3

Controlled Release from Erodible Slabs, Cylinders, and Spheres

H. B. HOPFENBERG

Department of Chemical Engineering, North Carolina State University, Raleigh, N.C. 27607

An extremely attractive class of controlled delivery devices is based upon the concept of an eroding host polymer which liberates an agent which is, potentially, active biologically. The agent may be dissolved, suspended, or dispersed within or chemically bonded to the host polymer. The device concept is based upon the premise that some zero-order process, either chemical, physical, or physico-chemical, will completely control the release kinetics. It is implicit, in the overall concept, that the rate determining process will occur at a boundary between essentially unaffected host polymer and previously swollen, degraded, or permeated material. The device functions ideally in the absence of boundary layers external to the device or within the previously degraded or swollen polymer. Specifically, it is assumed that diffusion of hydrolyzing or swelling water to the reaction site and elimination of active agent from this zone of reaction is extremely rapid compared with the rate determining process or processes occurring at this well defined boundary region.

Chemical relaxations controlling additive release from an implant device may be divided into two explicit categories. Neogi and Allan (1) have reviewed the concept of additives which are linked chemically to a host polymer whereby, consequent to placement, water penetrates the device hydrolyzing the chemical bond linking the would-be additive to the host polymer. It is assumed that migration of the liberated additive proceeds rapidly compared to the rate-determining chemical "relaxation" or "reaction" (2,3). Alternatively, chemically relaxing devices function as a consequence of chemical degradation of the host polymer, liberating biologically active compounds from the matrix of hydrolytically unstable host polymer (4-7). This concept requires, of course, that the degradation products of the host polymer be toxicologically acceptable to the organism or environment being treated by the delivery system.

The most simple physical relaxation might be dissolution of the host polymer thus liberating dissolved or suspended biologically active materials. If the dissolution proceeds at a constant

rate, a zero-order process would, therefore, ensue and controlled
and constant delivery might be anticipated.

In practice, erodible devices may actually be controlled by
more than one limiting mechanism. For instance, chemically eroding devices may be kinetically controlled by chemical reaction as
well as diffusion of either water to or by-product from the reaction site. Quite conceivably, the overall reaction constant
describing the rate-determining process may be an "apparent" constant which describes phenomenologically, a somewhat complex
overall mechanism. In any event, there are a wide variety of independent mechanisms that could result in controlled release of
additives from formed, erodible polymers. Although very stringent
physico-chemical requirements are imposed to obtain true "zero-
orderness;" a further, even more stringent geometrical requirement
is implicit in this particular device design.

For an erosion process which is, in fact, truly zero-order,
the eroding device will only deliver biologically active components at a controlled and constant rate if the device is a perfect
slab. Cooney has analyzed the somewhat related case of a surface-
controlled dissolution of pharmaceutical tablets and has suggested
various tablet geometries which would tend to stabilize the dissolution kinetics (8). The unified analysis presented here deals
with idealized delivery kinetics which would be expected from
eroding polymeric slabs, cylinders, and spheres which contain
dissolved, dispersed, or chemically bonded additive. Clearly, a
capsule-shaped device would be best described as a composite
cylinder and sphere and, therefore, the kinetics described here
should form the guidelines for rational device design and analysis.

Analysis

Analytical realtionships describing the kinetics of additive
release from erodible polymer formulations may be derived simply
if one assumes that there is a single zero-order process, characterized by a single rate constant, controlling the overall release
process. In general, this kinetic process might be characterized
by a rate constant, k_0, although it is not necessary to specify
the exact mechanism controlling the erosion process. Clearly this
erosion process could involve dissolution, swelling, chemical reaction of host polymer, or chemical reaction of ligands, binding
additive to a host polymer. Moreover, this phenomenological constant, k_0, could describe a process involving combinations of the
individual relaxations or, in special cases, could describe processes involving diffusion of reactant-water to or biologically
agent from the reaction zone. The models which are presented here
are useful for describing the kinetics of any erosion process regardless of the fundamental nature of the mechanism; however, the
models assume that the idealized release kinetics are not confounded by time dependent diffusional resistances internal to or
external from the eroding device.

Release Kinetics from Erodible Spheres. Consider the cross-section of a sphere undergoing erosion as presented in Figure 1. In the region $R \leq r \leq a$ erosion has already taken place and it is assumed that there are no diffusional resistances associated with the penetration of water, metabolites, or biologically active components within this region. In practice, this region may be totally eroded material as in the case of the dissolution or chemical degradation of the host polymer.

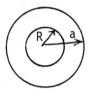

Figure 1. Cross-section of a spherical or cylindrical device which has eroded from position $r = a$ to a radial position R

Most importantly, however, the rate-determining relaxations--either chemical or physical relaxations which control the overall release kinetics--occur at position R at any specific time, t.
     If k_o is defined as the erosion constant which might have the units of $mg/hr-cm^2$, then the kinetic expression describing release from a sphere of radius a would be given by:

$$dM_t/dt = k_o 4\pi R^2 \qquad (1)$$

where M_t refers to the amount of biologically active material (mg) which is released from the device in a time t. The integral amount of biologically active material which is released from the device in time t, M_t will be given by the material balance:

$$M_t = (4\pi/3)C_o[a^3-R^3] \qquad (2)$$

where C_o refers to the uniform initial concentration of biologically active component which was originally dispersed or dissolved throughout the device prior to implantation and consequent exhaustion. C_o would be expressed in the consistent units; mg/cm^3.
     Since the rate determining relaxations which occur at the position R are carried out at an ever decreasing radius, corresponding to an ever decreasing area, a continuously decreasing release rate, dM_t/dt, results from a kinetic process which is, in fact, zero-order in a planar film geometry. If one substitutes the mass balance Equation (2), into the kinetic expression, Equa-

tion (1), one develops the following relationships consequent to the outlined algebraic simplifications:

$$\frac{d\,[4\pi C_0\,(a^3-R^3)]}{dt} = 3k_0\,4\pi R^2 \qquad (3)$$

Cancelling yields:

$$\frac{d(a^3-R^3)}{dt} = 3\frac{k_0}{C_0}\,R^2$$

differentiation and simplification provides:

$$dR/dt = (-k_0/C_0) \qquad (4)$$

Equation (4) justifies the intuitive notion that the relaxation front, positioned by the coordinate value R, moves toward the sphere center with a velocity equal to the relaxation constant, k_0, divided by the equilibrium additive concentration, C_0.

The algebraic relationship for R as a function of time is, therefore, given by

$$R = a - (k_0/C_0)t \qquad (5)$$

and is defined only for $0 \le t \le (C_0/k_0)a$.

Substituting (5) into (2) yields

$$M_t = \frac{4\pi C_0}{3}\,[a^3 - (a - \frac{k_0}{C_0}\,t)^3] \qquad (6)$$

and since

$$M_\infty = \frac{4\pi C_0 a^3}{3} \qquad (7)$$

where M_∞ is the amount of additive released consequent to exhaustion of the device, then:

$$M_t/M_\infty = 1 - [1 - \frac{k_0 t}{C_0 a}]^3 \qquad (8)$$

Equation (8) describes integral release kinetics whereby the fractional amount of additive released at time t (normalized to the amount of additive released at total exhaustion of the device), M_t/M_∞, does not increase linearly with time and therefore the device does not follow strict zero-order release kinetics. Accordingly, the rate of additive release decreases monotonically with time.

Release Kinetics from Erodible Cylinders. Consider the cross-section of a cylinder, perpendicular to the cylinder axis, undergoing erosion as described in Figure 1. Analogous to the spherical case, the region of $R \le r \le a$ is completely exhausted of additive which was originally distributed uniformly throughout the entire device at a concentration C_0. Conversely, at time t, in the region $0 \leq r \leq R$, there remains a uniform initial concentration of biologically active agent equal to C_0. There is, therefore, a discontinuity in concentration at the position r=R corresponding to the position at which the rate determining relaxations controlling delivery are occurring.

Employing the nomenclature k_0 to describe the relaxation constant, expressed in mg/hr-cm^2, the kinetic expression describing release from a cylinder of radius, a, is given by

$$dM_t/dt = k_0 2\pi RL \tag{9}$$

where L represents the length of the right cylinder. The amount of additive, M_t, released from the cylinder in time t will be given by

$$M_t = \pi[a^2 - R^2]LC_0 \tag{10}$$

Clearly, a continuously decreasing release rate, dM_t/dt results once again from a kinetic process which is, in fact, zero-order in planar film geometries. If one substitutes the mass balance Equation (10) into the kinetic expression, Equation (9), one develops the following equations consequent to the outlined algebraic simplifications:

$$d[\pi(a^2 - R^2)LC_0]/dt = k_0 2\pi RL \tag{11}$$

shich, upon cancelling, leads to

$$d[a^2 - R^2]/dt = k_0/C_0)2R \tag{12}$$

carrying out the differentiation, one obtains

$$dR/dt = -k_0/C_0 \tag{13}$$

Once again the intuitive notion is justified that the relaxation front, positioned by the coordinate value R, moves towards the cylinder center with a constant velocity equal to the relaxation constant k_0 divided by the equilibrium additive concentration C_0. The algebraic relationship for R as a function of time is therefore given by

$$R = a - (k_0/C_0)t \tag{14}$$

and is also defined only for

$$0 \leq t \leq (C_0/k_0)a \tag{15}$$

Substituting the previous equation into the original kinetic expression and recognizing that

$$M_\infty = \pi R^2 L C_0 \tag{16}$$

one obtains a result for the fractional amount of additive released, M_t/M_∞ by the following expression

$$M_t/M_\infty = 1 - [1 - k_0 t/C_0 a]^2 \tag{17}$$

Release Kinetics from Erodible Slabs. By inspection, one can write an expression for the fractional amount of additive released from a device as a function of the parameters k_0, C_0, a, and t given by Equation (18) where a is equal to the half-thickness of the slab:

$$M_t/M_\infty = k_0 t/C_0 a \tag{18}$$

An alternate form of this simple result would be

$$M_t/M_\infty = 1 - [1 - k_0 t/C_0 a] \tag{19}$$

One observes, therefore, that there is a simple unifying relationship describing additive release from spheres, cylinders, and slabs given by the expression:

$$M_t/M_\infty = 1 - [1 - k_0 t/C_0 a]^n \tag{20}$$

where n=3 for a sphere, n=2 for a cylinder, and n=1 for a slab. The symbol, a, represents the radius of a sphere or cylinder or the half-thickness of a slab.

Conclusions and Implications of the Analysis

The analytical models embodied in Equation 20 describe idealized release kinetics of additives from host polymers. The models assume that the rate determining relaxations are not confounded by diffusion of solubilizing, swelling or hydrolyzing water to the relaxation site nor by diffusional resistances involved with liberation of degradation by-products or biologically active agent from the zone of reaction. The kinetic responses resulting from slabs, cylinders, and spheres are compared. The derivations assume that the devices are physico-chemically identical, therefore, variation in overall release kinetics accrues soley from geometrical considerations, per se.

Constant delivery rate is only provided by slab-shaped devices. Delivery rates which decrease with time result from eroding cylinders and spheres even though the kinetic process providing the rate determining step is, in fact, zero-order.

These models are useful for calculating reaction or relaxation constant from integral release kinetics accruing from eroding spheres and cylinders. The true zero-orderness of an erosion mechanism can, in turn, be tested by comparing actual behavior with the models embodied in Equation (20). These models suggest that advanced device designs might provide for initial additive concentrations which are non-uniform thus compensating for the overall effects of device geometry. An approximation to perfectly zero-order kinetics afforded by the slab might be achieved by limiting the additive to the outer regions of spherical and cylindrical erosion-controlled delivery devices. Alternatively, more complex geometries involving hollow cylinders or cloverleaf shapes (8) will provide geometric compensation. Constant rate delivery will, therefore, result from these ideally functioning devices if they are not confounded by internal or external diffusional resistances. These more complex geometric entities will, in general, give rise to more serious boundary layer complications, however.

Literature Cited

(1) Neogi, A. N. and Allan, G. Graham, in "Controlled Release of Biologically Active Agents," ed. A. C. Tanquary and R. E. Lacey, pp. 195-224, Plenum Publishers, New York, 1974.

(2) Feld, W. A., Post, L. K., Harris, F. W., "Controlled Release from Polymers Containing Pesticides as Pendant Substituents," p. 113, Int'l. Control Release Pesticide Symp., Dayton, Ohio, 1975.

(3) Allan, G. G., Chopra, C. S., Neogi, A. N., and Wilkins, R. M., Nature (1971), 234, p. 349.

(4) Woodland, J. H. R., Yolles, S., Blake, D. A., Helrick, M., Myer, F. V., J. Med. Chem. (1973), 16, p. 897.

(5) Jackanicz, T. M., Nash, H. A., Wise, D. L., Gregory, J. B., Contraception (1973), 8, p. 227.

(6) Heyd, A., Kildsig, D. O., Banker, G. S., J. Pharm. Sci. (1969), 58, p. 586.

(7) Heller, J. and Baker, R. W., U. S. Patent #3, 811, 444 (May, 1974).

(8) Cooney, D. O., AIChE J. (1972), 18, p. 446.

Importance of Solute Partitioning on the Kinetics of Drug Release from Matrix Systems

T. J. ROSEMAN and S. H. YALKOWSKY

Pharmacy Research, The Upjohn Co., Kalamazoo, Mich. 49001

Controlled release drug-delivery devices provide a unique method to accurately meter the delivery rate of therapeutic agents to the patient. The dosage form is programmed to deliver drugs systemically or at their site of action in amounts that are needed to elicit the desired biological response. Controlled release offers greater convenience to the patient by reducing multiple dosing regimens and can provide more uniform blood concentrations of the drug than can be achieved with conventional routes of administration. This concept is illustrated in Figure 1 where sub-therapeutic and toxic dosing is eliminated by providing constant blood concentrations of the medicament (1).

Release rates are dictated by the design of the delivery system. Zero-order release occurs with reservoir devices which maintain a constant activity source of drug behind a rate controlling membrane. When the activity of the diffusing species is not constant, that is, it decreases with time, first order release rate profiles are expected. Monolithic devices containing dissolved or excess suspended drug yield release patterns which decline as the inverse of the square root of time (2). The drug properties and components of the delivery module must be carefully selected to provide the optimal release rate and yet assure acceptable physical and chemical stability of the system. Ideally, the drug should possess a short biological half-life and be relatively potent.

In general, researchers have elected to modify polymer properties to obtain the required release rate of the active species (3,4). Alternatively, the solute properties of the therapeutic agent can be favorably changed by making appropriate substituent modifications in the molecule. This last approach, which has received little attention, couples the pro-drug concept (5) into the design of the delivery system. Slight changes in the molecular structure of steroids, for example, can significantly alter their transport rates through silicone rubber (6,7). A systematic comparison of the data, however, is difficult because of variations in the design of the experiments among different investigators.

The purpose of this paper is to demonstrate the importance of lipophilic character, i.e., solubility behavior of the diffusing species, on the release mechanism. Esters of p-aminobenzoic acid are used as model compounds where alkyl chain length is systematically varied from the methyl to the heptyl ester. The in vitro release patterns are analyzed according to mathematical relationships which describe the kinetics of drug release from inert matrix systems.

The concept of controlled release is extended to a biological[a] system using vaginal rings containing medroxyprogesterone acetate[a]. The delivery system was designed to provide a continuous release of drug for extended time periods and is efficacious in inhibiting ovulation in humans (8). Serum drug concentrations and in vivo release profiles are quantitatively analyzed using the physical model approach. The relationship between in vitro and in vivo drug release kinetics is discussed.

EXPERIMENTAL

Synthesis of the propyl through heptyl esters of p-amino-benzoic acid were reported previously (9). The methyl, ethyl, and butyl esters were obtained commercially[b]. Purity of the esters were determined by gas-liquid[c] (GLC) chromatography. The chromato-grams exhibited a single peak. Melting points were in agreement with literature values (10). Medroxyprogesterone acetate had a labeled potency of 98% or greater. Compresssion distilled water and distilled in glass solvents were used throughout the study.

Preparation of Matrix Systems

Discs containing the appropriate ester of p-aminobenzoic acid were prepared by first levigating micronized drug into the mono-meric form of the silicone rubber[d]. After a uniform dispersion was obtained the mix was catalyzed with stannous octoate and placed into a specially designed circular dissolution holder having a depth of 0.25 cm and an exposed surface area of 10 cm^2 (Figure 2b). The holders were pressed against a plexiglass plate and the

---

[a] Provera, The Upjohn Company, Kalamazoo, MI 49001.
[b] Eastman, Rochester, NY 14650 (methyl and ethyl esters); Matheson, Coleman and Bell, Norwood, Ohio (butyl ester).
[c] Chromatographic conditions were: Hewlett Packard Model 402 Gas Chromatograph, 3% UCW-98, 80-100 mesh on Gas-Chrom Q (Applied Science Lab Inc., State Collete, PA 16801); 4 ft x 1/4 inch; detector - 270°C; column temperature for methyl to propyl was 120°C and for butyl to heptyl was 150°C; helium flow rate was 50 ml/min and hydrogen and air adjusted to maximize response.
[d] Silastic 382, Dow Corning, Midland, MI.

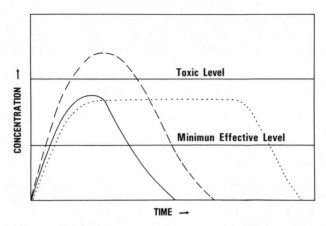

Figure 1.   Schematic representation of drug's blood concentra-
tion-time profile after oral administration (1). Key: —— standard dose; – – – – over dose; · · · · ideal dose.

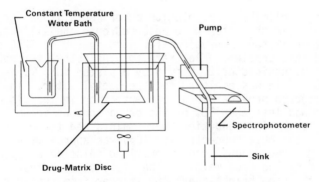

Figure 2a.   Sketch of complete dissolution apparatus

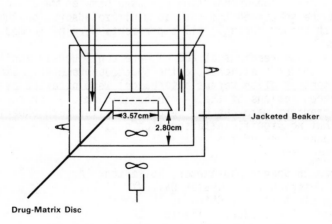

Figure 2b.   Detailed side view of dissolution cell

mix was cured at room temperature. Removal of the excess drug-
mix (flash) from the resultant disc of polymeric material was
facilitated by slightly undercutting the perimeter of the dissolution holder.

Vaginal rings (55 mm outside diameter and 36 mm inside diameter) containing 1% and 2% medroxyprogesterone acetate were prepared in a similar manner except that the mix was placed into
appropriately sized molds. Upon their removal, the rings were
deflashed.

Dissolution Procedure

An automated system was designed to measure the release of
the esters of p-aminobenzoic acid. A sketch of the apparatus is
shown in Figure 2a. Water (37°C) was pumped from a reservoir
through a 37°C controlled temperature dissolution compartment (100
ml), into a spectrophotometer [e], and then exited to a drain. The
path length of the spectrophotometric cell varied from 0.5 cm to
2.0 cm depending upon the release rate of the compound being
studied.

During preliminary dissolution experiments it was noted that
air bubbles from the water were adsorbed onto the silicone matrix.
Equilibration of the reservoir water containers, at 37°C overnight,
eliminated this problem. Flow rate for the methyl through hexyl
esters was maintained at 20 ml/min by a piston pump [f]. A flow
rate of 30 ml/min was employed for the heptyl ester. These rates
were selected to provide a drug concentration in the dissolution
media that was less than 10% of the drugs aqueous solubility.
Therefore ideal sink conditions were maintained throughout the
runs, i.e., the bulk concentration (C_B) was approximately zero.
A 300 R.P.M. synchronous motor [g] provided solution agitation below
the surface of the drug-matrix. The dissolution holder was adjusted to the same height above the stirrer from run to run. In
this way the hydrodynamics remained constant at all times. A
stainless steel tube connection was used between the dissolution
cell and the spectrophotometer, to minimize adsorption that could
occur with rubber tubing. All experiments were performed in
duplicate.

Absorbance readings at 285 nm were continuously monitored on
a chart recorder [h] attached to the spectrophotometer. Standard
curves (concentration versus absorbance) were obtained by pumping
known concentrations of the p-aminobenzoic acid ester through the
cell. Standards were checked before and after each experiment to
verify that no significant adsorption occurred in the pump or
tubing connections of the system.

---

[e] Beckman DB Spectrophotometer, Fullerton, CA.
[f] Fluid Metering Inc., Oyster Bay, NY 11771.
[g] Bodine Electric Co., Chicago, IL 60618.
[h] Beckman 10" recorder, Fullerton, CA.

Calculation of the Release Data

Figure 3 presents an example of the raw release data recorded from the spectrophotometer for 5% initial loading doses of the methyl and hexyl esters of p-aminobenzoic acid. The dissolution rates ($\frac{dQ}{dt}$) for a continuous flow system are expressed by the following equation (11):

$$\frac{dQ}{dt} = V \frac{dC}{dt} + FC \qquad \text{(Eq. 1)}$$

where:

V = volume in the dissolution compartment

dC/dt = change in concentration (C) with respect to time (t)

F = flow rate.

Integration of equation 1 from 0 to time, T, yields the cumulative amount of drug released (Q) per unit surface area as a function of time:

$$Q = VC_T + F \int_0^T Cdt \qquad \text{(Eq. 2)}$$

where; C_T is the solution concentration in the dissolution compartment at time, T.

RESULTS AND DISCUSSION

The mechanisms of drug release from inert polymeric matrix systems were reviewed by Baker and Lonsdale (2,12). Representative release rate-time profiles are shown in Figure 4. Zero-order, first-order, or time$^{-\frac{1}{2}}$ ($t^{-\frac{1}{2}}$) rate dependencies can be achieved depending upon the design of the delivery system. Reservoir devices, composed of a constant activity source of drug maintained behind a rate controlling membrane, provide release rates which are independent of time (zero-order). An exponential release pattern occurs when there is a non-constant source of drug in the reservoir and its thermodynamic activity decreases with time. Square root of time kinetics is predicted when the polymeric matrix contains molecularly dissolved drug, or suspended drug in equilibrium with dissolved drug. When only dissolved drug is present the square root of time function is operative during the first 60% of drug release which is then followed by a period of exponential decay. For the suspended or dispersed case where the total drug concentration is maintained at a value much greater than its solubility in the polymeric phase, the square root of time relationship is expected to be maintained throughout the time course of drug delivery.

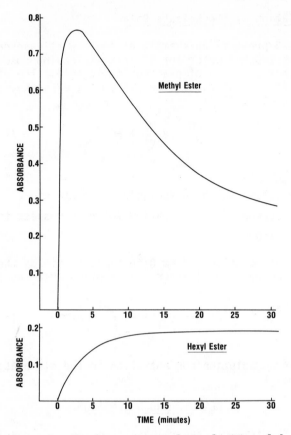

Figure 3.   Absorbance–time graphs for the 5% methyl and 5% hexyl esters of p-*aminobenzoic acid*

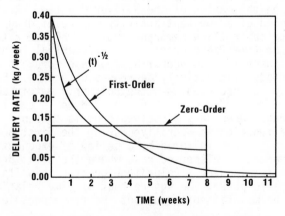

Figure 4.   Delivery rate profiles for different delivery systems (12)

It is possible, however, that a period of zero-order release may precede the square root of time dependence, yielding a triphasic release profile for the dissolved case and a biphasic release profile for the dispersed system. This type of behavior is exemplified when the diffusing species possesses a relatively high degree of lipophilicity, e.g., substances which have large partition coefficients (solubility in polymer/solubility in elution media) resulting in permeability rates through the matrix which are rapid compared to diffusion from the surface. The duration of the zero-order release period is dependent upon the initial drug loading dose, the resistance offered by the environmental diffusion layer, and the previously mentioned transport rate through the matrix phase. This situation is mathematically tractable and can be quantitatively expressed by use of appropriate physical-chemical parameters as described below.

Biphasic Release from Drug-Dispersed Matrix Systems

A schematic representation of the physical model for the release of steroids from an inert matrix system containing excess drug in suspension has been presented (13) and is shown in Figure 5. Initially the matrix contains homogeneously dispersed drug particles in equilibrium with dissolved drug. The release process is activated when the matrix comes into contact with the environmental fluid and a concentration gradient is established. At time, t, greater than zero, a depletion zone (ℓ) occurs in the matrix, across which subsequent diffusion occurs. At the moving front, the concentration of the drug is assumed to be equal to its equilibrium solubility in the polymeric phase. At the matrix-solution interface the concentration in the polymer is designated C'_s and the concentration in the aqueous solution is C'_a. In the environmental fluid, transport occurs across an aqueous boundary diffusion layer of thickness, h_a, into the bulk solution at a concentration of C_B.

With the assumptions that: (a) the dissolution of drug particles is fast compared to subsequent diffusion in the matrix; (b) a pseudo-steady state exists; (c) diffusion coefficients are constant for all species in a particular phase; (d) drug transport occurs through the matrix phase, and not pores; (e) the total drug concentration (A) is much greater than its solubility in the polymeric phase; and (f) "perfect sink" conditions are approximated, i.e. $C_B \cong 0$, the following general expressions were derived (13, 14) relating the amount released per unit surface area (Q) to time (t) for a planar matrix:

$$Q = \frac{-D_s h_a K A \varepsilon}{D_a \tau} + \left[\left(\frac{D_s h_a K A \varepsilon}{D_a \tau} \right)^2 + \frac{2 A D_s C_s \varepsilon t}{\tau} \right]^{\frac{1}{2}} \quad \text{(Eq. 3)}$$

where:

A = total concentration of drug in matrix (mg./cm.^{3})

D_a = diffusion coefficient in dissolution medium (cm.^{2}/min.)

D_s = diffusion coefficient in matrix phase (cm.^{2}/min.)

C_a = solubility in dissolution medium (mg./cm.^{3})

C_s = solubility in matrix phase (mg./cm.^{3})

K = partition coefficient ($C_s \backslash C_a$)

h_a = boundary diffusion layer (cm.)

ε = volume fraction

τ = tortuosity

Differentiating Q with respect to time yields the rate equation:

$$\frac{dQ}{dt} = \text{rate} = \frac{\alpha C_s}{2(\beta^2 K^2 + \alpha C_s t)^{\frac{1}{2}}} \qquad \text{(Eq. 4)}$$

where $\alpha = \dfrac{2AD_s \varepsilon}{\tau}$ and $\beta = \dfrac{D_s h_a A \varepsilon}{D_a \tau}$.

Two limiting cases of equations 3 and 4 result depending upon the magnitude of the $\beta^2 K^2$ term:

Case I Kinetics: $\beta^2 K^2 \gg \alpha C_s$

$$Q = \frac{D_a C_a t}{h_a} \qquad \text{or} \qquad \text{(Eq. 5)}$$

$$\frac{dQ}{dt} = \frac{D_a C_a}{h_a} \qquad \text{(Eq. 6)}$$

Case II Kinetics: $\beta^2 K^2 \ll \alpha C_s$

$$Q = \left(\frac{2AD_s C_s \varepsilon t}{\tau} \right)^{\frac{1}{2}} \qquad \text{(Eq. 7)}$$

$$\frac{dQ}{dt} = \left(\frac{AD_s C_s \varepsilon}{2t\tau} \right)^{\frac{1}{2}} \qquad \text{(Eq. 8)}$$

Case I represents a zero-order release process where the amount released is linearly related to time and thus the release rate is
independent of time. In this instance the major resistance to
release resides in the boundary diffusion layer. Case II is an
example of a matrix controlled kinetic process where Q is linearly
related to $(t)^{\frac{1}{2}}$ and dQ/dt decreases according to the inverse of
the square root of time. The Case II kinetic expression was originally derived by Higuchi (15).

In Vitro Release of Esters of p-Aminobenzoic Acid

A rigorous test of equations 3-8 can be accomplished by measuring the release of substances where the lipophilic character of
the diffusing species is altered in a systematic fashion, while
maintaining all other variables constant. A homologous series of
esters of p-aminobenzoic acid provides a means of incrementally
increasing the partition coefficient (C_s/C_a), thereby changing the
$\beta^2 K^2$ over at least six orders of magnitude. The β term is essentially insensitive to changes in K, as the terms A, h_a, ε, and τ
are fixed by the experimental design, and the diffusion coefficients are expected to be relatively constant over these moderate
changes in the molecular weight of the esters. The data is presented as the total amount of ester released with time and therefore equations 3, 5 and 7 are the relevant expressions. Since
equations 4, 6, and 8 are simply the derivatives of Q with respect
to time, analyses of the integrated expressions, i.e., 3, 5, and
7 are sufficient to test the theoretical concepts presented.

Figure 6 shows the Q vs. t plots for the methyl through heptyl
esters of p-aminobenzoic acid. A continuous release of each ester
from the silicone rubber matrix is noted, with the exact release
pattern being characteristic of the ester studied. At four hours,
release of the butyl ester was the highest being seven times
greater than the heptyl ester, which was released at the slowest
rate. By examining the release curves it is difficult to visually
correlate the overall release patterns to chain length because
the cross-over of the curves result from changes in the order of
release as time progresses. Equation 3, however, provides a
general expression for the release process for all of the esters
and also accounts for a transition period for Case I to Case II
kinetics. For example, at four hours, it can be shown that the
diffusion layer contribution reduces the total amount released by
no more than 15% for methyl through butyl esters. For times
greater than four hours, it is expected that Case II kinetics is
totally operative and at equal loading doses and diffusivities Q
is dependent upon C_s and not K. Absolute values of C_s are not
known but are approximated by the solubility of the esters in
silicone oil. Values for C_s are given in Table I, along with the
reported (10) aqueous solubilities and partition coefficients.
The order of release at four hours, i.e., butyl > propyl > ethyl >
methyl follows equation 7 using the silicone oil solubility data

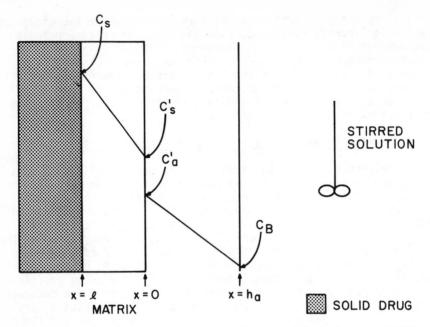

Figure 5. Hypothetical diagram for the matrix-boundary diffusion layer model (13)

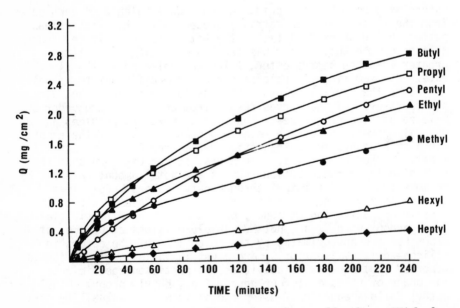

Figure 6.   Release of esters of p-*aminobenzoic from silicone rubber discs at 5% loading doses*

in Table I. Although the C_s values for pentyl through heptyl are high, the resistance across the diffusion layer is greater due to increasing K values and a transition period occurs, with Case I kinetics preceding the square root of time dependence.

Table I.   Solubility (mg./cm.^{3}) Data for Esters
of p-Aminobenzoic Acid (10)

Ester	Water (C_a)	Silicone Oil (C_s)	Partition Coefficient (K)
Methyl	3.82	0.79	0.208
Ethyl	1.68	1.38	0.817
Propyl	8.42×10^{-1}	2.31	2.75
Butyl	3.32×10^{-1}	3.44	1.03×10^{1}
Pentyl	9.32×10^{-2}	3.69	3.95×10^{1}
Hexyl	2.37×10^{-2}	2.48	1.05×10^{2}
Heptyl	5.88×10^{-3}	2.35	4.00×10^{2}

The pentyl ester represents the transitional chain length where a linear period of release is observed for about the first hour, followed by gradual curvature (Figure 6). For chain lengths greater than pentyl, Case I kinetics is followed and release is essentially independent of C_s for the four hour interval. The linear nature of the Q vs. t plot for the hexyl and heptyl esters support the use of equation 5. Substitution of the relevant physicochemical constants[i] into equation 3 provides an independent test of the theory. The theoretical plots are shown in Figure 7. Considering the assumptions in the model, the agreement of theory and data is quite acceptable.

Graphs of Q vs. (t)$^{1/2}$ are shown in Figures 8 and 9. Linear relationships are observed for the lower ester chain lengths. However a lag period occurs for all esters above methyl. This is evidenced by extrapolation of the linear portions to the x-axis. The time intercept increases as chain length increases exemplifying the transition of the kinetic schemes involved. The extreme curvature observed for the hexyl (see Figure 9) and heptyl esters is indicative of a Q vs. (t)$^{1/2}$ plot for a straight line. However,

---

[i] The values for the various parameters are listed in reference 14. The constant h_a in the present work was 34.9×10^{-4} cm. This was the average value calculated from the expression, $h_a = C_a D_a (dt/dQ)$ for the butyl, pentyl, and hexyl esters. The individual values were 42.5, 29.8, and 32.5×10^{-4} cm. for the respective esters.

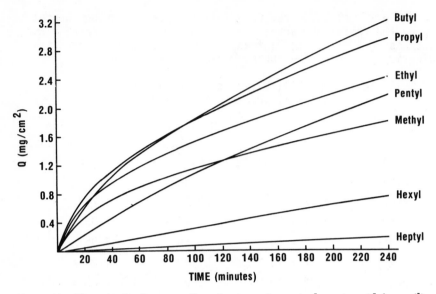

Figure 7.   *Theoretical release profiles of esters of* p-*aminobenzoic acid from silicone rubber discs at 5% loading doses*

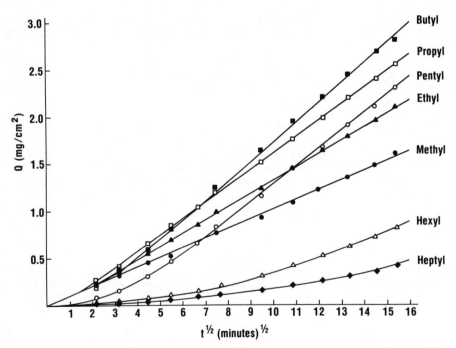

Figure 8.   *Plots of Q vs. (t)$^{1/2}$ for the esters of* p-*aminobenzoic acid from silicone rubber discs at 5% loading doses*

as a consequence of the insensitivity of this type of plot to the data, they appear linear at times greater than 2 hours. Therefore, it seems more instructive to evaluate the transition regions by calculating the time, t_{trans}, for which the resistance in the boundary diffusion layer and matrix are equal. This is given by the following expression [j] :

$$t_{trans} = \frac{3\beta^2 K^2}{\alpha C_s} \qquad \text{(Eq. 9)}$$

Time values for the esters are listed in Table II.

Table II.   Values of t_{trans} for a 5% Loading Dose of the Ester of p-Aminobenzoic Acid

Ester	t_{trans} (minutes)
Methyl	3.82×10^{-2}
Ethyl	3.37×10^{-1}
Propyl	2.28×10^{0}
Butyl	2.15×10^{1}
Pentyl	2.95×10^{2}
Hexyl	3.10×10^{3}
Heptyl	4.75×10^{4}

As chain length increases t_{trans} values increase dramatically, suggesting that the more lipophilic molecules will exhibit Case I kinetics for longer times.

Changes in the loading dose will alter the transition period according to equation 9. The influence of drug concentration is shown in Figure 10 for the methyl and butyl esters of p-aminobenzoic acid. Increasing the loading dose from 1% to 5% has no detectable influence on the time intercept for the methyl ester as the Q vs. $(t)^{1/2}$ plots are linear and pass through the origin. The x-intercept of the linear region for the butyl ester, however, increases due to a greater period of boundary diffusion layer control. The expected effect of loading dose on t_{trans} values is shown in Table III. Transition times are directly proportional to loading dose for a given ester and increase according to K^2 as alkyl chain length is extended. When matrix control is operative

---

[j] The helpful suggestions of Dr. D. Flanagan were appreciated on the calculation of t_{trans}. The values of β and α were 6.40×10^{-2} mg./cm.^{2} and 1.76×10^{-2} mg./cm.-min. respectively for a 5% w/w loading dose of the ester.

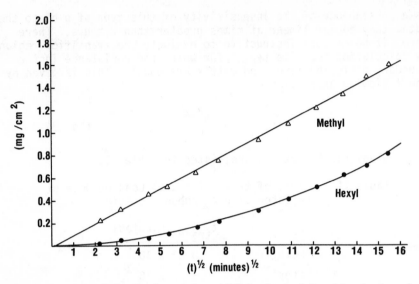

Figure 9.   Expanded scale plots of Q vs. $(t)^{1/2}$ for the methyl and hexyl esters of p-aminobenzoic acid at 5% loading doses

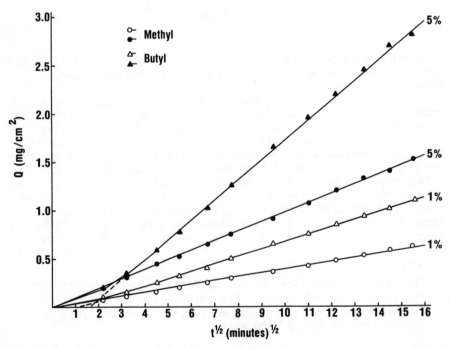

Figure 10.   Plots of Q vs. $(t)^{1/2}$ for the methyl and butyl esters of p-aminobenzoic acid at two loading doses

Table III.   Influence of Loading Dose on t_{trans} Values
for the Esters of p-Aminobenzoic Acid

Ester	Loading Dose	t_{trans} (minutes)		
		1%	5%	10%
Methyl		7.64×10^{-3}	3.82×10^{-2}	7.64×10^{-2}
Ethyl		6.74×10^{-2}	3.37×10^{-1}	6.74×10^{-1}
Propyl		4.56×10^{-1}	2.28×10^{0}	4.56×10^{0}
Butyl		4.30×10^{0}	2.15×10^{1}	4.30×10^{1}
Pentyl		5.90×10^{1}	2.95×10^{2}	5.90×10^{2}
Hexyl		6.20×10^{2}	3.10×10^{3}	6.20×10^{3}
Heptyl		9.50×10^{3}	4.75×10^{4}	9.50×10^{4}

(Eq. 7), the ratio of Q vs. $(t)^{\frac{1}{2}}$ slopes are dependent upon $(A)^{\frac{1}{2}}$ for a given compound. Calculated values for the ratio of the slopes (5%/1%) of the methyl and butyl esters are 2.46 and 2.73 respectively. These agree reasonably well with the theoretical ratio of 2.24. In contrast, when zero-order Case I kinetics applies, increasing the concentration over this range should have a minor effect on the amount released during the four hour time period of this study.

In Vitro Versus In Vivo Release Kinetics

The design of controlled release delivery systems requires the judicious selection of the drug and polymer in order to insure that in vivo release and subsequent absorption are in phase with the potency of the therapeutic agent. The results of the studies with p-aminobenzoates demonstrate the influence of solute properties on release. The drug release model, represented by equation 3, is sufficiently flexible to account for certain environmental factors which affect drug release. It has been reported for example that values of the boundary diffusion layer thickness from 250-500 x 10^{-4} cm. are not unreasonable in certain biological systems (16-18). This represents over a 10-fold increase in the resistance of the diffusion layer that was calculated for in vitro release of esters of p-aminobenzoic acid. Compounds such as the hexyl and heptyl esters which were released at zero order rates in vitro could show even longer periods of constant release during in vivo experiments. Theoretical release rate curves are shown in Figure 11 for the hexyl ester assuming h_a equals 500 x 10^{-4} cm. In vivo release is approximated by a zero order process for at least 20 days while the in vitro rate curve shows a transition from zero-order to square root of time kinetics. It is also noteworthy that the in vivo rates are less than the in vitro over the time scale employed. In contrast, the less lipophilic methyl ester shows a matrix controlled release profile (Figure 12) which is independent of the diffusion layer thickness.

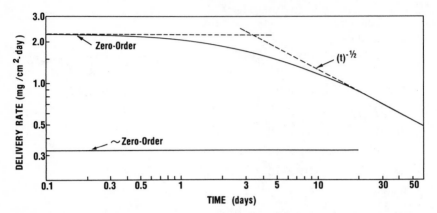

Figure 11.   Theoretical release rates of the hexyl ester of p-aminobenzoic acid from
silicone rubber. Key: upper curve—in vitro; lower curve—in vivo.

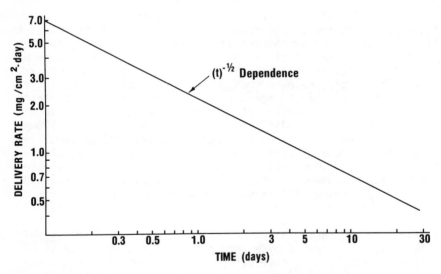

Figure 12.   Theoretical matrix-controlled release rates for the methyl ester of p-aminobenzoic acid from silicone rubber. Line represents both the in vitro and in vivo predictions.

A vaginal delivery system containing medroxyprogesterone acetate provides a medically useful example for the evaluation of these concepts under biological conditions. Vaginal rings, containing excess drug in suspension, are effective in inhibiting ovulation in humans (8,19). Figure 13 shows the in vivo release profile for over 126 days (six menstrual cycles). A period of linear release is evident during the first 21 days and then a gradual decrease occurs. At 21 days there is 30 per cent less drug released than under in vitro experimental conditions (7). Plots of Q' (mg. release/ring) vs. $(t)^{\frac{1}{2}}$ are illustrated in Figure 14. After an interval of initial curvature, linearity is observed. The time to reach this region is much greater for in vivo release, presumably due to a larger resistance to transport from the ring surface. For cylindrical geometry, plots of this type are valid when the fraction of drug released is less than 50% (7). The time period beyond this point is distinguished by the dotted line in the figure. The slopes of the linear regions of the in vitro and in vivo plots are parallel indicating that release is under matrix conrol (Case II) and is independent of the environmental conditions. The slope of the lines is 9.6 mg./$(day)^{\frac{1}{2}}$ and is in agreement with the independently calculated values of 10.9 and 11.2 mg./$(day)^{\frac{1}{2}}$ for the in vivo and in vitro runs respectively [k].

Medroxyprogesterone acetate blood concentrations are illustrated in Figure 15 for 1% and 2% w/w loading doses. The rings were inserted on the 5th day of the menstrual cycle and serum drug levels were assayed at one day intervals. Serum levels are characterized by an initial elevation one day after insertion to relatively constant serum levels which were maintained throughout the 21 days for both ring concentrations. The 2% ring, however, exhibits slightly higher values than the 1%. The constancy of the serum drug concentrations correlates with the linear release of drug (Figure 13) over this same time interval. The release data on this clinically tested delivery-system indicates that zero-order release was achieved for 21 days, even though square root of time kinetics was observed in vitro.

---

[k] Calculated from equation 7 using the following values from reference 7: C_S = 0.0874 mg./cm.^{3}; D_S = 2.50 x 10^{-5} cm.^{2}/min. For the in vitro experiment A = 15.2 mg./cm.^{3} and surface area = 36.3 cm.^{2} while the rings for the in vivo study possessed an A of 10.3 mg./cm.^{3} and a surface area of 42.7 cm.^{2}.

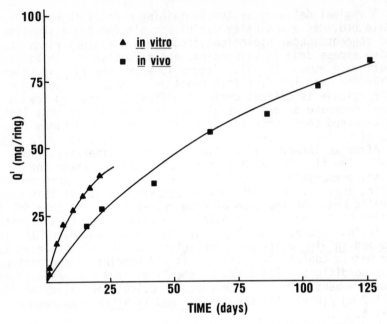

Figure 13.   Release of medroxyprogesterone acetate from vaginal rings

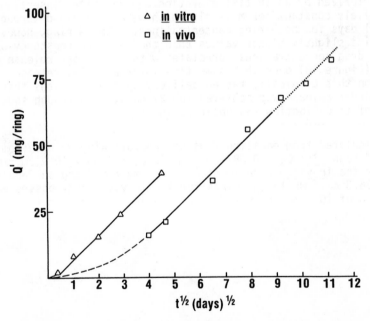

Figure 14.   Plots of Q' vs. (t)$^{1/2}$ for medroxyprogesterone acetate rings

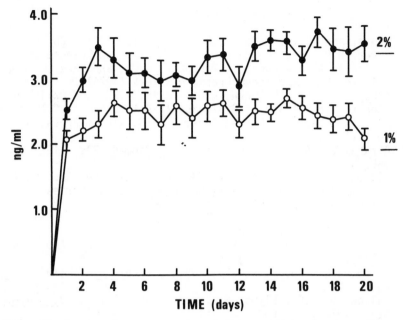

*Figure 15.   Serum medroxyprogesterone acetate concentrations from vaginal rings
(bars are ± SEM)*

ABSTRACT

Mathematical expressions derived on the basis of Fick's law of diffusion are applied to the study of the release of several model compounds from silicone rubber matrices. Ester chain length of a homologous series of p-aminobenzoic acid is systematically varied to illustrate the importance of the lipophilic character of the diffusing species. The time dependence of the release rate is shown to be dependent upon the partitioning and solubility of the diffusant, and expected square root of time profiles from in vitro experiments may lead to zero-order kinetics in vivo. Biological studies with a vaginal ring containing medroxyprogesterone acetate support this analysis as constant blood levels result even though a square root of time release dependence is observed in vitro.

ACKNOWLEDGMENTS

The laboratory assistance of Mrs. S.S. Butler and Ms. L.J. Larion was greatly appreciated. Blood samples were supplied by Dr. M. Thiery, University of Ghent, Belgium. Analyses of the medroxyprogesterone acetate rings were performed by the Physical and Analytical Chemistry unit of The Upjohn Company. Serum concentrations of medroxyprogesterone acetate were determined by Dr. D.G. Kaiser.

LITERATURE CITED

1. Hänselmann, B., and Voigt, R., Pharmazie (1971), 26, 57.
2. Baker, R.W., and Lonsdale, H.K., "Controlled Release of Bio-logically Active Agents," Tanquary, A.C., and Lacey, R.E., editors, P. 15, Plenum Press, New York (1974).
3. Akkapeddi, M.K., Halpern, B.D., Davis, R.H., and Balin, H., "Controlled Release of Biologically Active Agents," Tanquary, A.C., and Lacey, R.E., editors, P. 165, Plenum Press, New York (1974).
4. Abrahams, R.A., and Ronel, S.H., J. Biomed. Res. (1975), 9, 355.
5. Higuchi, T., and Stella, V., "Pro-drugs as Novel Drug Delivery Systems," American Chemical Society Symposium Series 14, Washington, D.C., 1975.
6. Sundaram, K., and Kincl, F.A., Steroids (1968), 12, 517.
7. Roseman, T.J., J. Pharm. Sci. (1972), 61, 46.
8. Mishell, D.R., Jr., Lumkin, M.E., and Stone, S., American J. Obstet. Gynecol. (1972), 113, 927.
9. Flynn, G.L., and Yalkowsky, S.H., J. Pharm. Sci. (1972), 61, 838.
10. Yalkowsky, S.H., Flynn, G.L., and Slunick, T.G., J. Pharm. Sci. (1972), 61, 852
11. Shah, A.C., and Ochs, J.F., J. Pharm. Sci. (1974), 63, 110.
12. Baker, R.W., and Lonsdale, H.K., "Proceedings International Controlled Release Pesticide Symposium," P.P. 9-39, Wright State University, Dayton, Ohio (1975).
13. Roseman, T.J., and Higuchi, W.I., J. Pharm. Sci. (1970), 59, 353.
14. Roseman, T.J., and Yalkowsky, S.H., J. Pharm. Sci. (1974), 63, 1639.
15. Higuchi, T., J. Pharm. Sci. (1963), 52, 1145.
16. Smulders, A.P., and Wright, E.M., J. Membrane Biol. (1971), 5, 297.
17. Winne, D., Biochim. Biophys. Acta. (1973), 298, 27.
18. Ho, N.F., APhA Acad. Pharm. Sci. Abstract Book (1972), 2 (2), 112.
19. Mishell, D.R., Jr., Contraception (1975), 12, 249.

Thermodynamics of Controlled Drug Release from Polymeric Delivery Devices

YIE W. CHIEN

Pharmaceutical Research Group, Development Department, Searle Laboratories, G. D. Searle & Co., Skokie, Illinois 60076

Introduction

Recent interest has centered on the idea of replacing daily administration of a drug with delivery devices that release a constant effective dose to target tissues via a controlled-release mechanism (1-10). The high permeability of silicone polymer to steroids has been widely applied to the development of drug-filled silastic capsules (11-22) and drug-impregnated silicone matrices (23-28) for long-acting hormonal contraception.

An in vitro drug elution system, which is simple and easy to construct and allows rapid characterization of the drug release mechanism, was introduced earlier from this laboratory (26). The application of such a system allowed characterization of the mechanism and rate of drug release in a much shorter period of time (26, 27, 29). The drug release profiles from silicone devices measured in such a system agreed with in vivo results collected in animals intravaginally (28) and subcutaneously (30-32).

In this report, the thermodynamics of controlled drug release from silicone polymer matrices will be fully analyzed both theoretically and experimentally.

Experimental

Silicone devices were prepared by thoroughly mixing 0.462 parts of Norgestomet[1] crystals, 8.538 parts of silastic 382 medical grade elastomer, and one part of silicone fluid 360[2] with a rotator[3] at 1000 rpm for five minutes. One drop (0.02 ml) of stannous octoate[2], as catalyst, was then incorporated and thoroughly mixed for another minute. The mixture was then delivered by a syringe pump[4] into Tygon tubing[5] (R-3603, I.D. 1/8 inch). The silicone polymer was allowed to cure overnight in an exhaust hood at room temperature. After proper crosslinking, the resultant silicone polymer matrix was removed from the Tygon mold and cut into the desired lengths for various studies.

The drug elution apparatus and the technique for determining

drug solubility in silicone polymer and in polyethylene glycol
400-water cosolvent combinations used in this investigation were
reported earlier (26). The assay of Norgestomet and other steroidal analogs was conducted using a spectrophotometer[6] at a λ max
value in the neighborhood of 240 nm.

Theoretical Analyses

It was reported earlier (29) that the release pattern of
drugs from a drug-dispersed polymer matrix can be defined by the
following two equations:

$$\delta m^2 + \frac{2(A-Cp)Dm\delta d\delta m}{(A-\frac{Cp}{2})Ds\bar{k}K} = \frac{2CpDm}{(A-\frac{Cp}{2})}t \qquad \text{(Eq. 1)}$$

$$Q = A\delta m \qquad \text{(Eq. 2)}$$

where Q is the cumulated amount of drug released from a unit surface area of polymeric device (mg/cm^2); A is the initial amount of
drug impregnated in a unit volume of polymer matrix (mg/cm^3); Cp
is the solubility of drug in the polymer phase (mg/ml); δd and δm
are the thicknesses (cm) of the hydrodynamic diffusion layer on
the immediate surface of the device and of the depletion zone,
respectively; Ds and Dm are the diffusivities (cm^2/sec.) of the
drug molecule in the elution solution and in the polymer matrix,
respectively; K is the partition coefficient of drug species from
polymer matrix to solution phase; $\bar{k}$ is a constant accounting for
the relative magnitude of the concentration gradients in both diffusion layer and depletion zone (29); and t is time.

The concentration profiles on a unit section of a polymeric
device are schematically illustrated in Figure 1. At the very
early stage of a drug elution study, the thickness of the drug depletion zone, δm, is so small that the following condition exists:

$$\delta m^2 \ll \frac{2(A-Cp)Dm\delta d\delta m}{(A-\frac{Cp}{2})Ds\bar{k}K} \qquad \text{(Eq. 3)}$$

So, Eq. 1 is reduced to:

$$\frac{2(A-Cp)Dm\delta d\delta m}{(A-\frac{Cp}{2})Ds\bar{k}K} = \frac{2CpDm}{(A-\frac{Cp}{2})}t \qquad \text{(Eq. 4a)}$$

or:

$$\delta m = \frac{\bar{k}DsKCp}{(A-Cp)\delta d}t \qquad \text{(Eq. 4b)}$$

Substituting Eq. 4b for the δm term in Eq. 2 gives:

$$Q = \frac{\bar{k}DsKCp}{\delta d}t$$

(Eq. 5a)

since the experiments were so designed that the initial amount of drug (A) incorporated into a unit volume of polymer matrix is much greater than the solubility (Cp) of the drug in this polymer; therefore $(A - Cp) \simeq A$.

We know (29) that Cs = KCp; so, Eq. 5a may be transformed to:

$$Q = \frac{\bar{k}DsCs}{\delta d}t$$

(Eq. 5b)

Eq. 5 indicates that at a very early stage of drug release dynamics, the partition-controlled process at the hydrodynamic diffusion layer is the rate-limiting step (Fig. 1). The rate of drug release at this initial state is defined by:

$$\frac{Q}{t} = \frac{\bar{k}Ds}{\delta d}Cs$$

(Eq. 6)

Taking the logarithm on both sides of Eq. 6 results in:

$$\log \left(\frac{Q}{t}\right) = \log K^1 + \log Cs$$

(Eq. 7)

where K^1, the constant of interfacial diffusion, is described by:

$$K^1 = \frac{\bar{k}Ds}{\delta d}$$

(Eq. 8)

If the constant of interfacial diffusion (K^1) is temperature-dependent and follows by the Arrhenius relationship of:

$$\log K^1 = \log K^1_0 - \frac{Ed,s}{2.303R} \cdot \frac{1}{T}$$

(Eq. 9)

where K^1_0 and Ed,s are the pre-exponential factor and the activation energy of interfacial diffusion, respectively.

It was established (33) that the mole fraction solubility ($\overline{Cs}$) of a solid drug in a real solution is also temperature-dependent and is defined by:

$$\log \overline{Cs} = -\log \gamma_s - \frac{\Delta Hf,s}{2.303RT}\left(\frac{Tm-T}{Tm}\right)$$

(Eq. 10a)

where γ_s is the activity coefficient of drug solute; $\Delta Hf,s$ is the energy required to increase the intermolecular distance in drug crystals, thus, allowing drug molecules to dissociate from the crystal lattice and to dissolve themselves into the solution structure; Tm is the temperature of melting point (on absolute scale); R is the gas constant; and T is the temperature of a given system (also on absolute temperature scale).

The solution process of a drug crystal in an elution medium can be visualized as consisting of two consecutive microscopic steps: (1) the dissociation of drug molecules from their crystal lattice and (2) the solvation of these dissociated drug molecules into a solution structure. The first step requires a dissociation energy and is a Tm-dependent process. The second step requires a solvation energy and is a T-dependent process. If it is the case, then, the energy term in Eq. 10a may be split to:

$$\log \bar{C}s = \log \frac{Cs}{Cs + Xs} = - \log \gamma_s + \frac{\Delta Hm}{2.303R} \cdot \frac{1}{Tm} - \frac{\Delta HT,s}{2.303R} \cdot \frac{1}{T}$$

(Eq. 10b)

where ΔHm is defined as the energy of dissociation which the drug molecules require to dissociate themselves from the crystal lattice structure and hence is dependent on the melting point (Tm) of the drug crystals; ΔHT,s is defined as the energy of solvation the drug molecules need to solubilize themselves into a solution structure and is dependent on the temperature of the solution system; and Xs is the mole fraction of the solvent molecules and is known as much greater than Cs, the solubility (concentration) of the drug solute.

In view of the facts that both terms of [log (Cs + Xs) − log γ_s] and ΔHm/2.303RTm are constant in a control condition, Eq. 10b may be simplified to:

$$\log Cs = constant - \frac{\Delta HT,s}{2.303R} \cdot \frac{1}{T}$$

(Eq. 10c)

Substituting Eqs. 9 and 10c into Eq. 7 gives a relationship that defines the effect of temperature on the rate of drug release under a diffusion layer partition-controlled process:

$$\log \left(\frac{Q}{t}\right) = constant - \frac{(Ed,s + \Delta HT,s)}{2.303R} \cdot \frac{1}{T}$$

(Eq. 11)

Eq. 11 suggests that a semilogarithmic relationship exists between the initial rate of drug release, Q/t, and the reciprocal, T^{-1}, of the temperature investigated. The magnitude of the temperature effect is illustrated by the sum of Ed,s, the activation energy for interfacial diffusion, and ΔHT,s, the energy of solvation.

On the other hand, after the lapse of a finite time, the thickness of the drug depletion zone, δm, becomes substantially greater; it results in:

$$\delta m^2 >> \frac{2(A - Cp) Dm\delta d}{(A - \frac{Cp}{2}) Ds\bar{k}K} \delta m$$

(Eq. 12)

so, Eq. 1 is reduced to:

$$\delta m = \left(\frac{2CpDm}{(A - \frac{Cp}{2})} t\right)^{\frac{1}{2}}$$

(Eq. 13)

Substituting Eq. 13 for the δm term in Eq. 2 gives:

$$Q = [2ADmCp]^{\frac{1}{2}} t^{\frac{1}{2}}$$

(Eq. 14)

since $(A - \frac{Cp}{2}) \simeq A$.

Eq. 14 implies that, after a finite period of drug elution, a matrix-controlled process becomes the predominant step in determining the mechanism of drug release from the drug-dispersed polymer matrix. Now, the cumulated amount, Q, of drug released from a unit surface area of a polymeric device is directly proportional to the square root, $t^{\frac{1}{2}}$, of time; and the release profile is thus defined by:

$$\frac{Q}{t^{\frac{1}{2}}} = [2ADmCp]^{\frac{1}{2}}$$

(Eq. 15)

Taking the logarithm of both sides of Eq. 15 gives:

$$2 \log \left(\frac{Q}{t^{\frac{1}{2}}}\right) = \log (2A) + \log Dm + \log Cp$$

(Eq. 16)

It was established (35) that the diffusivity of a drug in a polymer structure is defined by:

$$\log Dm = \log Dm° - \frac{Ed,m}{2.303R} \cdot \frac{1}{T}$$

(Eq. 17)

and the mole fraction solubility ($\log \bar{C}p$) of the same drug species in a polymer composition (33) may be defined as:

$$\log \bar{C}p = \log \frac{Cp}{Cp + Xp} = -\log \gamma_p - \frac{\Delta Hf,m}{2.303R} \left(\frac{Tm - T}{Tm}\right)$$

(Eq. 18a)

where Ed,m is the activation energy a drug molecule requires to diffuse in a polymer matrix; $\Delta Hf,m$ is the molar heat of fusion absorbed when the drug crystals melt into the polymer structure; γp is the activity coefficient of the drug solute in the polymer; Tm is the melting point temperature; and Xp is the mole fraction of the polymer composition. As discussed earlier, $\Delta Hf,m$ may also be split into two energy terms: ΔHm, the dissociation energy of the crystal lattice, and $\Delta HT,m$, the energy required for the solvation of drug molecules in the polymer structure. So, Eq. 18a may be described alternatively as Eq. 18b, shown below.

$$\log \bar{C}p = \log \frac{Cp}{Cp + Xp} = - \log \gamma_p + \frac{\Delta Hm}{2.303R} \cdot \frac{1}{Tm} - \frac{\Delta HT,m}{2.303R} \cdot \frac{1}{T}$$

(Eq. 18b)

or:

$$\log C_p = \text{constant} - \frac{\Delta H_T,m}{2.303R} \cdot \frac{1}{T} \qquad \text{(Eq. 18c)}$$

since both $[\log (C_p + X_p) - \log \gamma_p]$, ($\because X_p \gg C_p$), and $\frac{\Delta H_m}{2.303R\ T_m}$ terms are constant under controlled conditions.

Substituting Eq. 17 and 18c into Eq. 16 results in an expression which defines the temperature dependency of the drug release profile $(Q/t^{\frac{1}{2}})$ under the matrix-controlled process:

$$\log (Q/t^{\frac{1}{2}}) = \text{constant} - \frac{(E_d,m + \Delta H_T,m)}{4.606R} \cdot \frac{1}{T} \qquad \text{(Eq. 19)}$$

Eq. 19 indicates that a semilogarithmic relationship also exists between the steady-state drug release profile, $Q/t^{\frac{1}{2}}$, and the reciprocal, T^{-1}, of the temperature studied. Similar to Eq. 11, the magnitude of the temperature effect is also dependent on two energy terms: E_d,m, the activation energy for matrix diffusion, and $\Delta H_T,m$, the solvation energy for drug dissolution in a polymer matrix.

A comparison of Eq. 19 with Eq. 11 showed that the dependency of the drug release profile on temperature should be twofold greater in the diffusion-layer partition-controlled process than in the matrix-controlled process.

Results and Discussion

Controlled Drug Release from a Silicone Polymer Matrix: The release of Norgestomet, a potent progestin for estrus synchronization in heifers, from a silicone polymer matrix at an early stage of drug release (< 3 hours) is illustrated in Figure 2. Theoretical analyses conducted earlier suggested that this initial state drug release is predominately a partition-controlled process in the hydrodynamic diffusion layer (Figure 1) and a zero order drug release profile should be observed (as defined by Eq. 5). Apparently, the results collected at various temperatures agree with the theoretical expectation.

The rates of drug release (Q/t) at various temperatures can be calculated from the slope of the linear Q-t relationship (Fig. 2) as expected from Eq. 6. It was noted that the values of Q/t were dependent on the temperature of the drug elution system and increased approximately fourfold from 0.177 mcg/cm^2/min. to 0.672 mcg/cm^2/min. when the temperature was raised from 30°C to 50°C (Table I).

As time passed, the thickness (δm) of the drug depletion zone (Fig. 1) grew bigger and bigger. Soon the matrix-controlled process outweighed the partition-controlled process to become the rate-limiting step that dictated the whole course of controlled drug release from the polymer matrix system at steady-state.

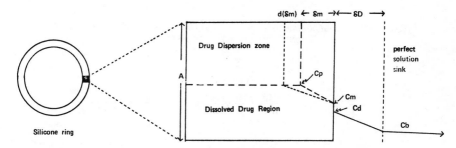

Figure 1. *Theoretical concentration profile existing in a drug dispersed silicone device in contact with a perfect solution sink.* (See text for the definition of A, Cp, Cm, Cd, Cb, δm and δd.)

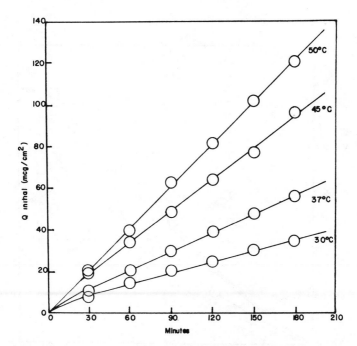

Figure 2. *Initial state release profiles of Norgestomet from a silicone polymer matrix at various temperatures. This linear relationship is defined by Eq. 5.*

Table I

Temperature Dependency of the Controlled Release of Norgestomet
from Silicone Polymer Matrix

Temperature (0°C)	(Q/t) initial (mcg/cm²/min.)	$\frac{(Q/t^{\frac{1}{2}})}{(mg/cm^2/day^{\frac{1}{2}})}$
30	0.177	0.593
37	0.300	0.809
45	0.502	0.950
50	0.672	1.028

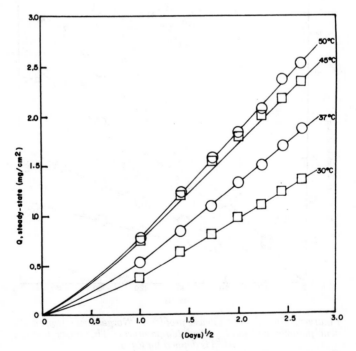

Figure 3. Steady-state release profiles of Norgestomet from a silicone polymer matrix at various temperatures. This linearity is defined by Eq. 14.

Under this new rate process, as expected from Eq. 14, the cumulated amount of drug released (Q) from a unit surface area of the polymeric device should become directly proportional to the square root of time ($t^{\frac{1}{2}}$). The results shown in Figure 3 illustrate this linear relationship. This $Q-t^{\frac{1}{2}}$ linearity was followed at all the temperatures studied. Following Eq. 15, the magnitude of $Q/t^{\frac{1}{2}}$ values can be estimated from the slope of the linear $Q-t^{\frac{1}{2}}$ plots (Fig. 3). It was noted that the $Q/t^{\frac{1}{2}}$ values were also temperature dependent and increased approximately twofold from 0.593 mg/cm^2/day$^{\frac{1}{2}}$ to 1.028 mg/cm^2/day$^{\frac{1}{2}}$ when the temperature of the elution solution was raised from 30°C to 50°C (Table I).

As the temperature of the drug elution system increased from 30°C to 50°C, the magnitude of the initial release rate, (Q/t) initial, was enhanced approximately fourfold while the slope ($Q/t^{\frac{1}{2}}$) of Q vs. $t^{\frac{1}{2}}$ profile was increased only approximately two times. This observation agreed with the earlier theoretical analyses (compare Eq. 11 with Eq. 19). It appears to be due to the differences in their energy requirements between partition-controlled and matrix-controlled processes.

Eq. 11 indicates that a semilogarithmic relationship should exist between the values of (Q/t) initial and the reciprocal of the temperatures. Eq. 19 implies that a similar relationship exists between the values of ($Q/t^{\frac{1}{2}}$) and the reciprocal of the temperatures (Fig. 4). It appears that the magnitude of (Q/t) values is more sensitive to variations in the temperature of the drug elution system than $Q/t^{\frac{1}{2}}$ data. Following Eqs. 11 and 19, the magnitudes of the composite energies required for the controlled release of Norgestomet under partition-controlled and matrix-controlled processes can be computed from the slopes of this Arrhenius-type relationship (Table II). The results suggested that the matrix-controlled release process required a composite energy term (10.30 Kcal/mole) which is 2.37 Kcal/mole lower than that (12.67 Kcal/mole) required for the release of drug under the partition-controlled process.

Comparisions made between Eq. 11 and Eq. 19 pointed out that the difference in energy requirements between partition-controlled and matrix-controlled processes could possibly be due to either the difference in the energy of activation (Ed,s for interfacial diffusion and Ed,m for matrix diffusion) and/or the difference in the solvation energy for drug solubilization (ΔHT,s for elution solution and ΔHT,m for polymer phase). This question may easily be answered by measuring the magnitudes of solvation energy required for the solution of a drug in an elution medium (ΔHT,s) and in polymer phase (ΔHT,m). These measurements can be carried out simply by studying the temperature-dependency of the solubility of Norgestomet in a polyethylene glycol-water combination and in a silicone polymer.

Eqs. 10b and 18b can be simplified to the following equations to define the effect of temperature on the mole fraction solubility

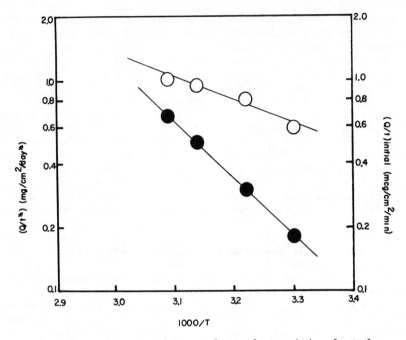

Figure 4. Temperature dependency of the steady-state (○) and initial state release (●) profiles of Norgestomet from a silicone polymer matrix. Data are from Table I.

Table II

Comparison on the Energy Requirements
For the Release of Norgestomet Under
Matrix-controlled and Partition-controlled Processes

Processes	Energy Requirements*
Matrix-controlled	(Ed,m + ΔHT,m) = 10.30 Kcal/mole
Partition-controlled	(Ed,s + ΔHT,s) = 12.67 Kcal/mole

*Calculated from Figure 4 following Eqs. 11 and 19 respectively of Norgestomet in solution medium and in silicone polymer:

$$\log \bar{C}s = \text{constant} - \frac{\Delta HT,s}{2.303R} \cdot \frac{1}{T}$$ (Eq. 10d)

$$\log \bar{C}p - \text{constant} - \frac{\Delta HT,m}{2.303R} \cdot \frac{1}{T}$$ (Eq. 18d)

where constant $= \frac{\Delta Hm}{2.303R \ Tm} - \log \gamma_s$ (or γ_p) for the same drug species.

Both Eqs. 10d and 18d imply·that the mole fraction solubility ($\bar{C}s$ or $\bar{C}p$) of Norgestomet is exponentially dependent on the reciprocal, T^{-1}, of the temperature tested. These linear semilogarithmic relations are illustrated in Figure 5 for solution solubility and in Figure 6 for polymer solubility. From the slope of these linearities, the solvation energy for the solution of Norgestomet in various polyethylene glycol-water cosolvent systems and in pure water may be estimated (Table III). The solvation of Norgestomet in pure water (as an elution medium) required a solvation energy ($\Delta HT,s$) of 5.88 Kcal/mole. The addition of various volume fractions of polyethylene glycol into the aqueous elution medium significantly improved the aqueous solubility of Norgestomet (Fig. 5). It also resulted in an increase in the magnitude of $\Delta HT,s$ by approximately 2.36 Kcal/mole. It was also observed that the solution of Nortestomet in silicone polymer required a solvation energy ($\Delta HT,m$) of 6.60 Kcal/mole (Fig. 6).

Subtracting this $\Delta HT,m$ value from the result we reported earlier (Table II) on ($Ed,m + \Delta HT,m$), the activation energy (Ed,m) for the diffusion of Norgestomet in silicone polymer matrix may easily be estimated. A value of 3.70 Kcal/mole was obtained. Similarly, the activation energy (Ed,s) for the interfacial diffusion of Norgestomet in a polyethylene glycol-water cosolvent system may also be calculated. For example, in an elution medium containing 75% v/v polyethylene glycol 400, the magnitude of Ed,s value was estimated to be 3.85Kcal/mole. This Ed,s value (3.85 Kcal/mole) is very close to the Ed,m value (3.70 Kcal/mole) for the diffusion of Norgestomet in silicone polymer matrix. This calculation suggests that the differences in energy required for partition-controlled and matrix-controlled processes (Table II) are obviously due to the difference in the solvation energy required for drug solubilization. The solubilization of Norgestomet in a 75% v/v polyethylene glycol solution required a solvation energy ($\Delta HT,s$ = 8.82 Kcal/mole) that was 2.22 Kcal/mole more than for solubilization in a silicone polymer ($\Delta HT,m$ = 6.60 Kcal/mole).

Dissociation Energy of Crystal Lattice (ΔHm): Earlier in the analyses of the influences of temperature on the release profiles of Norgestomet from silicone polymer matrix (Eqs. 11 and 19) and the mole fraction solubilities (Eqs. 10d and 18d) of Norgestomet in elution medium and silicone polymer, the magnitude of ΔHm, the

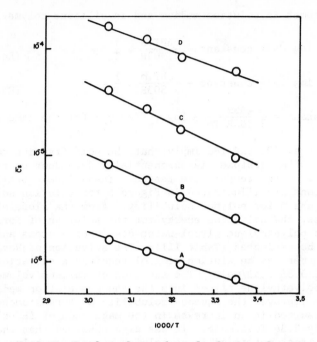

Figure 5. Semilogarithmic relationship between the mole fraction solubility ($\overline{C_s}$) of Norgestomet in various polyethylene glycol 400–water combinations and the reciprocal of the temperature (T^{-1}). Key: A, pure water; B, 20% v/v polyethylene glycol 400; C, 40% v/v polyethylene glycol 400; D, 60% v/v polyethylene glycol 400.

Table III

The Solvation Energy ($\Delta HT,s$) Required for the Dissolution
of Norgestomet in Various Elution Media

Elution Media	$\Delta HT,s$ (Kcal/mole)
H_2O	5.88
Polyethylene Glycol-H_2O Combinations	
20% v/v PEG 400	7.69
40% v/v PEG 400	9.73
60% v/v PEG 400	6.71
75% v/v PEG 400	8.82
	$\overline{\chi}$ (±S.D.) 8.24 (±1.32)

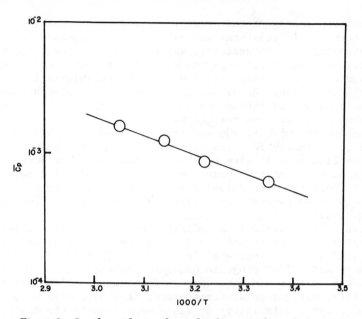

Figure 6.   *Semilogarithmic relationship between the mole fraction solubility ($\overline{Cp}$) of Norgestomet in silicone polymer and the reciprocal of the temperature (T^{-1}). ΔHT, m value was calculated to be 6.60 kcal/mole.*

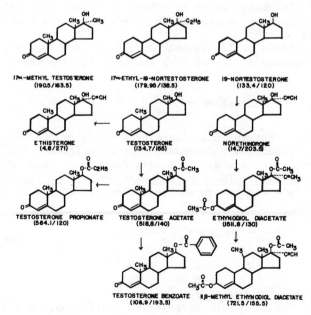

Figure 7.   *Chemical structure and polymer solubility (in mg/l.)/melting point (°C) of testosterone derivatives*

dissociation energy of the crystal lattice, was treated as a constant term. This treatment was well justified because the same drug species, i.e. Norgestomet, was studied throughout the tests. Now, however, it is necessary to determine how much this ΔHm term contributed to the energy required for the solubilization of drug particles in either the silicone polymer or the polyethylene glycol-water cosolvent system and then for the release of Norgestomet molecules from silicone polymer matrix.

Inspection of Eqs. 10b and 18b indicated that this ΔHm value can be conveniently measured by studying the dependency of the mole fraction solubilities of a homologous series of Norgestomet analogs on their melting point temperatures (Tm). The measurements of mole fraction solubility were required to be conducted at a constant temperature, for example, 37°C was applied for the present analyses.

The effect of chemical modifications on the melting point temperature and the solubility in silicone polymer at 37°C was investigated and is illustrated in Figures 7 (for testosterone derivatives), and 8 (for progesterone derivatives), and 9 (for estradiol derivatives). In most cases, if the chemical modification lowered the melting point temperature, it should also have increased polymer solubility; it was exemplified by the acetylation of Norethindrone to Ethynodiol diacetate (Fig. 7). The acetylation of both 3-keto and 17-hydroxy groups in Norethindrone lowered the Tm value by 73.5° and enhanced the Cp value by more than ten times. On the other hand, if the chemical modification raised the melting point temperature, it decreased polymer solubility; the addition of 11β-methyl group to ethynodiol diacetate, which elevated Tm by 25.5° and decreased Cp by more than two times, is a typical example.

If variations of log γ_p and $\Delta HT,m/2.303RT$ values are small among a homogenous series of drug analogs, Eq. 18b may be reduced to:

$$\log \bar{C}p = \text{constant} + \frac{\Delta Hm}{2.303R} \cdot \frac{1}{Tm} \qquad \text{(Eq. 20)}$$

which suggests that the mole fraction solubility ($\bar{C}p$) of a drug species is exponentially dependent on the reciprocal (Tm^{-1}) of its melting point temperature. This semilogarithmic relationship is illustrated in Figure 10. The correlation between log $\bar{C}p$ and Tm^{-1} after a multiple regression analysis, for all the 27 steriods is expressed by:

$$\log \bar{C}p = -10.249 + \frac{3.085}{Tm} \qquad \text{(Eq. 21)}$$

N	R	S^2
27	0.85	0.15

The results of a high correlation coefficient (R = 0.85) and

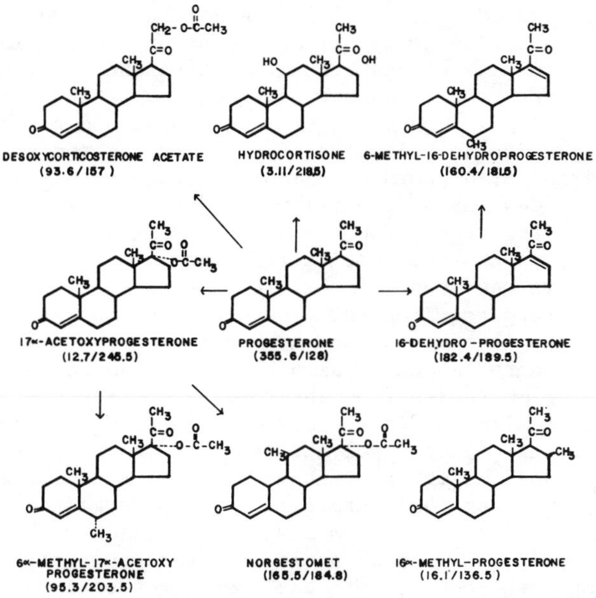

Figure 8. Chemical structure and polymer solubility (in mg/l.)/melting point of progesterone derivatives

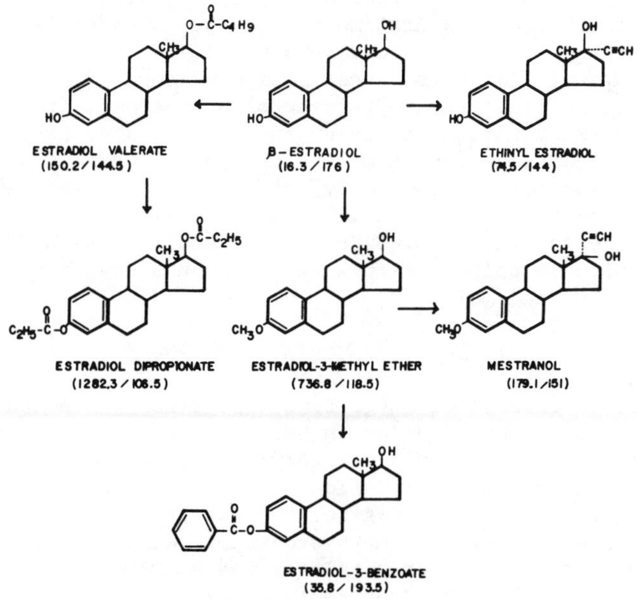

Figure 9.   Chemical structure and polymer solubility (in mg/l.)/ melting point (°C) of estradiol derivatives

a low residual variance (S^2 = 0.15) imply that the mole fraction
solubility of steroids is highly dependent on their melting point
temperature. In view of the relation established earlier on the
dependency of the drug release profiles (Eqs. 5a and 15) on polymer solubility (Cp), it appears that Eq. 20 should provide a useful application in the selection of drug analogs and in the chemical modification of a pharmacologically active agent for the development of a desirable drug delivery system.

From the slope ($\Delta Hm/2.303R$ = 3.085) in Figure 10, the dissociation energy of crystal lattice (ΔHm) was calculated to be 14.12
Kcal/mole. This magnitude of ΔHm (14.12 Kcal/mole) is the additional energy term required for the release of Norgestomet from a
silicone polymer matrix. In summary, the steady-state release of
Norgestomet requires a ΔHm value of 14.12 Kcal/mole for the dissociation of drug molecules from their lattice structure, a $\Delta HT,m$
value of 6.60 Kcal/mole for the dissolution of drug molecules in
their surrounding silicone polymer, and a Ed,m value of 3.70 Kcal/
mole for their diffusion in silicone matrix. A sum of 24.42 Kcal/
mole is necessary for the overall release of Norgestomet, under a
matrix-controlled process, from a silicone device at 37°C.

In Figure 10, all the 27 analogs of testosterone, progesterone and estradiol series were analyzed together in view of the
minor structural difference in their basic steroidal ring systems
(Figs. 7-9). This all-together treatment was justified by the
result expressed by Eq. 21. These analogs may also be classified
into three families following their structural characteristics
(Figs. 7-9) and analyzed separately (Table IV). It appeared that
the differences in the magnitudes of the ΔHm values between various
families (13.06 to 16.79 Kcal/mole) and the combined T-P-E family
(14.12 Kcal/mole) were not very substantial.

In summary, from this investigation we concluded that mechanistically, the steady-state release of Norgestomet from the silicone polymer matrix requires three energy-activated processes:
(1) The dissociation of drug molecules from a crystal lattice requires a dissociation energy (ΔHm) of 14.12 Kcal/mole; (2) the
dissolution of drug molecules in silicone polymer requires a solvation energy ($\Delta HT,m$) of 6.60 Kcal/mole; and (3) the diffusion of
drug molecules in polymer matrix requires an activation energy
(Ed,m) of 3.70 Kcal/mole.

Abstract

The controlled release of Norgestomet (SC-21009), a potent progestin for estrus synchronization in heifers, from a drug-dispersed
silicone polymer matrix-type delivery device was investigated in a
perfect sink in vitro drug elution system. The results indicated
that the initial state of drug release was predominately a partition-controlled process in the hydrodynamic diffusion layer and
that the steady-state of drug release was mainly a matrix-
controlled process in the drug depletion zone. Theoretical

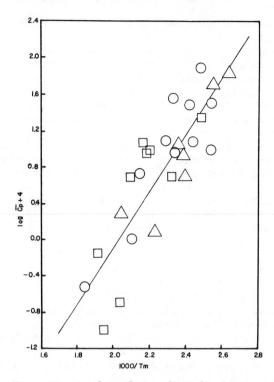

Figure 10. Semilogarithmic relationship between the mole fraction solubility ($\overline{C}p$) *of testosterone* (○), *progesterone* (□) *and estradiol* (△) *derivatives in silicone polymer and the reciprocal of the melting point temperature* (Tm^{-1}) *as expected from Eq. 20. A value of 14.12 kcal/mole was obtained for* ΔHm.

Table IV

Statistics and Thermodynamics of log $\overline{C}p$ vs. Tm^{-1} Relationship

Steroids	log $\overline{C}p$ vs. Tm^{-1} Relationships (Eq. 20)	ΔHm (Kcal/mole)
Testosterone family	log $\overline{C}p$ = -9.631 + $\frac{2.855}{Tm}$ N (11), R (0.87), S^2 (0.11)	13.06
Progesterone family	log $\overline{C}p$ = -11.469 + $\frac{3.668}{Tm}$ N (9), R (0.79), S^2 (0.23)	16.79
Estradiol family	log $\overline{C}p$ = -11.763 + $\frac{3.644}{Tm}$ N (7), R (0.94), S^2 (0.04)	16.68
Combined T-P-E family	log $\overline{C}p$ = -10.249 + $\frac{3.085}{Tm}$ N (27), R (0.85), S^2 (0.15)	14.12

analyses suggested that these two processes of drug release should result in Q vs. t and Q vs. $t^{\frac{1}{2}}$ release profiles respectively. Experimental observations agreed with these analyses. Mathematical models were also derived to search for the energy terms required for these two energy-activated processes. The results revealed that, mechanistically, the controlled release of Norgestomet from the matrix-type delivery device required three energy-activated steps: (1) The dissociation of drug molecules from a crystal lattice required a dissociation energy (ΔHm) of 14.12 Kcal/mole; (2) The dissolution of drug molecules in a silicone polymer (steady-state) or in an elution medium (initial state) required a solvation energy of 6.60 and 8.82 Kcal/mole, respectively; and (3) The diffusion of drug molecules in a polymer matrix (steady state) or in a solution phase (initial state) required an activation energy of 3.70 and 3.85 Kcal/mole, respectively. The dissociation energy was determined using 27 analogs of testosterone, progesterone and estradiol families.

References

(1)   Nakano, M.; J. Pharm. Sci.; (1971) 60 571

(2)   Long, D. M., Jr. and Folkman, J.; U.S. pat. 3,279,996 (Oct 18, 1966); through Chem. Abstr.; (1967) 66 5759g

(3)   Folkman, J., Reiling, W. and Williams, G.; Surgery; (1969) 66 194

(4)   Folkman, J., Long, D.M., Jr. and Rosenbaum, R.; Science; (1966) 154 148

(5)   Folkman, J. and Long, D.; Ann. N.Y. Acad. Sci.; (1964) 111 857

(6)   Siegel, P. and Atkinson, J.; J. Appl. Physiol.; (1971) 30 900

(7)   Bass, P., Purdon, R. and Wiley, J.; Nature; (1965) 208 591

(8)   Powers, K. G.; J. Parasitol.; (1965) 51 53

(9)   Clifford, C. M., Yonker, C. E. and Corwin, M. D.; J. Econ. Entomol.; (1967) 60 1210

(10) Wepsic, J. G.; U.S. pat. 3,598,127 (Aug. 10, 1971)

(11) Kincl, F. A., Benagiano, G. and Angee, I.; Steroids; (1968) 11 673

(12) Cornette, J. C. and Duncan, G. W.; Contraception: (1970) 1 339

(13) Lifchez, A. S. and Scommegna, A.; Fert. Steril.; (1970) 21 426

(14) Mishell, D. R. and Lumkin, M. E.; ibid.; (1970) 21 99

(15) Croxatto, H., Diaz, S., Vera, R., Etchart, M. and Atria, P.; Amer. J. Obstet., Gynecol.; (1969) 105 1135

(16) Chang, C. C. and Kincl, F. A.; Fert. Steril.; (1960) 21 134

(17) Kratochvil, P., Benagiano, G. and Kincl, F. A.; Steroids; (1970) 13 505

(18) Dzuik, P. J. and Cook, B.; Endocrinology; (1966) 78 208

(19) Schumann, R. and Taubert, H. D.; Acta Biol. Med. Germ.; (1970) 24 897

(20) Tatum, H. J., Coutinho, E. M., Filho, J. A. and Santanna, A. R. S.; Amer. J. Obstet. Gynecol.; (1969) 105 1139
(21) Tatum, H. J.; Contraception; (1970) 1 253
(22) Benagiano, G., Ermini, M., CHang, C. C., Sundaram, K. and Kincl, F. A.; Acta Endocrinol.; (1970) 63 29
(23) Haleblian, J., Runkel, R., Mueller, N., Christopherson, J. and Ng, K.; J. Pharm. Sci.; (1971) 60 541
(24) Duncan, G. W.; U.S. pat. 3,545,439 (Dec. 8, 1970)
(25) Roseman, T. J. and Higuchi, W. I.; J. Pharm. Sci.; (1970) 59 353
(26) Chien, Y. W., Lambert, H. J. and Grant, D. E.; ibid.; (1974) 63 365
(27) Chien, Y. W. and Lambert, H. J.; ibid.; (1974) 63 515
(28) Chien, Y. W., Mares, S. E., Berg, J., Huber, S., Lambert, H. J. and King, K. F.; ibid.; (1975) 64 1776
(29) Chien, Y. W., Lambert, H. J. and Lin, T. K.; ibid.; (1975) 64 1643
(30) Chien, Y. W.; American Pharmaceutical Association, 122nd Annual Meeting in San Francisco, April 19-24, 1975, Vol. 5, No. 1, pg. 125
(31) Chien, Y. W., Conference on "Drug Therapy and Novel Delivery Systems"; cosponsored by Battelle Memorial Institute and University of Washington, Seattle, Washington, April 29-May 1, 1974
(32) Chien, Y.W., Rozek, L. F. and Lambert, H. J.; American Chemical Society Symposium on "Controlled Release Polymeric Formulations"; New York, N.Y., April 7-9, 1976
(33) Martin, A. N., Swarbrick, J. and Cammarata, A.; "Physical Pharmacy". Lea and Febiger, Philadelphia, 1969, Chapter 12
(34) Barrer, R. M.; Nature; London (1937) 140 106
(35) Crank, J. and Park, G. S.; "Diffusion in Polymers", Academic Press, New York, N.Y., 1968, Chapters 2 and 3

Footnotes

1. Searle Laboratories, Division of G. D. Searle & Co., Box 5110, Chicago, Illinois 60680
2. Dow Corning Corp., Midland, Michigan 48640
3. Cole-Parmer Instrument, Chicago, Illinois 60680
4. Sage Instruments, Model 341, Cambridge, Massachusetts 02139
5. Norton, Inc., Akron, Ohio 44309
6. Coleman Model 124D Spectrophotometer, Sicentific Products, McGaw Park, Illinois 60085

Acknowledgments

Appreciation is extended to Ms. D. M. Jefferson for her technical assistance and to Drs. W. Han, J. H. Lambert, H. K. Lee and T. K. Lin for their constructive peer review. The author also wishes to thank Ms. B. Sullivan for her assistance in manuscript preparation.

6

Controlled Release of Desoxycorticosterone Acetate from Matrix-Type Silicone Devices: In Vitro–In Vivo Correlation and Prolonged Hypertension Animal Model for Cardiovascular Studies

YIE W. CHIEN and HOWARD J. LAMBERT

Pharmaceutical Research Group, Development Department, Searle Laboratories, G. D. Searle & Co., Skokie, Ill. 60076

LEONARD F. ROZEK

Cardiovascular Group, Biological Research Department, Searle Laboratories, G. D. Searle & Co., Skokie, Ill. 60076

Introduction

"Metacorticoid" hypertension, induced by the chronic administration of desoxycorticosterone acetate to rats in conjunction
with NaCl loading, simulates both pathologically and physiologi-
cally the syndrome of essential hypertension as seen in man (1).
To induce experimental hypertension in rats to evaluate anti-
hypertensive activity of various drugs, requires either daily injections of a DCA suspension or implantation of a DCA-containing
wax pellet (2) while maintaining the rats on saline. The first
technique produces a consistent onset of metacorticoid hypertension within 21 to 28 days but requires considerable daily injection time which may be hazardous for the animals. The second
technique usually results in wide variations in hypertension onset
because of inconsistent release rates of DCA from the wax matrix.
Recent reports (3-6) from this laboratory have demonstrated
that the release of steroids may be substantially prolonged and
their release profiles may be controlled at programmed levels by
homogeneously impregnating the steroids in a matrix-type silicone
polymer device (3). With this approach the intravaginal absorption of ethynodiol diacetate, a progestin, from a vaginal silicone
device was remarkably sustained (6). The same drug delivery
system was also used for the subcutaneous administration of DCA to
rats and hypertension was successfully initiated and maintained
(7).

In this investigation both the in vitro and in vivo release profiles of DCA from matrix-type silicone devices were measured and their relationship was analyzed. The time profiles for the production of metacorticoid hypertension in rats as well as the dose-response relationship were also studied.

Experimental

Preparation of Matrix-type Silicone Device: Desoxycortico-sterone acetate[1] (0.5-2.0 g.) was accurately weighed and thoroughly incorporated into 10.0 g. of Silastic 382 medical grade elastomer[2] by a mixer[3] at 1,000 r.p.m. for 5 minutes. One g. of Silastic 360 medical fluid[2] was added and thoroughly mixed for 2 minutes. One drop of stannous octoate[2], as catalyst, was then incorporated and thoroughly mixed for another minute. The mixture was then delivered by a syringe pump[4] into Tygon tubing[5] (I.D. 3/16", O.D. 5/16"). The silicone polymer was allowed to cure overnight in an exhaust hood at room temperature. After cross-linking, the resultant silicone device was removed from the Tygon mold and cut into desired lengths for various studies.

In vitro Drug Release Studies: The system used for in vitro drug release studies was reported previously (3). In the present investigation, 16 cm. lengths of the silicone devices were mounted in the arms of a plexiglas holder in a circular shape. The holder was then rotated at a constant speed (81 r.p.m.) in an elution medium (150 ml. of 75% v/v polyethylene glycol 400[6] in water) at 37°C. 50 ml. of the elution medium was sampled daily and replaced with the same quantity of drug-free elution medium (which was also maintained at 37°C). The sample was then assayed spectrophotomet-rically at a λmax of 240 nm. The daily amount of DCA released and the mechanisms of drug release were then analyzed using a computer program.

In vivo Drug Release Studies: Sixty male Charles River CD[R] strain rats (with an average weight of 130 to 190 gm. and an age of 4 to 6 weeks) were used in this investigation. A control group (implanted with placebo devices) was examined in parallel with the treated group (implanted with drug-containing device). The systolic blood pressure of each rat was indirectly determined using a programmed electrophygmomanometer[7] at the onset of the study and thereafter at weekly intervals throughout the investigation.

Following the determination of initial blood pressure, the rats were anesthetized with ether. A one cm. cutaneous incision was made in the dorsal thoracic area of each rat. After the formation of a subcutaneous tunnel with forceps, a 3 cm. length of the silicone device was inserted. The incision was closed with wound clips and the rats were then returned to their cages for recovery.

Both control and treated groups were maintained on a normal laboratory rat diet with a 1% saline fluid ration for the duration of the study.

At scheduled intervals, 5 to 7 rats were randomly selected from the treated group for removal of the silicone devices. After the measurements of systolic blood pressure, the devices were removed and their residual DCA content was completely extracted with methanol and assayed spectrophotometrically.

The placebo devices were removed from the control group at the end of each study following the final reading of systolic blood pressure and heart rate.

Subcutaneous Bolus Injection: Forty Charles River CD[R] (male, 28 days old) strain rats were randomly assigned to 5 equal groups. Systolic blood pressure was determined via a caudal plethysomograph[8] with recorder. On Day 0, all animals were weighed and blood pressures measured. All animals were then placed on a fluid ration of 1% NaCl and the assigned treatments were begun and continued for 28 days. A final set of values was obtained on Day 35 to determine the persistence and severity of blood pressure changes following discontinuation of the DCA treatments. DCA was administered daily S.C. in a volume of 1 ml./kg. of a suspension in 0.5% aqueous Tween 80 solution. The concentration of DCA was adjusted so that each group received 0, 0.2, 1.0, 2.0 and 5.0 mg./ kg., respectively. Mean group blood pressures and body weights were measured on Day 0, 7, 14, 28 and 35. Statistical significance of the differences between the means was determined using Student's t test at the 95% level of confidence ($p < 0.05$).

Results and Discussion

Subcutaneous Bolus Injection: The time course for the elevation of systolic blood pressure after daily subcutaneous bolus injections is shown in Figure 1. The initial mean systolic pressure (Day 0) prior to DCA administration did not differ significantly among groups. Blood pressures of the control group increased from 97($\pm$3) to 151($\pm$6) mm. Hg during the investigation. This increase was apparently due to the intake of 1% NaCl solution. Meanwhile, the increase in the blood pressures of Groups D and E (with daily doses of 1.0 and 0.2 mg./kg., respectively) was not significantly different from the values seen in the control group. On the other hand, the blood pressures of Groups A and B, which received a higher DCA dose (5.0 and 2.0 mg./kg./day, respectively), increased at a greater rate than the control group. These two groups (A and B) exhibited statistically higher mean values of systolic blood pressure in comparison with the control group after 21 and 28 days of DCA administration. The data also suggested that the magnitude of the elevation of systolic blood pressure for these two groups was dose-dependent, i.e., the 5 mg./kg. group showed a greater pressure elevation than the 2 mg./kg. group.

After termination of DCA administration on Day 28, the systolic blood pressure of Group B gradually returned to a level that was statistically insignificant from the control. Group A, which received the highest dose of DCA, did not return to the level of the control group in this investigation.

Thus, a minimum daily dose of 2 mg./kg. can produce a statistically significant elevation of systolic blood pressure within 21 days.

Subcutaneous Implantation of DCA-silicone Devices

(A) <u>In vitro Release of DCA from Silicone Devices</u>: The <u>in</u>

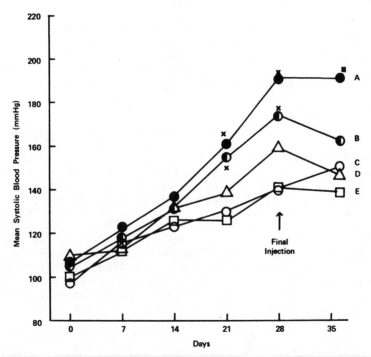

Figure 1. Time course and dose dependency of the elevation of the mean systolic blood pressure (mmHg) of rats (which were randomly divided into five groups with eight rats in each group) after daily subcutaneous injection of desoxycorticosterone acetate suspension for 28 days. Daily dose levels (mg/kg): (A) 5.0, (B) 2.0, (C) 0 (control); (D) 1.0; and (E) 0.2. Symbol (*) indicates a significant difference (p < 0.05) in the values of systolic blood pressure between treated and control group. For a clear illustration, the standard error (≤ 5%) for each data point was not shown.

vitro release pattern of desoxycorticosterone acetate (DCA) from a
matrix-type silicone device is illustrated in Figure 2. The cumulative amount (Q) of DCA released from a unit surface area of the
silicone device increased in proportion to the days of elution in
a solution medium, but not in a linear relationship manner. This
curved Q-t release pattern is very similar to our earlier observations for ethynodiol diacetate (3), a progestin for oral contraception. It was previously established (3-6) that this matrix-
controlled process is defined by the following expression:

$$Q = \sqrt{Dm(2A-Cp)Cp}\ t \qquad\qquad\qquad\text{(Eq. 1)}$$

where Q is the cumulative amount of DCA released from a unit surface area of a silicone device; A is the initial amount of DCA
homogeneously impregnated in a unit volume of polymer matrix; Dm
is the apparent diffusivity of DCA in a polymer structure; Cp is
the maximum solubility of DCA in silicone polymer; and t is time
(in days).

Eq. 1 indicates that the cumulative amount of DCA released
from a unit surface area of a silicone device, (Q) should be a
linear function of the square root of time ($t^{\frac{1}{2}}$). That is, a
linear relationship should be observed when one plots Q against $t^{\frac{1}{2}}$
(Fig. 3). The slope of this Q-$t^{\frac{1}{2}}$ linearity is defined as:

$$\frac{Q}{t^{\frac{1}{2}}} = \sqrt{Dm(2A-Cp)Cp}$$

$$\qquad\qquad\qquad\qquad\qquad\text{(Eq. 2)}$$

Eq. 2 suggests that for a given drug (whose Dm is a constant
value at a given condition) the magnitude of $Q/t^{\frac{1}{2}}$ value, the slope
of a Q-$t^{\frac{1}{2}}$ plot, is dependent on the square root of (2A-Cp)Cp.
That is, for a given drug (whose solubility in a polymer, Cp, is
constant at a given temperature) the greater the amount (A) of
drug incorporated in a polymeric device, the higher the value of
$Q/t^{\frac{1}{2}}$ that will result. This $Q/t^{\frac{1}{2}}$ vs. $[(2A-Cp)Cp]^{\frac{1}{2}}$ relationship is
demonstrated in Figure 4. A slope ($Dm^{\frac{1}{2}}$) of 0.207 cm./$day^{\frac{1}{2}}$ with
intercept at the origin was obtained. The linear relationship
(Fig. 4) implies that, if one incorporates more DCA into a silicone device to extend its duration of treatment, it will also result in a higher value of $Q/t^{\frac{1}{2}}$ and hence, a greater amount of drug
released at a given time.

The magnitude of Dm, the effective diffusivity of DCA in the
polymer structure, can be calculated from the slope ($Dm^{\frac{1}{2}}$) of the
linear $Q/t^{\frac{1}{2}}$ vs. $[(2A-Cp)Cp]^{\frac{1}{2}}$ plot (Fig. 4). A value of 4.94×10^{-7}
cm^2/sec. results. This value of diffusivity (4.94×10^{-7} cm^2/sec.)
is slightly higher than the diffusivity (3.79×10^{-7} cm^2/sec.) of
ethynodiol diacetate in the same matrix system (3). Considering
the difference in molecular volume between DCA and ethynodiol diacetate, this difference in their diffusivity is expected.

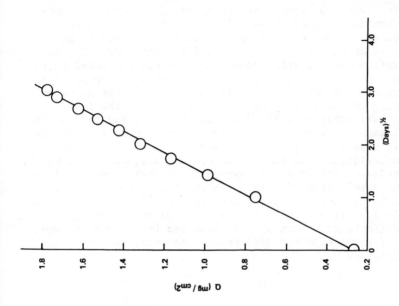

Figure 3. Linear relationship between the cumulative amount (Q) of desoxycorticosterone acetate released from a unit surface area of silicone device and the square root of time ($t^{1/2}$) as defined in Equation 1.

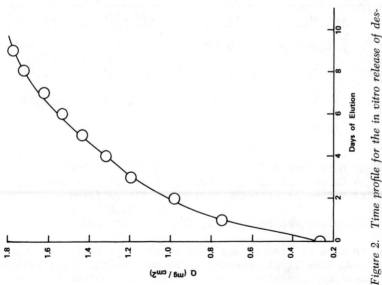

Figure 2. Time profile for the in vitro release of desoxycorticosterone acetate (A = 64.91 mg/cm³) from matrix-type silicone device at 37°C. Q is the cumulative amount of drug released from a unit surface area of device.

(B) In vivo Release of DCA from Silicone Devices and Dose-Response Relationships: Ormsbee and Ryan (7) prepared silicone devices with four dose levels of DCA (Table I, Column 1). Sub-cutaneous implantation of these silicone devices in rats for 11 weeks produced a dose-dependent elevation of the systolic blood pressure similar to that shown in Figure 1. Unfortunately, no release profile was reported and no analysis was conducted on the in vitro and in vivo releases of DCA from this matrix-type of de-livery device. However, these analyses are useful for a better understanding of the in vitro-in vivo correlation, the dose-response relationship of DCA-induced hypertension and for the fur-ther development of a suitable silicone device to deliver an op-timal daily dose of DCA for a programmed duration of treatment. In this investigation, we have tried to estimate, following Eq. 2, the magnitudes of $Q/t^{\frac{1}{2}}$ for the four silicone devices prepared in Ormsbee and Ryan's study (Table I, Column 4). From these $Q/t^{\frac{1}{2}}$ values (with unit surface area), the apparent $Q/t^{\frac{1}{2}}$ values for each silicone device (with a surface area of 8.604 cm.^{2}) may also be calculated (Table I, Column 5). As expected from Figure 4, the magnitude of these expected $Q/t^{\frac{1}{2}}$ values increased as the dose levels increased.

Table I

Calculation on the Expected Values of $Q/t^{\frac{1}{2}}$
from Silicone Devices Loading with
Various Doses of Desoxycorticosterone Acetate

Dose		(c) $[(2A-Cp)Cp]^{\frac{1}{2}}$	$Q/t^{\frac{1}{2}}$	(d)
mg/kg (a)	mg/rat (b)	$(mg/cm^3)^{\frac{1}{2}}$	$mg/cm^2/day^{\frac{1}{2}}$	$mg/day^{\frac{1}{2}}$
10	1.44	0.599	0.124	1.067
50	7.20	1.356	0.281	2.418
100	14.4	1.921	0.398	3.424
500	72.0	4.30	0.890	7.658

(a) Data from Reference 7
(b) Calculated values. Average body weight = 144 gm/rat
(c) Volume of silicone device = 0.815 cm^3/device,
            Cp = 0.1047 mg/cm^3
(d) Calculated from Eq. 2, $(Dm)^{\frac{1}{2}}$ = 0.207 cm/day$^{\frac{1}{2}}$

The results of Ormsbee and Ryan's study (7) suggested that the 100 mg/kg dose level appeared to be most suitable for inducing metacorticoid hypertension in rats. From the apparent $Q/t^{\frac{1}{2}}$ value (3.424 mg/day$^{\frac{1}{2}}$) in Table I, the total quantity of DCA released

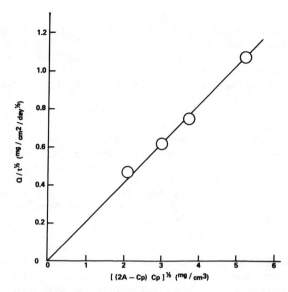

Figure 4. Linear relationship between $Q/t^{1/2}$ and $[(2A\text{-}Cp)Cp]^{1/2}$ as defined by Equation 2. Slope $(Dm^{1/2})$ = 0.207 $cm/day^{1/2}$.

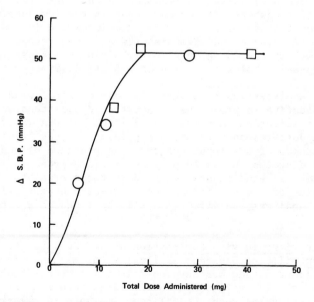

Figure 5. Relationship between ΔS.B.P. (the difference in the mean systolic blood pressure between treated and control groups) at Day 28 and the total dose of desoxycorticosterone acetate administered by ○ daily bolus injection and □ silicone device implantation

from this dose level (100 mg/kg) in a silicone device over 77-day
subcutaneous implantation ($t^{\frac{1}{2}}$ = 8.77 days$^{\frac{1}{2}}$) was estimated to be
30.03 mg. This amount of DCA is equivalent to a daily subcutane-
ous bolus injection of 390 mcg/rat/day for 77 days, which is essentially equal to the minimum daily dose of 2 mg/kg (or 400 mcg/
200 g) established earlier (Fig. 1) in which the average body
weight of rats was 196.3 gm.

In their examination, Ormsbee and Ryan (7) also observed that
a 500 mg/kg dose of DCA did not elevate systolic blood pressure
much more than the 100 mg/kg dose. Using the same calculation
applied earlier, this dose level (500 mg/kg) in a silicone device
should deliver DCA at a level equivalent to a daily subcutaneous
bolus dose of 1023.3 mcg/rat/day for 56 days. (All the animals
died before this date.) This dose level (1023.3 mcg/rat/day)
again was very close to the 1,000 mcg/rat/day (or 5 mg/kg/day) established earlier (Fig.1). These analyses show dose-response
similarities between silicone device implantation and daily bolus
injections.

To compare the relative efficacy of producing metacorticoid
hypertension in rats using these two techniques of DCA administration, an effort was made to correlate the differential systolic
blood pressure (the differences in the mean values of systolic
blood pressure between treated and control groups) on Day 28 to
the total dose of DCA administered by either daily bolus injection or silicone device implantation (Fig. 5). Obviously, both
methods of DCA administration resulted in the same trend of dose-
response relationships. It appears that in the low dose regimen,
the differential systolic blood pressure increased in proportion
with the total dose of DCA administered and then reached a plateau
at approximately the 18 mg dose level. This 18 mg dose is equivalent to a daily bolus injection of DCA of 642.9 mcg/rat/day for
28 days.

These analyses indicate that silicone device implantation was
equally effective in producing metacorticoid hypertension as the
daily bolus injection, although the delivery of DCA was different.
The common dose-response relationship (Fig. 5) that resulted from
the two methods of DCA input suggests the presence of a slow rate
step which dictates the whole process of blood pressure elevation.
More fundamental studies are required in these areas for a better
understanding of the DCA-induced metacorticoid hypertension.
Additional analyses and discussion will be found in a later
section.

(C) In vitro-In vivo Correlation of the Subcutaneous Release
of DCA from Silicone Devices: Following the mechanistic analyses,
a 3 cm silicone device was developed in the present study for 100-
day treatment. Its volume and surface area were smaller (65.6 and
56.3%, respectively) than the silicone implants (5 cm) prepared by
Ormsbee and Ryan for 77-day application (7). The incorporation of
a dose of 78.49 mg of DCA into this 3 cm delivery device resulted

in a drug concentration (A = 146.9 mg/cm^3) substantially greater than the Ormsbee-Ryan implant (A = 88.3 mg/cm^3) with DCA loading of 500 mg/kg. In vitro elution studies of this 3 cm silicone device have given a $Q/t^{\frac{1}{2}}$ value of 1.072 mg/cm^2/day$^{\frac{1}{2}}$. This is equivalent to an apparent $Q/t^{\frac{1}{2}}$ value of 5.194 mg/day$^{\frac{1}{2}}$ from a silicone device with a surface area of 4.845 cm^2. This magnitude of $Q/t^{\frac{1}{2}}$ value (5.194 mg/day$^{\frac{1}{2}}$) is in between the values resulting from Ormsbe-Ryan implants with DCA dose levels of 100 mg/kg and 500 mg/kg (Table I, Column 5). Implantation of this 3 cm silicone device ($Q/t^{\frac{1}{2}}$ = 5.194 mg/day$^{\frac{1}{2}}$) may avoid the outcome observed in the case of high dose (500 mg/kg) Ormsbee-Ryan implants. Ormsbee and Ryan reported (7) that all of the rats that received the silicone devices with 500 mg/kg dose level were dead by Week 8.

Subcutaneous implantation of these 3 cm silicone devices in the dorsal thoracic area of 60 rats for 14, 28, 43, 56, 97 and 104 days has resluted in a release profile (Fig. 6) very similar to the $Q-t^{\frac{1}{2}}$ relationship (Fig. 3) observed in the in vitro study under sink conditions. Following Eq. 2, the in vivo $Q/t^{\frac{1}{2}}$ value was calculated from the data in Figure 6 as 1.025 mg/cm^2/day$^{\frac{1}{2}}$. This magnitude of $Q/t^{\frac{1}{2}}$ value is 4.4% lower than the in vitro $Q/t^{\frac{1}{2}}$ value (1.072 mg/cm^2/day$^{\frac{1}{2}}$) reported earlier (Fig. 3).

For the analysis of in vitro-in vivo relationship, the desoxycorticosterone acetate molecules released from a silicone device are presumed to dissolve at first in the tissue fluid surrounding the implanted device before they diffuse through various biological barriers (cell layers or membrane laminates) to reach the capillary blood vessels, which maintain a perfect biological sink by hemoperfusion, in the thoracic area. In such a case, the rate of drug permeation (dQ'/dt) across a unit surface area of the biological barrier (with an aqueous diffusion layer on each side of the barrier) should be directly proportional to the drug concentration (Co) in the tissue fluid (as the driving force for drug permeation) and inversely proportional to the total diffusional resistance (ΣR) (6) which the desoxycorticosterone acetate molecules encounter along the way as they penetrate through the biological barrier:

$$\frac{dQ'}{dt} = \frac{Co}{\Sigma R}$$

(Eq. 3)

The total diffusion resistance (8) is the sum of the diffusional resistances as follows:

$$\Sigma R = Rt + \sum_{i=1}^{i=n} R_{bi} + Rc$$

(Eq. 4)

where Rt and Rc are the diffusional resistances across the aqueous diffusion layers on the tissue side and on the circulation side of the barrier, respectively; and ΣR_{bi} is the apparanet (gross) diffusional resistance across the i layers of biological barrier.

Eq. 4 is equivalent to:

$$\Sigma R = \frac{\delta t}{D_t K_{bi/\ell}} + \sum_{i=1}^{i=n} \frac{\delta bi}{D_{bi} K_{i/i-1}} + \frac{\delta c}{D_c K_{c/bi}} \qquad \text{(Eq. 5)}$$

where δ, D, and K represent the thickness, diffusivity and partition coefficient across two contacting phases, respectively; and the subscripts b, t and c stand for biological barriers and the aqueous diffusion layers on the tissue and the circulatory hemoperfusion sides of the barriers, respectively.

The instantaneous rate of drug release at time $\underline{t}$ may be derived by differentiating Eq. 1 with respect to time:

$$\frac{dQ}{dt} = \frac{1}{2}\sqrt{\frac{Dm(2A-Cp)Cp}{t}} \qquad \text{(Eq. 6)}$$

The rate of drug permeation (dQ'/dt) should be equal to the rate of drug release (dQ/dt) at a steady state. Equating Eq. 3 with Eq. 6 yields Eq. 7:

$$2Co(t)^{\frac{1}{2}} = \Sigma R[Dm(2A-Cp)Cp]^{\frac{1}{2}} \qquad \text{(Eq. 7)}$$

Eq. 7 suggests that the concentration (Co) of desoxycorticosterone acetate in the tissue fluid surrounding the implanted silicone device decreases with the square root of time $(t^{\frac{1}{2}})$ as the drug molecules diffuse actively to a sink; that is, under a matrix-controlled process (where the release of drug from the silicone matrix is a rate-limiting step), the magnitude of $2Co(t)^{\frac{1}{2}}$ is a constant since both ΣR and $[Dm(2A-Cp)Cp]^{\frac{1}{2}}$ are constants under controlled conditions. Eq. 7 also indicates that the magnitude of Co is directly proportional to the magnitude of the total diffusional resistance (ΣR) when the same silicone device is implanted in a different animal or a different tissue of the same animal (a different value of ΣR is expected). Therefore, the greater the magnitude of ΣR, the higher the value of Co since the absorption of the desoxycorticosterone acetate is inhibited. The value of ΣR can be calculated from Eq. 8:

$$\Sigma R_{\text{(in vivo)}} = \frac{2Co(t)^{\frac{1}{2}}}{[Dm(2A-Cp)Cp]^{\frac{1}{2}}_{\text{in vivo}}} = \frac{2Co(t)^{\frac{1}{2}}}{(Q/t^{\frac{1}{2}})_{\text{in vivo}}} \qquad \text{(Eq. 8)}$$

provided that the drug concentration (Co) in the tissue fluid is measurable.

In the in vitro elution studies, the elution medium was maintained at sink conditions throughout the experiment. In this case, only the thickness of the hydrodynamic diffusion layer $(\delta\ell)$ exists between the surface of the silicone device and the bulk of the elution medium.

Eq. 4 may be reduced to:

$$\Sigma R \text{ in vitro} \bullet R_\ell = \frac{\delta\ell}{D\ell} \qquad\qquad\qquad \text{(Eq. 9)}$$

where $K_{\ell/\ell} = 1$ and Eq. 7 becomes:

$$\Sigma R \text{ in vitro} = \frac{2C_0(t)^{\frac{1}{2}}}{(Q/t^{\frac{1}{2}}) \text{ in vitro}} \qquad\qquad \text{(Eq. 10)}$$

Currently, mearuring or calculating the ΣR in vivo value (Eqs. 4 and 8) can be done only with a great deal of difficulty. Extensive instrumentation has to be applied and many approximations have to be assumed. Under such conditions, however, the prediction of in vivo release profiles from an in vitro study can be done without knowing the magnitude of ΣR in vivo value, by establishing an in vitro-in vivo relationship (6). This relationship may be established by studying the mechanisms and the rates of drug release under both in vitro and in vivo conditions using the same type of drug delivery system. It was exemplified by the intravaginal absorption studies of ethynodiol diacetate in rabbits (6). A proportionality can be established by comparing ΣR in vivo (Eq. 8) with ΣR in vitro (Eq. 10). It yields:

$$\frac{\Sigma R \text{ in vivo}}{\Sigma R \text{ in vitro}} = \frac{(Q/t^{\frac{1}{2}}) \text{ in vitro}}{(Q/t^{\frac{1}{2}}) \text{ in vivo}} \qquad\qquad \text{(Eq. 11)}$$

The magnitudes of $(Q/t^{\frac{1}{2}})$ in vitro and $(Q/t^{\frac{1}{2}})$ in vivo for the controlled release of desoxycorticosterone acetate from silicone devices (matrix-type) were determined as 1.072 mg/cm^2/day$^{\frac{1}{2}}$ (Fig.3) and 1.025 mg/cm^2/day$^{\frac{1}{2}}$ (Fig. 6), respectively. Using Eq. 11, the ratio of ΣR in vivo/ΣR in vitro was estimated to be 1.046. It suggests that the total diffusional resistance the desoxycorticosterone acetate molecules have to overcome during their subcutaneous absorption in the thoracic area is only 1.046 times the total diffusional resistance they encounter in the parallel in vitro elution study.

The magnitude of an in vivo release profile, $(Q/t^{\frac{1}{2}})$ in vivo, from in vitro release data, $(Q/t^{\frac{1}{2}})$ in vitro, can be predicted by using the following equation:

$$(Q/t^{\frac{1}{2}})\text{in vivo} = (Q/t^{\frac{1}{2}})\text{in vitro} \bullet \frac{\Sigma R \text{ in vitro}}{\Sigma R \text{ in vivo}} \qquad \text{(Eq. 12)}$$

In this study, the magnitude of $(Q/t^{\frac{1}{2}})$ in vivo (1.025 mg/cm^2/day$^{\frac{1}{2}}$) for the subcutaneous release of desoxycorticosterone acetate from an implanted silicone device can be related to its in vitro $Q/t^{\frac{1}{2}}$ value (1.072 mg/cm^2/day$^{\frac{1}{2}}$) by a factor (ΣR in vitro/ΣR in vivo) of 0.956. This proportionality (0.956) was found very useful in the translation of in vitro data to in vivo drug release

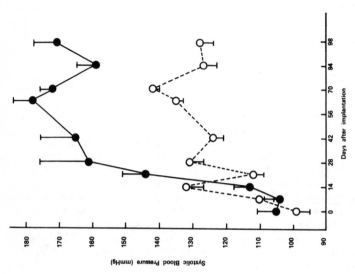
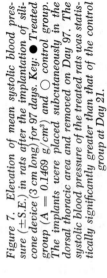

Figure 7. Elevation of mean systolic blood pressure (±S.E.) in rats after the implantation of silicone device (3 cm long) for 97 days. Key: ● Treated group (A = 0.1469 g/cm³) and ○ control group. The implants were placed subcutaneously in the dorsal thoracic area and removed on Day 97. The systolic blood pressure of the treated rats was statistically significantly greater than that of the control group at Day 21.

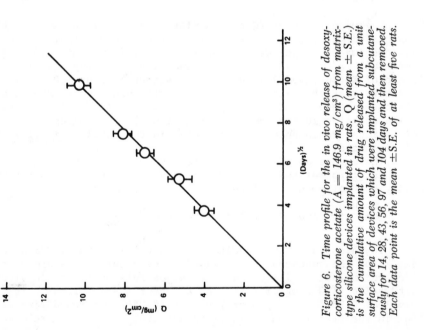

Figure 6. Time profile for the in vivo release of desoxycorticosterone acetate (A = 146.9 mg/cm³) from matrixtype silicone devices implanted in rats. Q (mean ± S.E.) is the cumulative amount of drug released from a unit surface area of devices which were implanted subcutaneously for 14, 28, 43, 56, 97 and 104 days and then removed. Each data point is the mean ±S.E. of at least five rats.

profiles as long as the in vitro drug elution studies were conducted under controlled conditions (where ΣR in vitro is constant).

Eq. 12 is a useful working equation for the future development of a suitable long-acting delivery system. As soon as this
relationship is established, the proportionality of ΣR in vitro/
ΣR in vivo can be applied to translate all the short-term in vitro
drug release results (7-day release data in this investigation) to
long-term in vivo studies (104-day subcutaneous absorption in this
investigation). It is so convenient that only the in vitro elution experiments are required to formulate a desirable long-
acting delivery device for delivering an optimal dose for a programmed duration of treatment.

(D) Prolonged "Metacorticoid" Hypertension: One of the
primary objectives of this study was to investigate the possibility of producing a reproducible, prolonged "metacorticoid" hypertension by subcutaneous implantation of single DCA-containing
silicone device. Figure 7 is a typical result, demonstrating the
development of long-acting hypertension in rats by such a method
of desoxycorticosterone acetate delivery.

It was noted that the systolic blood pressure of both treated
and control rats was elevated substantially after the implantation
of either DCA-containing silicone device or placebo. Possibly
this was caused by the daily intake of normal saline. At Day 21,
however, the elevation of systolic blood pressure in the treated
rats was significantly greater statistically than that in the control group. This hypertension state was maintained and prolonged
for 76 days until the silicone implants were withdrawn on Day 97.
This long-acting experimental hypertension model should facilitate
a routine evaluation program of anti-hypertensive drugs.

In conclusion, this investigation has demonstrated that a
perfect in vitro-in vivo relationship exists for the controlled
release of desoxycorticosterone acetate from a matrix-type silicone device. The subcutaneous implantation of such a polymeric
drug delivery system in rats has yielded a reproducible, long-
acting "metacorticoid" hypertension which should facilitate the
evaluation of anti-hypertensive drugs.

Abstract

The controlled release pattern of desoxycorticosterone
acetate (DCA) from matrix-type silicone devices was fully investigated in a "perfect sink" in vitro drug elution system. The
effect of the drug content on the release profile was examined and
the effective diffusivity of desoxycorticosterone acetate was determined. The 104-day subcutaneous implantation of a 3 cm DCA
device in each of 60 rats provided excellent in vivo correlation
of drug release predicted in vitro and a prolonged metacorticoid
hypertension. The elevation of systolic blood pressure was initiated at Day 21 and sustained for an additional 77 days. The

Dose-response relationship for systolic blood pressure elevation was analyzed and compared with that observed after a daily bolus injection.

Literature Cited

(1) Stanton, H. C. and White, J. B.; Arch. Int. Pharmacodyn.; (1965) 154 351
(2) Sturdevant, F. M.; Ann. Intern. Med.; (1958) 49 1281
(3) Chien, Y. W., Lambert, H. J. and Grant, D. E.; J. Pharm. Sci.; (1974) 63 365
(4) Chien, Y. W. and Lambert, H. J.; ibid.; (1974) 63 515
(5) Chien, Y. W., Lambert, H. J. and Lin, T. K.; ibid.; (1975) 64 1643
(6) Chien, Y. W.; Mares, S. E.; Berg, J.; Huber, S.; Lambert, H. J. and King, K. F.; ibid.; (1975) 64 1776
(7) Ormsbee, H. F., III and Ryan, C. F.; ibid.; (1973) 62 255
(8) Scheuplein, R. J.; J. Theoret. Biol.; (1968) 18 72

Footnotes

1. Searle Chemicals, Inc., P.O. Box 8526, Chicago, Illinois
2. Dow Corning Corp., Midland, Michigan 48640
3. Cole-Parmer Instrument, Chicago, Illinois 60680
4. Sage Instruments, Model 341, Cambridge, Massachusetts 02139
5. Norton, Inc., Akron, Ohio 44309
6. MC/B Manufacturing Chemists, Norwood, Ohio 45212
7. Narco Biosystems, Inc., Model PE-300, Houston, Texas 77017

Acknowledgment

The authors wish to express their appreciation to Ms. D. M. Jefferson, Mr. K. G. Roller and Ms. L. Zeitlin for their technical assistance and also to Ms. B. Sullivan for her manuscript preparation.

Interfacing Matrix Release and Membrane Absorption— Analysis of Steroid Absorption from a Vaginal Device in the Rabbit Doe

G. L. FLYNN, N. F. H. HO, S. HWANG, E. OWADA, A. MOLOKHIA, C. R. BEHL, W. I. HIGUCHI, T. YOTSUYANAGI, Y. SHAH, and J. PARK

The University of Michigan, College of Pharmacy, Ann Arbor, Mich. 48109

The vaginal route of administration of drugs for contraceptive purposes has been clinically proven to be an effective means of therapeutic delivery of the chemical drug entities. Both protestational steroids (1) and prostaglandins (2) have been successfully used vaginally. It has been suggested by those involved in this research that the vaginal route may provide a means of avoiding systemic toxicities of the contraceptive agents while at the same time realizing their full contraceptive potentials. In part this suggestion is based on presumed local or regional action of the contraceptives. But even if the action is systemic certain advantages over other modes of administration accrue. The vaginal route provides for continuous administration and thereby, under properly controlled conditions, ultra-efficient use of the therapeutic agents. In other words, the vaginal route may be used as a source of continuous "infusion" of drug to avoid surging and ebbing of blood levels associated with the use of oral dosage forms (tablets and capsules) which are administered as discrete, discontinuous doses. Moreover, the perieum venous plexus, which "drains" the vaginal tissue and rectum, flows into the pudental vein and ultimately into the vena cava, which circumnavigates the liver on first pass. This is in marked contrast to the gastrointestinal blood supply which "drains" into the portal vein and passes directly through the liver before being turned into the general circulation. Thus, so-called first pass effects in the liver are avoided by the vaginal route. Drugs efficiently metabolized in the liver often do not escape intact to the general system upon oral administration. Both progesterone and β-estradiol are poorly bioavailable orally and it has been speculated that this inefficiency is attributable to a liver first pass effect. Therefore, vaginal administration may be of real consequence with the natural contraceptive steroids.

In order to realize the full potential of the vaginal route of administration, one must be able to design and program physicochemical systems (vehicles or devices) to deliver the therapeutic agents which they contain to the general circulation at a

specified, optimal rate. At a minimum both the rate of presentation of the drug to the device-vaginal membrane interface and the
rate of uptake by the vaginal membrane must be considered. Most
of the work on the drug delivery capabilities of unique vaginal
delivery systems has focused on the former aspect, that is, on
the device drug release characteristics. It has generally been
assumed that release from the device will be the principal rate
controlling factor and that the vaginal wall and contiguous
hydrodynamic boundary are relatively unimportant. Until recently,
this remained an assumption only as there were no quantitative
data on the permeability of the tissue nor any mechanistic understanding of its barrier properties. These problems are now being
fruitfully explored in our laboratories (3,4,5). Furthermore,
Roseman (6) provides a strong clue that this assumption may be
tenuous as he has demonstrated that the absorption of the contraceptive steroid, medroxyprogesterone-17-acetate (Provera), suspended in a cylindrical polydimethylsiloxane (Silastic) matrix
is significantly controlled in the initial release period by a
"boundary layer" existing between the surface of the device and
the general tissue circulation (diffusional sink). The boundary
layer "thickness" chosen to fit the data was several times larger
than the true hydrodynamic boundary layer observed in in vitro
release studies. The possibility exists that some of the boundary layer diffusive resistance in vivo can be assigned to the
vaginal membrane.

A completely predictive analysis of the drug delivery capabilities of a vaginal formula or device must necessarily include
simultaneous assessment of the release and the membrane uptake
and transport components. The latter is comprised of two distinct
contributions which are physically assignable to a true boundary
layer of moisture between the device and the vaginal surface and
the tissue or membrane itself. The absorption of drugs vaginally
in principal may be regulated by any or all of the above phases
depending on the relative resistances of the respective strata.
To be more specific, the absorption from a device is a process
dependent on several definable sequential steps. If the device
is a suspension matrix, the steps are dissolution of the finely
divided solid particles in the matrix into the matrix continuum,
diffusion through the matrix to the matrix surface, partitioning
into and diffusion across the fluid boundary layer (moisture)
between the device and the vaginal wall, permeation of the surface vaginal tissue (vaginal epithelium) and, lastly, uptake and
distribution by circulating blood and lymph at some distance in
the tissue.

In the present studies we have developed methods whereby
the permeability of the vaginal membrane can be independently
quantitatively assessed. This, coupled with the independently
determined matrix release characteristics allows for the development of a comprehensive model based upon diffusion through a series barrier composed of right concentric cylinders. The model

suggests that the rate controlling step in the absorption process will vary with the vaginal residence time of the device and it relates the relative rate determining capacity of a step to the physicochemical properties of the diffusant (drug), the device, the aqueous boundary layer and the vaginal membrane. Experiments have been performed in which the in vivo release of progesterone is followed from a thin cylindrical suspension matrix wrapped around an inert solid core, using residual analysis as a measure of the amount absorbed. This constitutes a third and confirmatory experimental stage and, taken together, the separate experimental approaches of assessment of in vitro matrix release, assessment of the actual membrane permeability and assessment of in vivo release put the bioavailability question in a most practical context.

Thus, as a part of a continuing systems analysis of the vaginal delivery of drugs, the results of studies on membrane permeability of the rabbit vagina, in vitro release from a silicone polymer matrix, in vivo absorption from the matrix and the composite physical model and equations are brought together and integrated in this report. A rigorous description is presented for the drug release and absorption process.

Theoretical Development of the Model

A physical picture of a cylindrical matrix device in the vaginal cavity is given in Figure 1. The important features are the receding boundary layer in the device as the drug is eluted with time, an aqueous boundary layer between the device and the vaginal surface and a vaginal membrane composed of a lipid continuum with interspersed "pores" or an aqueous shunt pathway. The drawing is highly schematic and not meant to suggest either the actual construction of the membrane (real pores) or actual dimensions of the parts. The essential features of the membrane, parallel lipid and aqueous pathways, have been demonstrated in previous permeability experiments with the n-alkanols.

Following T. Higuchi (7) and Roseman and W. Higuchi (8), it is assumed that the drug in the matrix is finely divided and uniformally distributed such that matrix dissolution is not a rate determining factor and a sharp boundary is maintained between the suspension phase and the eluted region within the device which recedes into the device as time passes. The drug is assumed to have a finite solubility in the matrix, C_S, and a total concentration per unit volume including the undissolved solids much greater than C_S and indicated by A. The drug is assumed to reach the matrix surface by diffusion through the matrix continuum rather than pores and end diffusion is neglected. Under these conditions an activity gradient for the drug will be established beginning at the receding boundary interface within the device and essentially terminating at the outer reaches of the vaginal microcirculation where the drug is picked up and

systemically diluted. This gradient is depicted in Figure 1 as
a discontinuous concentration gradient from matrix to blood.

Assuming a quasi steady-state at all times, the fluxes in
the matrix, aqueous diffusion layer and vaginal membrane will be
instantaneously equivalent and may be mathematically represented
by:

$$J_{matrix} = - \frac{2\pi h D_e (C_s - C_s')}{\ln a/a_o} \tag{1}$$

$$J_{aq} = 2\pi h a_o \frac{D_{aq}}{h_{aq}} (C_a - C_b) \tag{2}$$

$$J_{membrane} = 2\pi h a_m \left[\frac{\alpha D_o C_o}{h_m} + \frac{(1-\alpha) D_p C_p}{h_m} \right] \tag{3}$$

where h is the length of the cylinder; D_e is the effective diffusion coefficient in the matrix; a, a_o and a_m are the radial dimensions of the receding boundary in the matrix, the cylinder and
vaginal membrane surface, respectively; h_{aq} and h_m are the thicknesses of the aqueous diffusion layer and the vaginal membrane;
D_{aq}, D_o and D_p are the diffusion coefficients in the aqueous
layer, the lipid phase of the membrane and the aqueous pores
respectively, α is the volume fraction of the lipid biophase of
the membrane; C_s and C_s' are the solubility of the drug in the
matrix and concentration at the surface on the matrix side; C_a
and C_b are the concentrations in the aqueous layer at the matrix
surface and membrane surface and C_o and C_p are the concentrations
in the membrane at the interface of the lipid, pores and aqueous
layer. The radial receding boundary a is, for a given set of
diffusional parameters, a function of the total amount of drug
in the matrix A, and time of release. It is taken as the sharp
interface between the suspension depleted zone in the matrix with
the remainder of the matrix (8). Since the polymer matrix often
contains fillers and other obstructions to diffusion, the effective diffusion coefficient in the matrix is described by:

$$D_e = \frac{\varepsilon D}{\tau} \tag{4}$$

where D is the intrinsic diffusion coefficient, ε is the porosity
and τ is a factor accounting for non-linearity of the "average"
diffusional path called the tortuosity. The partition coefficients of the drug for the polymer matrix-water (K_s) and lipid
biophase-water (K) are defined as follows:

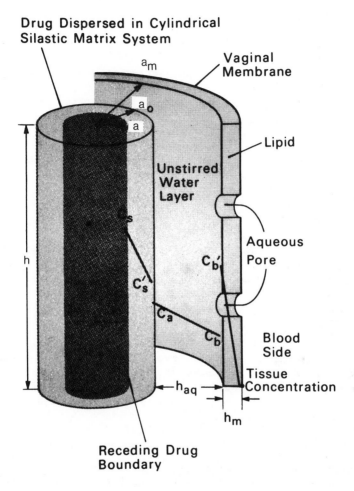

Figure 1. Schematic of a cylindrical matrix device in the vaginal lumen

$$K_s = \frac{C_s'}{C_a} \tag{5}$$

$$K = \frac{C_o}{C_b} = \frac{C_o}{C_p} \tag{6}$$

The continuity of flow across the series of barriers in the quasi steady-state is given by:

$$J_{matrix} = J_{aq} = J_{membrane} \tag{7}$$

Combining equations 1, 2, 3, 5, 6 and 7 yields:

$$J_{matrix} = \frac{2\pi h D_e C_s}{\frac{D_e K_s}{a_o}\left(\frac{1}{P_{aq}} + \frac{1}{P_m}\right) - \ln (a/a_o)} \tag{8}$$

where P_{aq} is the permeability coefficient across the aqueous diffusion layer or is the reciprocal diffusional resistance across this phase:

$$P_{aq} = \frac{D_{aq}}{h_{aq}} \tag{9}$$

and P_m is the complex permeability coefficient across the membrane or is the sum of the permeability coefficients of the parallel lipid and aqueous pathways:

$$P_m = P_o + P_p = \frac{\alpha D_o K}{h_m} + \frac{(1-\alpha)D_p}{h_m} \tag{10}$$

The membrane and diffusion layer phases can be approximated as planar resistances in series as the thicknesses of these regions are small in comparison to the vaginal cavital dimensions (9). The receding boundary on the other hand must be characterized in terms of its actual (cylindrical) geometry.

The flux out of the matrix is a function of the rate of change in the thickness of the receding boundary. Accordingly, if $A \gg C_s'$;

$$J_{matrix} = \frac{dQ}{dt} = -2\pi h A a \frac{da}{dt} \tag{11}$$

where Q is the amount of drug released, h is the length of the cylinder, a is the radial coordinate of the receding boundary and t is the time.

Combining Eqs. 8 and 11 and integrating between $a = a_0$ at $t = o$ and $a = a$ at $t = t$, the change in the receding boundary with time is:

$$\left[\frac{D_e K_s}{2a_0} \left(\frac{1}{P_{aq}} + \frac{1}{P_m}\right) + \frac{1}{4}\right]\left(a_0^2 - a^2\right) + \frac{a^2}{2} \ln (a/a_0) = \frac{D_e C_s}{A} t \qquad (12)$$

Based on equation 11 the amount and also the fraction of drug released are:

$$Q = \pi h A(a_0^2 - a^2) \qquad (13)$$

$$\frac{Q}{\pi a_0^2 hA} = \left[1 - (\frac{a}{a_0})^2\right] \qquad (14)$$

It follows upon incorporation of Eq. 13 into Eq. 12 that:

$$\frac{1}{2\pi hA}\left[\frac{D_e K_s}{a_0}\left(\frac{1}{P_{aq}} + \frac{1}{P_m}\right) + \frac{1}{2}\right] Q + \frac{1}{2}(a_0^2 - \frac{Q}{\pi hA}) \ln\sqrt{1 - \frac{Q}{\pi h a_0^2 A}}$$

$$= \frac{D_e C_s}{A} t \qquad (15)$$

or

$$\left[\frac{D_e K_s}{a_0}\left(\frac{1}{P_{aq}} + \frac{1}{P_m}\right) + \frac{1}{2}\right] Q + (\pi h a_0^2 A - Q) \ln\sqrt{1 - \frac{Q}{\pi h a_0^2 A}}$$

$$= (2\pi h D_e C_s) t \qquad (16)$$

Several simplified forms of Eqs. 12 and 16 may be specified for particular boundary conditions. At relatively early time periods $a/a_0 \simeq 1$ and:

$$\ln a/a_0 \simeq \frac{a}{a_0} - 1 \qquad (17)$$

Thus, Eq. 12 becomes:

$$\left[\frac{D_e K_s}{2a_o} \left(\frac{1}{P_{aq}} + \frac{1}{P_m}\right) + \frac{1}{4}\right] (a_o^2 - a^2) - \frac{a^2}{2a_o} (a_o - a) = \frac{D_e C_s}{A} t \tag{18}$$

Also, when:

$$\frac{Q}{\pi h a_o^2 A} << 1.0 \tag{19}$$

it follows that:

$$\frac{1}{2} \ln \left(1 - \frac{Q}{\pi h a_o^2 A}\right) \stackrel{\sim}{\sim} - \frac{Q}{2\pi h a_o^2 A} \tag{20}$$

With some rearrangement of terms, Eq. 15 reduces to a quadratic expression for this latter condition:

$$\frac{Q^2}{2\pi h a_o^2 A} + \frac{D_e K_s}{a_o} \left(\frac{1}{P_{aq}} + \frac{1}{P_m}\right) Q = (2\pi h D_e C_s) t \tag{21}$$

After differentiating with respect to time, the rate of drug released from the matrix per unit area is:

$$\frac{1}{2\pi h a_o} \frac{dQ}{dt} = \frac{dQ'}{dt} = \frac{D_e C_s A}{\sqrt{\left[D_e K_s \left(\frac{1}{P_{aq}} + \frac{1}{P_m}\right)\right]^2 + 4D_e C_s At}} \tag{22}$$

For cases where either the hydrodynamic boundary layer or vaginal membrane are rate controlling Eq. 22 becomes:

$$\frac{dQ'}{dt} = \frac{C_s P_{aq} P_m}{K_s (P_{aq} + P_m)} \tag{23}$$

and the release is zero order. When the receding boundary has progressed sufficiently to establish the matrix controlled case:

$$\frac{dQ'}{dt} = \frac{1}{2} \sqrt{\frac{D_e C_s A}{t}} \tag{24}$$

which is the typical square root of time dependency for such systems. Considering Eqs. 22, 23 and 24, it can be seen that the rate (or flux) changes from the non-matrix-controlled case to the matrix-controlled case with time as the resistance in the receding boundary increases. The practical question is not so much whether a device is diffusion layer-vaginal membrane controlled or matrix controlled but, how long can or will the zero order release be sustained in vivo for, in any protracted usage period, matrix control is inevitable.

General Nature of the Vaginal Mucosal Barrier

The absorption of chemicals into the systemic circulation via the vaginal route has been known to occur for about a century. Early reports of vaginal absorption were associated with human toxicities and deaths from vaginally administered, turn of the century products containing mercury, arsenic and other poisons. These occurrences are reviewed by Macht (10). Later, attention was turned to the possibilities of the vaginal tract as a site for drug administration for systemic effects (11). For the most part clinical or pharmacological evidence for absorption was obtained and absorption was only qualitatively demonstrated. Until very recently in our laboratories, no systematic studies of vaginal absorption were performed and nothing mechanistic was known about the barrier. The perfusion apparatus used in these studies is schematically shown in Figure 2 where a rib-cage perfusion cell is connected to the perfusate reservoir, pump, and an assemblage for flushing out the vagina prior to initiating a run. The operation of this system has been previously described (3). In Figure 3 a schematic diagram of the cell in place in the doe's vaginal cavity is shown. The cell is implanted surgically and a given rabbit is useful for studies for a period of roughly a week after recovery from the operation. In our initial studies with model permeants, the n-alkanols and the n-carboxylic acids, which were chosen because of regularly altering physicochemical properties, we were able to show that the vaginal barrier was, operationally, similar to other moist mucosal barriers. It is permeable to non-electrolytes and ions, shows a partitioning dependency with certain compounds and is of sufficiently low diffusional resistance that the hydrodynamic fluid boundary layer in series in perfusion experiments comes into play very early as one ascends a homologous series. These features are displayed in Figure 4 where the sigmoid shaped curve for the n-alkanols permeating the rabbit vaginal membrane are shown. These are presented as the ratio of the permeability coefficient of any arbitrary n-alkanol to that of methanol. Actually both absolute and relative rates of absorption of an alkanol and methanol were simultaneously obtained in each experimental run by using two different radiolabels (^{3}H and ^{14}C) on the simultaneously administered species. Stirring effects using a magnetically operated stirrer placed on a center shaft in the perfusion cell were used to unequivocally demonstrate the existence of a significant hydrodynamic boundary layer barrier. The "pore" route or parallel aqueous pathway through the membranous structure is exhibited as

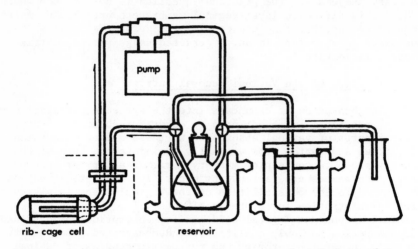

Figure 2.   Schematic of the perfusion system showing the cell, the circulating pump, the perfusate reservoir, and, on the right, the system for flushing out the cell and lines

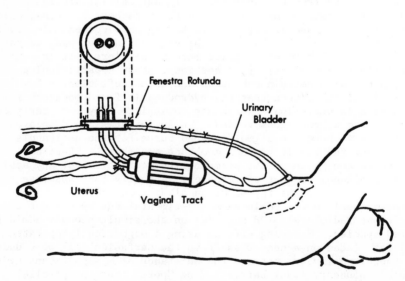

Figure 3.   Diagram of the perfusion cell in place in the rabbit vaginal lumen

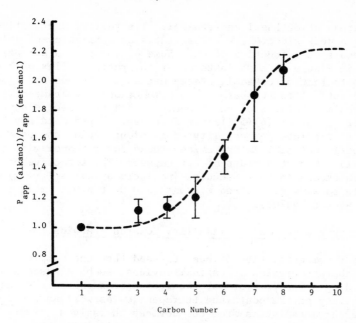

Figure 4. Relative permeability of the n-alkanols *(methanol = 1) as a function of alkyl chain length*

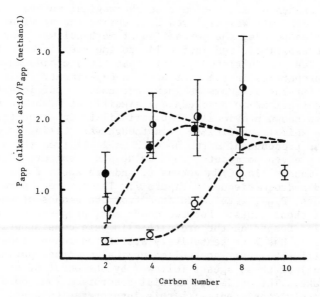

Figure 5. Relative permeability of the n-alkanoie *acids at pH = 3 (●), pH = 6 (◐) and pH = 8 (○). The dotted lines in this figure and Figure 4 are theoretical curves based on a bifunctional membrane in series with an aqueous stratum.*

the plateau at methanol and ethanol. Its reality was confirmed
using the weak electrolyte carboxylates as permeants and doing
experiments as a function of pH. Some of these data are presented in Figure 5, also in terms of the ratio of flux of the
species to that of co-administered methanol. The dashed lines
are theoretical curves based on a bifunctional membrane-diffusion
layer model. Details of these analyses are presented elsewhere
in papers in print (4)(5)(12) or in press. These data may be converted to absolute permeability coefficients using the permeability coefficient of 1.7×10^{-4} cm/sec found for methanol with a standard deviation on the order of 0.4 cm/sec. The effective boundary
layer thickness in these studies (no intravaginal stirring) was
found to be several hundred microns (250 μ or 0.025 cm is taken
as the average value).

Studies on the Vaginal Permeability Towards Steroids

In the introduction it was stressed that the complete operational characteristics of vaginal devices, such as suspension
matrix drug delivery systems, requires assessment of the vaginal
permeability of the contained therapeutics as well as the in vitro
release characteristics from the devices themselves. There are
circumstances where the former can be rate limiting and, in any
case, the barrier properties of the vaginal tissues establish an
upper limit on the amounts of drug which can be systemically delivered. For these reasons we began studies to characterize the
permeation rates of steroids across the vaginal mucosa. The rib-
cage perfusion cell was employed but, unlike the previous studies
with model compounds, the permeation of methanol was assessed in
a separate experiment run just prior to the steroid experiment.
This practice was initiated just in case the steroids changed the
membrane properties in the course of an experiment. This was not
a concern for the alkanols as they were used in sufficiently di-
lute concentrations to preclude any significant membrane effects.
It had been shown previously that variability in sequential runs
in a given animal was minimal even though variability between
animals was pronounced, often as much as ± 50% from the average
value for a given permeant. The raw uptake data were plotted in
the usual manner, log C/C_0 versus t, and are shown for progesterone and hydrocortisone in Figure 7. The apparent permeability
coefficients, P_{app}, were calculated from the slopes of the linear
regions of these plots. For two compounds, progesterone and
estrone, intercepts on the ordinate axis were consistently observed. This has been tentatively attributed to an almost completely diffusion layer controlled vaginal membrane partitioning
(or binding) of these agents followed by the onset of steady-
state uptake. The estimated initial absorption rate data are
quantitatively consistent with this interpretation considering
the extreme hydrophobic natures of progesterone and estrone and
a P_{aq} value based on an effective boundary layer thickness of

approximately 250 μ (0.025 cm) and D_{aq} values of about 7×10^{-6} cm^2/sec. The data for the four steroids are tabulated in Table I.

TABLE I

Vaginal Permeability Parameters
of Several Steroids

Steroid	$P_{app} \times 10^4$ (cm/sec)[1]	$P_m \times 10^4$ (cm/sec)[2]
Progesterone	1.92	6.1
Esterone	2.05	7.6
Hydrocortisone	0.48	0.58
Testosterone	0.59	0.75
Methanol (control)[3]	2.06	--

1. From the slope of the steady-state portion of the curves as found in Figs. 6 and 7.

2. Calculated from

$$\frac{1}{P_{app}} = \frac{1}{P_{aq}} + \frac{1}{P_m}$$

assuming no pore diffusion ($P_p = 0$) and based on $h_{aq} \simeq 250$ μ and $D_{aq} = 7 \times 10^{-6}$ cm^2/sec.

3. Average value with steroids.

The diffusion layer thickness is an estimate based on the alkanols studied which were performed at the same perfusion rate. The steroid diffusivity in water is an estimate based on Sutherland-Einstein calculation. The most significant aspect of these data is the near boundary layer control observed for progesterone and estrone. These two steroids apparently have little problem partitioning into and diffusing across the vaginal membrane. On the other hand, hydrocortisone and testosterone, two considerably more polar steroids, are primarily held back by the membrane and diffuse across a several hundred micron thick effective diffusion layer with relative ease. Pore permeation was discounted as studies on the gastrointestinal membrane indicate such large molecules do not gain access to the aqueous channels.

In Vitro Matrix Release

In order to get basic diffusional parameters of some select steroids in an experimental matrix system for later predictive analysis, the release of two steroids, progesterone and hydrocortisone, was followed from polydimethylsiloxane (Silastic[R] 382) sheeting using two different procedures. In the first procedure the exsorption of radiolabeled steroid was followed from sheeting

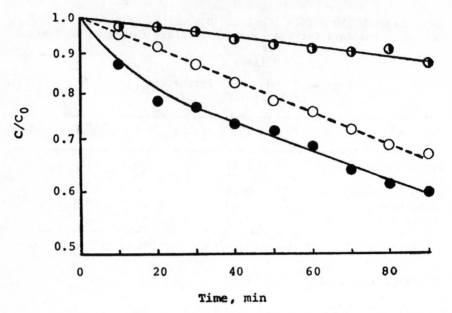

Figure 6. Vaginal absorption of estrone, ●; testosterone, ◑; and the reference compound, methanol, ○

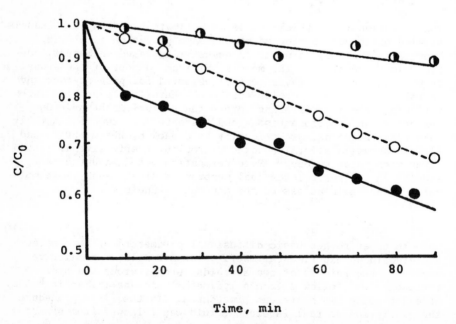

Figure 7. Vaginal absorption of progesterone, ●; hydrocortisone, ◑; and methanol, ○

which had been saturated with the tagged compound by long immersion in saturated aqueous solutions. Membrane sheeting, 500 microns thick, was made for the purpose in the following manner. Six drops of stannous octoate catalyst* was mixed thoroughly with 30 gms of Silastic 382 elastomer base** in a glass container for two minutes. The mixture was pressed between two flat teflon-coated steel plates (4x6 inches) and cured for 24 hours at room temperature. These plain membrane sheets were then cut into convenient sizes for steroid uptake and release studies. The plain silastic membranes (5.2 x 5.2 cm^2) were allowed to equilibrate with a saturated aqueous steroid solution containing both tritium-labeled and cold material. Equilibrium was ascertained by taking samples at various time intervals for assay by liquid scintillation counting. The steroid-loaded membranes were rinsed with distilled water and wiped with an absorbing tissue. Release of the radiolabeled compound into 0.1 M, pH 6.0 isotonic phosphate buffers was followed.

The experimental setup employed in the release experiments is shown in Figure 8. The membrane was cemented to a glass base and an open cylinder bolted to the upper surface to make a cup-like container. The system above the membrane surface was jacketed for temperature control. Release was followed into the buffer solution overlayered over the membrane. One ml samples were taken at predetermined intervals and replaced with fresh solvent. The data were corrected for the diluting effect of the sampling and replacement procedure.

The second procedure involved release of cold steroid from suspensions of the steroids in polydimethylsiloxane. Sheeting was prepared as previously but, before adding the catalyst, the steroid was carefully levigated into the fluid silicone polymer in a fashion to assure uniform distribution. Micronized steroid was used here to eliminate particle size effects on the release process. The 1.5% progesterone suspension film was prepared, for example, by incorporating 0.75 gm of progesterone into 50 gm of the elastomer. After thorough distribution, 15 drops of the catalyst were added and the mass was compressed as before to a thickness of 500 microns. Rectangular strips of the sheeting were cut to dimensions of 3.3 cm x 6.3 cm and wrapped around glass posts made to be the same size as the rib-cage permeation cell. These were glued to the glass surface so that only the upper surfaces (and edges) were exposed when placed in the eluting solution. The total membrane area, neglecting the edges, was 20.7 cm^2. A photograph of the matrix apparatus is shown in Figure 9. The membrane devices were mounted and immersed in a bath and 37°C water was continuously metered into the bath with the overflow draining into a laboratory sink. The continuous flushing maintained a sink condition for the exsorption process. A stirrer

---

*Catalyst M, Dow Corning, Midland, Mich.
**Silastic 382 Elastomer Base, Dow Corning, Midland, Mich.

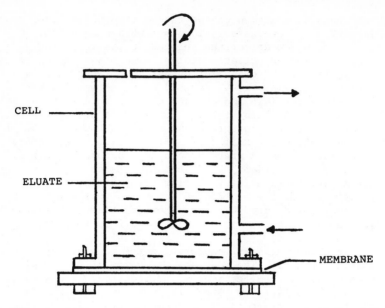

CELL

ELUATE

MEMBRANE

Figure 8.   *Apparatus for the release of steroids from saturated polydimethyl-*
siloxane matrices

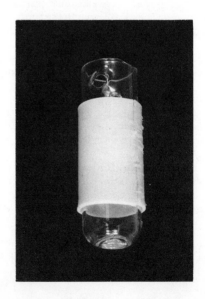

Figure 9.   *The suspension ma-*
trix release membrane device

was placed in the bath to keep the aqueous contents fully mixed
and to minimize the effective aqueous diffusion layer. Release
in this case was followed by analysis of residual progesterone
(or hydrocortisone) in the Silastic membrane. Devices prepared
identically from the same membrane suspension were periodically
removed from the bath, cut into smaller pieces (2 to 5) and then
each piece was weighed, extracted three times with methylene
chloride for an hour each time and brought to a 100 ml volume.
Samples were taken from the latter and assayed spectrophotometrically. The procedure worked well with progesterone but was inadequate for hydrocortisone due to problems of incomplete extraction. The release device was prepared in the described fashion
for two reasons. Firstly, the device was prepared to be an exact
prototype of a system later to be used as an intravaginal implant
in the rabbit doe. Secondly, the thin film was used in order
that significant percentages of release would be obtained in
reasonable periods of time. Since release was by difference or
by residual analysis, significant percentages had to be released
to get accurate data. A solid cylindrical device would have required the assessment of small differences between the initial
loading and the residual loading unless extremely long and, from
the standpoint of in vivo studies, impractical times had passed.
    The kinetic data from the flat solution matrix system were
analyzed according to non-steady-state diffusion from a semi-
infinite slab. The eluting buffer was vigorously stirred to
minimize the effective hydrodynamic boundary layer and a quasi-
steady-state flux across the aqueous diffusion layer was assumed.
The method of Suzuki, Higuchi and Ho (13), who have solved the
appropriate equation using a finite difference technique, was
employed to strip the operative diffusional coefficients from the
data, with the assistance of a digital computer. Partition coefficients were obtained from the equilibrium situation and from
independent partitioning studies. The diffusional parameters
found for progesterone were in very close agreement with those
published by Roseman and Higuchi (8) for a polydimethylsiloxane
suspension system and we used the literature values, which were
regarded as reliable, in subsequent analyses. These values and
those obtained for hydrocortisone are provided in Table II.
    The suspension matrix data were analyzed according to the
Roseman and Higuchi model using the equations provided in the
theoretical section. The data were compared with theoretical
curves based on the equations derived for the matrix diffusion
layer model. These studies were not used to evaluate parameters
per se, but to confirm that the system would release steroids in
a predictable fashion. Data for the 1.5% suspension membrane are
tabulated in Table III and plotted in Figures 10 and 11. These
data are presented in detail to indicate the good reproducibility
of the assay procedure and the apparent uniformity of distribution of solids obtained (zero time data). In Figure 11 these
data are plotted as the percent released as a function of time.

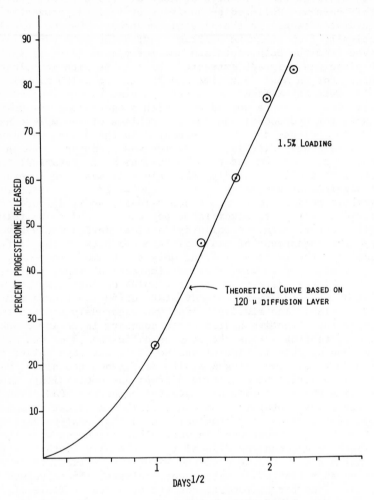

Figure 10. Progesterone release from the 1.5% loaded matrix as a function of the $\sqrt{t}$. Extrapolation of the linear portion of the curve yields an x-intercept of $\approx 0.5 \sqrt{day}$ which corresponds to about 6 hr for the onset of $\sqrt{t}$ dependency.

TABLE II

Values of Physical Parameters Used in the
Simulation Studies and in the
In Vivo Vaginal Absorption in the Rabbit

Parameters	Progesterone*	Hydrocortisone
Structure		
Solubility in matrix, C_s, mg/ml	0.572	0.014
Solubility in H_2O C_{aq}, mg/ml	0.0114	0.28
Diffusion coefficient in matrix, D_e, cm^2/sec	4.5×10^{-7}	4.5×10^{-7}
Diffusion coefficient in H_2O, D_{aq}, cm^2/sec	7×10^{-6}	7×10^{-6}
Silastic/H_2O partition coefficient, K_s	50.2	0.05***
Permeability coefficient** of rabbit vaginal membrane P_m, cm/sec	7×10^{-4}	5.8×10^{-5}

Silastic cylinder
Radius, a_o, cm   1.0
Height, h, cm   6.0

Steroid concentration
A, mg/ml   15; 50; 100

Aqueous diffusion layer thickness, h_{aq}, cm 10^{-2}; 5×10^{-2}, 10^{-1}

*Physical constants of progesterone in Silastic 382 such as C_s, C_{aq}, D_e, K_s were determined previously by Roseman and Higuchi (8).

**P_m of progesterone and hydrocortisone were obtained from vaginal abosrption studies.

***K_s of hydrocortisone was determined with Silastic 382.

TABLE III

Release of Progesterone from a 1.5%
Suspension Matrix Membrane at 37°C

Membrane Weight	Time (Days)	Absorbance	Progesterone in Membrane	%* Remaining
(gm)			(mg/gm)	
0.5545	0	0.435	15.14	100
0.5308	0	0.435	15.81	100
0.5419	0	0.440	15.67	100
0.4576	0	0.375	15.74	100
0.7735	1	0.460	11.49	76.6
0.8490	1	0.500	11.40	76.0
0.8920	1	0.520	11.30	75.3
0.7013	1	0.405	11.12	74.1
0.8833	2	0.365	7.93	52.8
0.9158	2	0.400	8.41	56.0
0.9078	3	0.265	5.52	36.8
0.7874	3	0.290	7.01	46.7
0.8490	3	0.270	6.03	40.2
0.8566	3	0.275	6.09	40.6
0.9262	4	0.175	3.49	23.3
0.8906	4	0.164	3.41	21.9
0.8370	5	0.125	2.89	17.9
0.7847	5	0.100	2.22	15.6
0.9180	5	0.130	2.55	17.0
0.8961	5	0.125	2.50	16.7

* The % released is obviously 100 - % remaining.

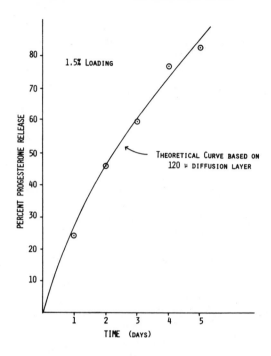

Figure 11. Release of progesterone as a function of time for a 1.5% loading

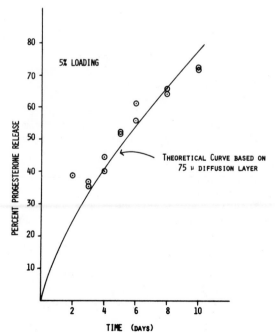

Figure 12. Release of progesterone as a function of time for a 5% loading

The curve through the data is a theoretical line based upon the parameters found in Table II and the equations presented in the theoretical section. A 120 µ thick diffusion layer was found to best fit these data, which seemed a reasonable value based on the experimental design. These same data are plotted as % released versus the square root of time $(t^{1/2})$ in Figure 10. It can be seen that, after an initial lag period, the release entered matrix control and the expected linearity as a function of $t^{1/2}$ was observed. An interesting feature of the method is that it allowed for assessment of the boundary layer controlled period ($\sim$ 6 hours based on the abscissal intercept) which would not have been possible using a solid device coupled with a residuals assay technique (% remaining assay). The slope of the linear region in the $t^{1/2}$ plot was compared with the expected theoretical slope and found to be within 5% of theory. These procedures were repeated using a membrane with a 5% loading with equally good results. The data from the more concentrated device are given in Figure 12. The curve through these data is a theoretical line and includes a diffusion layer of 75 microns. On reproducing these results an average operative diffusion layer (all studies) in the experimental setup was found to be 100 µ. Overall the experiments proved that the device, which was designed to be implanted in the rabbit vagina, was predictable in its release characteristics, at least in so far as progesterone is concerned. Studies with hydrocortisone are continuing. Reproducible extraction of this steroid remains a problem. The actual release _in vivo_ with the latter compound will be performed in monkeys as animal sacrifice is not necessary with this animal.

Simulation Analysis

Using the results of the _in situ_ vaginal absorption of the steroids in the rabbit, the _in vitro_ physicochemical characterization of the steroids with the polymeric membrane, the _in vitro_ release kinetic studies of steroids from the silicone rubber matrix (theoretical in the case of hydrocortisone) and the physical model, a rigorous theoretical analysis of drug delivery from an implanted device is possible. Simulations of the simultaneous release of progesterone from a cylindrical polydimethylsiloxane matrix and vaginal absorption serves as a prototype for assessing the concurrent physicochemical roles of the membrane, aqueous diffusion and receding boundary layers. Another prototype steroid used in these simulation studies is hydrocortisone. The values of the physical parameters of progesterone and hydrocortisone and the cylinder used in the analysis are found in Table II. The size assumed for the cylinder is the same as that of the rib-cage cell used previously.

The flux per unit area of the cylinder versus time profiles for progesterone are shown in Figures 13 and 14 for different aqueous diffusion layer thicknesses and initial concentrations

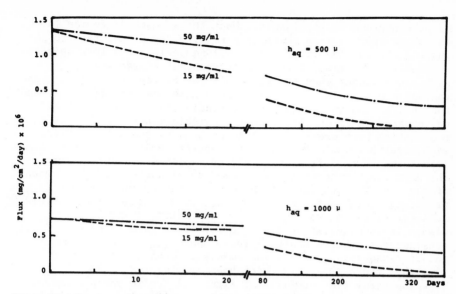

Figure 13.   Quasi steady-state rate of release of progesterone as a function of time when there is a 500μ (upper curves) and 1000μ (lower curves) aqueous boundary layer for 1.5% and 5% membrane loadings

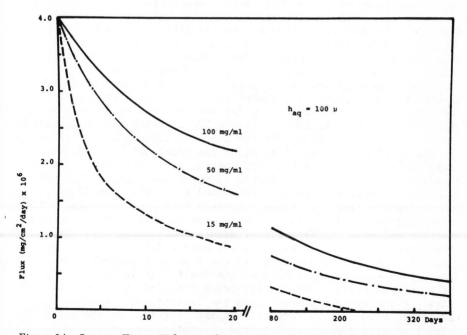

Figure 14.   Same as Figure 13 but for the case where the effective boundary layer thickness is only 100μ

of progesterone in the matrix. When the aqueous diffusion layer is 500 to 1000 microns thick (Figure 13), the fluxes tend to be invariant with time for relatively long periods and then decrease gradually with time. This time independent characteristic is maintained longer when the aqueous layer between the cylinder and vaginal membrane is quite thick (1000 µ as compared to 500 µ) and the initial loading steroid concentration is also high (50 mg/ml as compared to 15 mg/ml). The mechanistic interpretation is that the initial zero order rate is determined by the aqueous diffusion layer barrier. Initially the matrix resistance is many times less than the resistance of these thick fluid boundary layers. The high loading concentrations tend to slow the rate of movement of the receding boundary of the drug in the cylindrical matrix by providing a high effective reservoir concentration in the matrix. At later times the rate changes to the matrix-controlled mechanism. It is significant that the rate in Figure 13 remains fairly constant for about 6 months. Thus, one might expect the metering out of reasonably constant increments of drug in that period of time when there is a very thick boundary layer.

The early time profiles of Figure 14 are in sharp contrast to those in Figure 13. Here the aqueous diffusion layer thickness is 100 microns, which would be a more likely situation when the progesterone containing polymer cylinder forms a snug fit with the membrane of the vaginal tract. In fact, even this might be an exaggerated estimate. The rate is essentially matrix-controlled. Again, an effect of the loading concentration on the rate is observed. With the 100 mg/ml total concentration the early time periods are more influenced by the diffusion layer than that at lower concentrations. At low concentrations the release of the steroid from the matrix is the predominant rate-controlling factor once the cylinder is inserted into the vagina.

In Figures 15 and 16 the predicted total amounts of progesterone released from the cylinder (6 cm long and 2 cm diameter) as a function of time are shown for various loading concentrations (100, 500 and 1000 microns). In the 500 and 1000 micron diffusion layer situations in Figure 15 the initial slopes are unaffected by the loading concentrations since the transport kinetics are diffusion layer-controlled. The initial rates are zero order as predicted in Eq. 23. Because the 15 mg/ml concentration cannot sustain the diffusion-controlled period as long as the 50 mg/ml concentration case, the slope decreases with time until the total drug delivery capacity is depleted. The initial steroid concentration and size of the cylinder determine the drug capacity. The curves in Figure 16 with the 100 micron diffusion layer are indicative of the situation where the transport mechanism is essentially matrix controlled at the onset. It is interesting to point out that, other factors being constant, the total delivery capacity is dependent upon the loading concentration as expected; however, the total time taken in releasing the total amount of drug depends on both the concentration and transport mechanism.

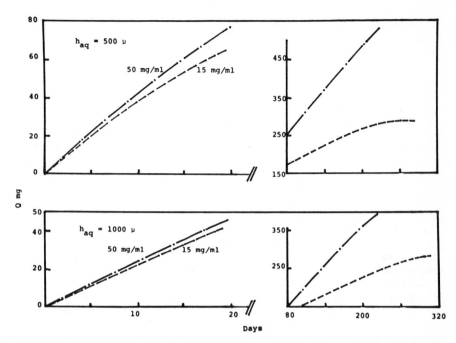

Figure 15.   Amount of progesterone released as a function of time for 1.5% and 5% loaded matrices operating with boundary layers of 500μ (upper) and 1000μ (lower) thicknesses

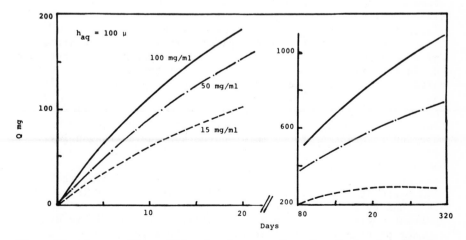

Figure 16.   Same as Figure 15 but for the case where the effective boundary layer thickness is only 100μ

The predicted changes in the receding boundary zone thickness with time at various concentrations of progesterone and aqueous diffusion layer thicknesses are shown in Figures 17 and 18. This zone of depleted drug would be translucent as compared to the opaque core of the drug-matrix suspension. According to Roseman and Higuchi (8), the measurement of this zone with time gives one a rapid estimation of the amount of drug released with time. For a fixed diffusion layer thickness the radial thickness of the zone increases more rapidly with time with the lower concentration. In general, the rate of change in zone thickness is rapid when the progesterone concentration is low and the diffusion layer is small.

In Figures 19-21 a similar analysis is provided for hydrocortisone. As can be seen in Figure 19 by the rapid fall in the fluxes with time, the overall transport kinetics are mechanistically controlled by the release of hydrocortisone from the polydimethylsiloxane cylinder at concentrations of 50 and 100 mg/ml and aqueous boundary layers of 100 and 500 microns thick. From the eighth day the fluxes decrease very slowly and, perhaps from a practical viewpoint, may be considered to be fairly constant between the 10th and 80th day. For a given concentration of 50 or 100 mg/ml, the initial flux per unit area of the cylinder is 1.5×10^{-6} for the 100 micron diffusion layer case and 1.15×10^{-6} for the 500 micron layer case; however, the fluxes converge in 6 hours. The corresponding time changes in the total amount of drug released from the matrix and the receding boundary zone thickness are found in Figures 20 and 21 respectively.

A comparison between the progesterone and hydrocortisone simulation studies gives an interesting mechanistic insight into the transport processes involved. The flux per unit area of the cylinder versus time profiles in Figure 22 typifies the differences in the transport mechanisms of progesterone and hydrocortisone. The concentration is fixed at 50 mg/ml, but the diffusion layer thickness is varied from 100 to 1000 microns. If one considers only the aqueous diffusion layer and the vaginal membrane, one finds that for progesterone the resistance of the diffusion layer is equal to that of the vaginal membrane when the diffusion layer thickness (h_{aq}) is 100 microns and is ten-fold greater when h_{aq} is 1000 microns. Correspondingly, for the more polar hydrocortisone the resistance of the diffusion layer is 12-fold less than that of the vaginal membrane when h_{aq} is 100 microns and the resistances are about equal when h_{aq} is 1000 microns. Thus, in general, the transport of progesterone across the aqueous and membrane layers tend to be more on the aqueous diffusion layer-controlled side and the transport of hydrocortisone is more vaginal membrane controlled.

When one now brings in the steroid-polymer device, the additional resistance in the matrix, which increases with the retreating boundary and is in series with the aqueous layer and vaginal membrane resistances, must be considered. With the large matrix-aqueous partition coefficient (K_S) for progesterone, the change

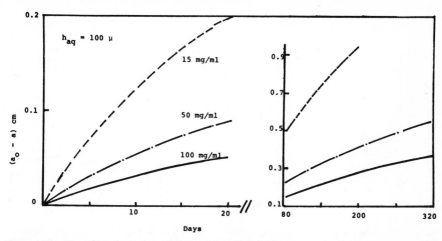

Figure 17.   Receding boundary differential radial thickness as a function of time for progesterone matrices containing 1.5%, 5%, and 10% loadings and operating with a boundary layer of 100μ thickness

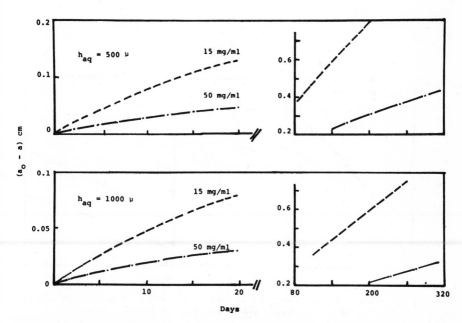

Figure 18.   Same as Figure 17 but for the cases where the effective boundary layer thicknesses are 500μ (upper) and 1000μ (lower) and for 1.5% and 5% loadings

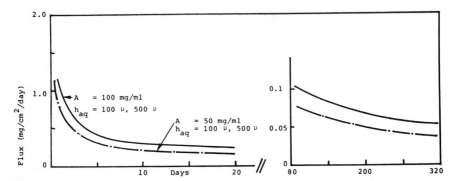

Figure 19. *Theoretical rate release curves for hydrocortisone at 5% and 10% loadings. The flux is essentially invarient for boundary layer thicknesses ranging from 100 to 500μ.*

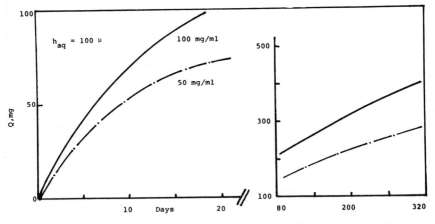

Figure 20. *Cumulative amount of hydrocortisone released as a function of time at 5% and 10% loadings and for a 100μ effective boundary layer*

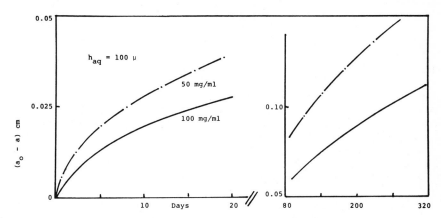

Figure 21. Differential radial thickness of the receding boundary with time for hydrocortisone at 5% and 10% loadings and for a boundary layer of 100μ thickness

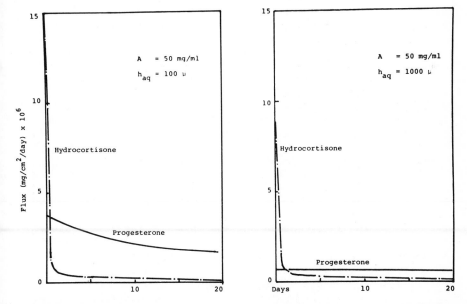

Figure 22. Comparison of progesterone and hydrocortisone release rates at 5% loading for a 100μ diffusion layer (left) and a 1000μ diffusion layer (right) over the initial 20-day period

in the net flux with time is largely influenced by the aqueous
diffusion layer in the first 20 days. In comparison, with the
small K_s of 0.05 for hydrocortisone the net flux changes quite
rapidly with time from vaginal membrane control to matrix control.

In Vivo Release from an Implanted Device

In order to complete the picture, in so far as possible,
matrix release studies were performed in living animals (rabbit
doe) using implanted vaginal devices containing progesterone and
hydrocortisone. The devices were designed to be identical in
radial dimensions and overall length to the perfusion cell used
in early studies to obtain the basic vaginal membrane permeability data. These were surgically implanted by entering the abdominal wall and opening the upper end of the vaginal chamber, a
procedure fully analogous to that used to insert the permeation
cell (3). The animals were stitched closed marking the t=0 for
the individual runs. Each data point represents a separate
rabbit.

A schematic drawing of the device along with the dimensions
of the attached matrix membrane is shown in Figure 23. These dimensions are close to but not exactly the same as the dimensions
of the matrix membranes used in the in vitro suspension matrix
release case. On a predetermined schedule rabbits with the devices in place were sacrificed and the devices recovered. The
membrane wrapping was removed and rinsed with water to clear away
surface debris. The membranes were then sectioned into 3 or 4
pieces, which were weighed and then analyzed as previously described. The absorbance at 240 nm of the extract, properly diluted, was measured and the residual steroid calculated. Because
of previous difficulties, great care was taken to remove the
hydrocortisone fully from the membrane. The raw data from these
studies are given in Table IV for devices loaded respectively
with 1.4% progesterone, 4.7% progesterone and 5.1% hydrocortisone.
These data are graphically presented in Figures 24 and 25 as %
released as a function of time and amount released as a function
of the square root of time ($t^{1/2}$) respectively. The percentage
compositions indicated on the plots are round numbers.

It is obvious considering these data that release for progesterone is for the most part matrix-controlled. This is indicated
for the 4.7% progesterone containing device by the curvature in
the release versus time plot (Figure 24) and the linearity in the
$t^{1/2}$ plot. The intercept on the abscissa for the 4.7% progesterone $t^{1/2}$ plot near the origin is consistent with the early
onset of matrix control or a relatively insignificant membrane-
boundary layer effect. Analysis of the data according to the
model, assuming matrix control, indicates that the observed release is in reasonable agreement with prediction (Table V). At
the 4.7% loading the predicted slope of the steady-state portion
of the $t^{1/2}$ relationship should be 1.1 mg/cm^2/$\sqrt{day}$ and the

TABLE IV

In Vivo Steroids Release from Silastic Membrane (1 mm thick) in the Rabbit Vagina

a. 1.4% Progesterone

Time Day	Steroid % in Membrane	Release %	Q (mg/cm^2)
0	1.37		
2	0.272	80.1	1.32
3	0.134	90.2	1.48
∞	0	100	1.64

b. 4.7% Progesterone

0	4.71		
2	3.11	34.0	1.95
4	2.20	53.3	3.01
6	1.53	67.5	3.82
∞	0	100	5.65

c. 5.1% Hydrocortisone

0	5.06		
4	5.09	(-0.6)	neg.
9	4.91	3.0	0.18
16	4.73	6.5	0.39
∞	0	100	6.07

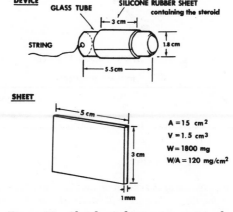

Figure 23. Sketch of the in vivo matrix device and dimensions of the wrapped membrane matrix

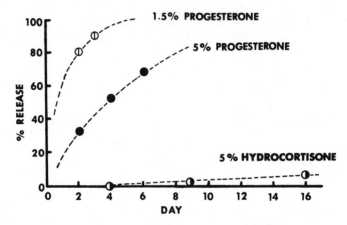

Figure 24.   In vivo release of progesterone and hydrocortisone as
a function of time and matrix loading

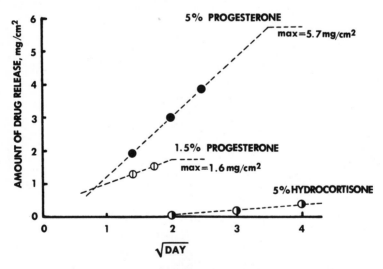

Figure 25.   In vivo release of progesterone and hydrocortisone as a function
of √t and matrix loading. The plot indicates early onset of matrix control
for progesterone.

TABLE V

Experimental and Model Predicted Release
"Rates" of Progesterone and Hydrocortisone In Vivo

Steroid	Initial Amount per Unit Volume (mg/ml)	Mg Released/cm^2/$\sqrt{\text{day}}$	
		Experimental*	Predicted**
Progesterone	47	1.8	1.1
	14	0.5	0.59
Hydrocortisone	51	0.21	0.18

* Determined from the slope of Q' versus $\sqrt{t}$ plot.

** Matrix-controlled case: $dQ'/d\sqrt{t} = \sqrt{D_e C_s} A$.

observed value is 1.8. The agreement is somewhat better for the
two point 1.47% data, 0.59 predicted versus 0.5 observed. It is
recognized that the data are limited; regardless, the in vitro and
theoretical predictions are substantially confirmed by the behavior of the device in vivo.

The case of hydrocortisone appears somewhat different. The
in vivo data for this steroid suggest a long lag time till the onset of matrix control, possibly as much as four days. Thereafter
the data appear linear on the $t^{1/2}$ plot suggesting matrix control.
Again, processing these data as $t^{1/2}$ quasi-steady-state yields
good agreement between experiment and theory. The predicted release in matrix control based on the parameters in Table II is
0.18 mg/cm^2/$\sqrt{\text{day}}$ and the experimental value is 0.21. Thus, the
data suggest that these two structurally similar compounds
(steroids) behave fundamentally differently in terms of release
from polydimethylsiloxane matrices over the first several days
the devices are in place. It should be pointed out that this difference is, in retrospect, predicted in the simulation analysis.
The device inserted in the rabbit was made to form a snug fit
against the wall of the vaginal cavity. This snugness precludes
any significant thickness to the aqueous boundary layer. It was
shown that progesterone is controlled early on by the aqueous
boundary layer and that the vaginal membrane offers relatively
little diffusional resistance. Thus, if snug fitting reduces the
effective hydrodynamic boundary layer, the release from the device
will very rapidly enter matrix control. Conversely, the principal
early determinant of absorption in the case of hydrocortisone is
the vaginal membrane itself, not the boundary layer (Table I).
Thus, the onset of matrix control should be normally delayed as
snug fitting the device should have negligible effect on the membrane. The in vivo data are consistent with this interpretation.

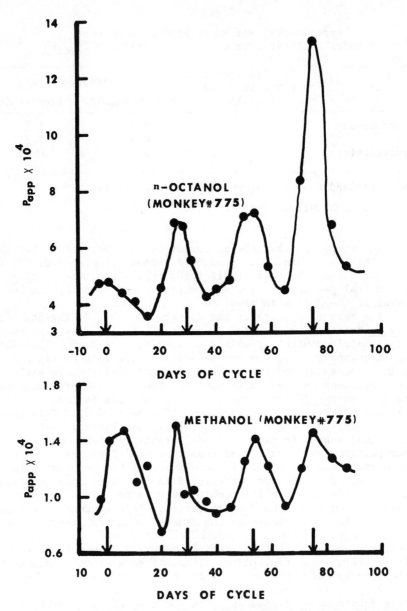

Figure 26. *Plot of the apparent permeability coefficients of* n-*octanol (upper) and methanol (lower) as a function of time and estrus cycle. The arrows indicate the time of observed menstruation.*

Primate Studies—New Concepts

The in vivo release studies in the rabbit were terminated for
two reasons, experimental costliness and some early breakthroughs
in similar studies in the primate species, the Rhesus monkey. Ultimately the aim of the research is to benefit the human female
and, since the rabbit doe does not exhibit an estrus cycle but
ovulates in response to physical (sexual) contact with the male,
it does not show the typical cyclical membrane changes associated
with the rhythmic pattern of hormones of the sexual cycle. Therefore, studies were begun in a more typical species and a species
for which the data might be directly extrapolatable to the human
case. The female Rhesus was chosen as its estrus patterns are
very like the menstrual patterns of the human female.

The vaginal cavity of the Rhesus, like the human, is accessible from outside, allowing the direct insertion of a perfusion
permeability cell and matrix devices, obviating the need for
surgical implantation. This has eliminated extremely difficult
elements in the studies, the surgical procedure and the ultimate
animal sacrifice, and for this reason studies have progressed
rapidly with the primate species. The early results unequivocally
demonstrate that the vaginal membrane permeability varies cycli-
cally with the estrus cycle (Figure 26). This is true for methanol, which has a membrane controlled permeability, and octanol,
which is controlled by diffusing across the aqueous strata of the
total barrier. The latter observation suggests that the aqueous
strata resistance not only includes the hydrodynamic boundary
layer but also the tissue's aqueous regions, which of course also
thin and thicken in response to estrogen secretions. Overall the
monkey's vaginal permeability is slightly less than that of the
rabbit at its highest (immediately following menstruation) and
several-fold smaller at ovulation (between cycles).

With regard to the use of matrices and other release devices,
the monkey data gathered to date add several new features. These
include the nonconstancy of the membrane permeability as a function of the menstrual cycle and the increased membrane resistance
found in the primate species. Studies, either underway or planned, are being aimed at accessing the significance of these factors on steroid absorption and drug delivery from dosage systems.

Literature Cited

1. Mishell, D.R., Jr., Lumkin, M.E. and Stone, S.; Amer. J. Obstet.
   Gynecol. (1972); 113: 927.
2. Nuwayser, E.S. and Williams, D.L.; Adv. Expt. Med. Biol. (1974);
   47: 145.
3. Yotsuyanagi, T., Molokhia, A., Hwang, S.S., Ho, N.F.H., Flynn,
   G.L. and Higuchi, W.I.; J. Pharm. Sci. (1975); 64: 71.
4. Hwang, S.S.; "Systems Approach to the Study of Vaginal Drug Absorption in the Rabbit", University of Michigan Thesis, 1975.

5. Hwang, S.S., Owada, E., Yotsuyanagi, T., Suhardja, L., Ho,
   N.F.H., Flynn, G.L. and Higuchi, W.I.; J. Pharm. Sci., submitted for publication, February 1975.
6. Roseman, T.J.; Adv. Expt. Med. Biol. (1974); $\underline{47}$: 99.
7. Higuchi, T.; J. Pharm. Sci. (1963); $\underline{52}$: 1145.
8. Roseman, T.J. and Higuchi, W.I.; J. Pharm. Sci. (1970); $\underline{59}$:
   353.
9. Flynn, G.L., Ho, N.F.H., Higuchi, W.I. and Kent, J.; J. Pharm.
   Sci. (1976); $\underline{65}$: 154.
10. Macht, D.I.; Pharmacol. Pathol. (1918); $\underline{10}$: 509.
11. Rock, J.R., Baker, H. and Bacon, W.; Science (1947); $\underline{105}$: 13.
12. Hwang, S.S., Owada, E., Suhardja, L., Ho, N.F.H., Flynn, G.L.
    and Higuchi, W.I.; J. Pharm. Sci., submitted for publication,
    April 1976.
13. Suzuki, A., Ho, N.F.H. and Higuchi, W.I.; J. Pharm. Sci.
    (1970); $\underline{59}$: 644.

Controlled Release of Biologically Active Agents

SEYMOUR YOLLES, THOMAS LEAFE, MARIO SARTORI, MARY TORKELSON, and LAIRD WARD

Department of Chemistry, University of Delaware, Newark, Del. 19711

FRED BOETTNER

Rohm and Haas Co., Springhouse, Pa. 19477

Previous papers from this laboratory have dealt with the development of a system for delivery of drugs at controlled rates, over a long period of time (1,2), and with the release rates of narcotic antagonists (2,4,5) and anticancer agents (3) from composites with polymers. The influence of the (a) nature of the polymer, (b) molecular weight of the polymer and (c) form of the composites on the release rates was also investigated (2,6).

This paper reports the results of recent investigations relative to in vivo and in vitro release rates of progesterone (Δ^4-pregnene-3,20-dione), β-estradiol (estra-1,3,5 (10)-triene-3,17-diol) and dexamethasone (9-fluoro-11 β, 17,21-tri-hydroxy-16α-methylpregna-1,4-diene-3,20-dione) from poly(lactic acid) (PLA) composites.

Experimental

All countings were performed with liquid scintillation spectrometers[1]. The counting solution consisted of a mixture of 2,5-diphenyloxazole (22.0 g), 1,4-bis[2-(4-methyl-5-phenyloxazolyl)]benzene (0.4 g), and Triton X 100® [2] (a nonionic wetting agent) (1000 ml) diluted to 4000 ml with toluene in the in vivo experiments. Aquasol® [3] was used as a

---

1. Packard Tri-Carb model 3003 (Packard Instruments, Downers Grove, IL) was used in the in vivo experiments, and a Beckman LS-100 (Beckman Instruments, Fullerton, CA) was used in the in vitro experiments.
2. Rohm and Haas, Philadelphia, PA
3. New England Nuclear Corp., Boston, MA

scintillation liquid in the in vitro experiments.

Preparation of Progesterone-PLA Chips.

Unlabeled progesterone[4] (0.61 g), ^{14}C-progesterone[3]
(3.5 ml benzene solution), poly(lactic acid),
prepared as in ref. (2) (1.05 g) and tributyl
citrate (0.09 g) were dissolved in dichloromethane
(150 ml). The solvent was flashed off under reduced
pressure and the residue, wrapped in aluminum foil,
was melt-pressed[5] at 170° under a total load of 3
metric tons for 30 sec. (shims 0.90 mm thick were
used) to produce films of uniform thickness in which
no imperfection due to air or gas was observed.
The films were ground in a cooled CRC Micro-Mill(TM) [6]
The particles obtained were screened, and fractions
of an average size of 0.45-0.25 mm were collected.
The specific radioactivity was 0.052 mCi/g.
Unlabeled composites were prepared in the same way,
except that ^{14}C-progesterone was not added.

Preparation of Progesterone-PLA Beads.

Solution
A. To Acrysol(R) A-5[2] (24% solution) (16 g) was
added a solution of CM-cellulose 9M31F(R) [7] (1.7%
solution) (41 g) in 550 ml distilled water, prepared
the night before. After adjusting pH to 10.3-10.4
with a 50% sodium hydroxide solution, a solution of
Pharmagel(R) [8] (0.4 g) in 50 ml water, 2 drops of
Triton X 155[2] and 10 g of dichloromethane were added
and stirred at 50°C just before use. Solution B.
PLA (9 g) [prepared as in ref. (2)] was added to a
mixture of methanol (8 ml) and dichloromethane
(125 g) while stirring, and just before mixing with
solution A, a solution of progesterone (partially
tagged as in the preparation of the chips) in
methanol and dichloromethane was added.

Solution A was placed in a one liter, round
bottom, 3-neck-flask, equipped with paddle stirrer.
Solution B was added while stirring (120-130 rpm)
and passing nitrogen over the surface of the liquid.
The reaction mixture was heated to 60-65° over 1-2 hr.
period. (If agglomerates are noticed, agitation is
increased to 170-175 rpm.) After cooling to r.t.,

---

4.   Sigma Chem. Co., St. Louis, MO
5.   Carver laboratory press model C
6.   The Chemical Rubber Co., Cleveland, OH
7.   Hercules Inc., Wilmington, DE
8.   Kind and Knox Gelatin Co., Cherry Hill, NJ

the beads were collected by filtration and washed with water. A yield of about 9 g of beads was obtained. The beads obtained were screened and fractions of an average size 0.42-0.25 mm were collected. The specific activity of the composite was 0.0358 mCi/g.

Annealed beads were obtained by heating beads prepared as above at 150-160° for 10 secs. in a rotating tube.

Preparation of Estradiol-PLA Chips.

A mixture of β-estradiol[4] (3.01 g), tributyl citrate (0.76 g), poly(lactic acid) (11.25 g) and dichloromethane (350 ml) was stirred at r.t. Solvent was evaporated under vacuum at 60° and the residue worked up as described above for the preparation of progesterone-PLA chips.

Preparation of Dexamethasone-PLA Chips.

A mixture of dexamethasone[4] (3.01 g), tributyl citrate (0.76 g), poly(lactic acid) (11.26 g) and dichloromethane (250 ml) was stirred at r.t. Solvent was evaporated under vacuum at 60° and the residue worked up as previously described for the preparation of progesterone-PLA chips. A 10% composite was prepared similarly.

Experiments In Vivo. A) Implantation Method.

These experiments were performed on groups of three or five beagle type mongrels, weighing approximately 10 Kg, by implanting suspensions in methylcellulose of 28.6 mg of progesterone-PLA (A.I. 35%) per Kilo-animal when non-annealed beads were used, and 68.5 mg of progesterone-PLA (A.I. 35%) per Kilo-animal when chips were used.

The following implanting procedure was used: progesterone-PLA composite (beads or chips) was placed in the barrel of a 5 ml plastic syringe and methylcellulose solution in physiological saline added while shaking until an even distribution of the composite particles throughout the methylcellulose was obtained. This suspension was injected subcutaneously posterior to the shoulder in the back region of either side. Urine samples were collected and radioassayed by standard liquid scintillation counting technique (see ref. (2)).

B)   Control Experiments on Urinary Excretion
Radioactivity.   In order to determine the relationship of urinary excretion radioactivity to actual
release of progesterone from implanted composites
with PLA, control experiments were performed.   A
solution of 0.1 + 0.02 g of tagged progesterone,
sans PLA, in methylcellulose was implanted subcutaneously into 5 dogs and the radioactivity of urine
monitored daily.   An average of 29% of the implanted
drug was recovered in urine during the 30 day test.
In the supposition that the remaining 71% consisted
of material released through other ways, the values
of the progesterone released in urine have been
corrected by multiplying them by the factor 3.45
(= 100/29).
C)   Blood Level of Drug by Radioimmunoassay.
The Radioimmunoassay (RIA) technique described in
ref. (7) and (8) was used for the determination of
the blood level of progesterone and dexamethasone
in dogs and of estradiol in wethers.   In the tests
with progesterone, composites containing 15% and 30%
A.I., as a 30% suspension in methylcellulose, were
injected into bitches.   Doses of 15, 60 and 240 mg
of progesterone for animal were used and the blood
levels of progesterone were determined daily by RIA
techniques.

In the tests with estradiol, composites of PLA
containing 20% estradiol were injected as a 30%
suspension in methylcellulose.   Doses of 16 mg of
estradiol were used and the blood levels measured
daily by RIA techniques.

In the tests with dexamethasone, composites of
PLA containing 10% and 20% A.I. were injected as suspension in methylcellulose.   Doses of 16 mg of
dexamethasone per animal were used and the blood
levels measured daily as above.

Experiments In Vitro.   The release rates of
progesterone-PLA composites were also determined in
vitro by dialyzing samples of composite with Ringer's
solution.   The dialysis cell[9] consisted of two
Plexiglass blocks 5 x 5 x 1.5 cm with hemi-
spherical chambers separated by a lamb skin membrane.
The following procedure was used: the assembled
dialysis cell was placed on a magnetic stirrer and
one of the needle inlets in the lower half of the
cell was connected to a pump (peristaltic) capable

---

9.   National Scientific Co., Cleveland, OH

of delivering 10 ml/hour of Ringer's solution
(pH 7.0). The other side of the lower half of the
cell (other exit needle) was connected to a tube
leading to a 500 ml graduated receiver for sample
collection. The pump was started and the lower half
of the cell was filled with dialyzing fluid (Ringer's
solution), being careful to remove all air bubbles
from below the surface of the membrane. (This
insures contact between dialyzing fluid and the
whole membrane surface.)

Dialyzing fluid (1-2 ml), which remained static
through the experiment, was placed in the upper half
of the cell. Composite sample, such as beads or
chips, was added through a 5 mm hole in the top of
the cell and while stirring the upper chamber was
filled to capacity by means of a fine tipped eye-
dropper (Pasteur dropper). Samples of dialysis
effluent were collected every 24 hrs. (250 ml/day)
and the radioactivity determined by standard
technique.

Counting solutions were prepared by dissolving
one ml of dialysis effluent in 10 ml of scintillation
solution. The counts found were corrected for
(a.) background (subtract 14,875 dpm/ml; previously
determined by counting four different 1 ml samples
of the Ringer's solution); (b.) for recorded counting
efficiency. Dividing counts found minus background
by fractional efficiency gave the corrected dpm/ml.
Total dpm/day was obtained by multiplying dpm/ml by
the total sample volume. The sample size and type
are given in Table I. Calculations for %/day were
made as follows:

$$\%/day = \frac{Total\ dpm/day}{Total\ dpm\ in\ cell} \times 100$$

Table I. Type of Composite and Sample Size

Type of Composites	Sample Size, g	dpm in cell
chips	.0345	3,069,150
chips	.0399	3,100,230
film	.0653	5,073,810
film	.0669	5,198,130
non-annealed beads	.0364	2,706,822
non-annealed beads	--	--
annealed beads	.0433	3,441,200
annealed beads	.0414	3,290,200

Results and Discussion

The in vivo tests with ^{14}C-progesterone-PLA
chips, injected as methylcellulose suspensions in
dogs, show that the cumulative amount of drug
released during an 82 day period averaged 79% of
the administered dose. Of this amount, only an
average of 23% was recovered in urine. The daily
amount of progesterone released (see Fig. 1) averaged
2.5% of the dose during the first 10 days after
implantation, decreased gradually to about 1% of
dose during the following 30 days and then remained
relatively constant at about 0.6% for the duration
of the test.

When non-annealed beads instead of chips were
used, the release rates were similar to those
obtained by implanting a suspension of neat ^{14}C-
progesterone. Almost 100% of the administered dose
was released from the composites in about 45 days,
and of this amount only about 30% was found in the
urine. The daily amount of progesterone released
after reaching a maximum of about 13% of the dose
during the first two days after implantation decreased
gradually to 1% of dose during the following 18 days
and then remained at 0.2-0.5% of the dose during the
following 23 days (Fig. 1). This behavior indicates
that the non-annealed beads, due to their macro-
reticular type of structure, provide the drug with
ample opportunity to diffuse rapidly through the
polymer matrix.

In the in vivo tests by RIA with progesterone
chips (30% A.I.), blood levels of progesterone of
3 ng/ml for a period of 21 days (Fig. 2) were
obtained when doses of 240 mg in PLA chips were
injected in bitches. The blood level then decreased
to 0.7 ng/ml during the following days and remained
fairly constant at about this level for the duration
of the tests (60 days). These concentrations are
above the normal progesterone levels found in control
tests. Similar release profiles were obtained in
tests performed by injecting 15 and 60 mg of progesterone in PLA chips of 30% A.I. Blood levels of
about 0.8 ng/ml were found during the first 25 days
after injection, decreasing to lower than 0.6 during
the following 30 days of the test. In tests with
progesterone composites (15% A.I.), a blood level
of 2.8 ng/ml was reached in the first day when doses
of 240 mg were injected; then the blood level

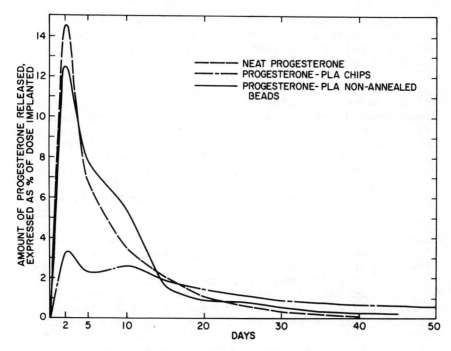

Figure 1.   *In vivo daily release of* ¹⁴*C-progesterone*

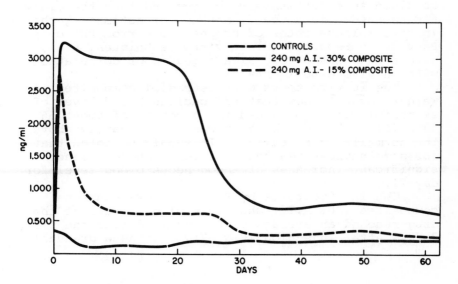

Figure 2.   *Daily level of progesterone in blood*

decreased to about 0.5 ng/ml in 25 days following a slope similar to that obtained with a 30% composite. As expected, the higher loading dose afforded the higher blood level.

The in vitro releases of progesterone from ^{14}C-progesterone-PLA composites, as beads, chips and films, were determined by the membrane dialysis technique described above. The results reported in Fig. 3 show that progesterone is released faster from PLA composites in form of non-annealed beads than from composites as chips or films. The daily release from non-annealed beads began at a rate of about 4% during the first 2 days, then decreased gradually and remained at about 3% for the duration of the test (20 days). The daily release from chips started at about 2.5% in the first 3 days and decreased to about 1.1% during the following 7 days. Composites in form of films released progesterone at the very low rates of about 1%/day in the first day and 0.3%/day for the duration of the test (13 days).

A considerably reduced release of progesterone from beads was obtained by heating the beads at 150-160° for 10 seconds (Fig. 4). By this treatment the release rate of progesterone became similar to that from composites in form of chips.

Comparison of these in vitro results with those obtained in the above described in vivo tests by the implantation method show (Fig. 5) that the release rates of ^{14}C-progesterone from chips, determined by the dialysis technique, are similar to those obtained in experiments with dogs and that the dialysis technique is a useful method for estimating the in vivo release rates of progesterone from PLA chips. Previously reported (2) in vitro techniques, e.g., with a Raab extractor, always gave poor correlations with in vivo experiments.

The in vivo tests with estradiol composites in wethers by RIA show that efficacious blood level of estradiol can be obtained for a period of about 55 days (Fig. 6). Weight gain was significantly above the normally expected (9). It should be noted that for some unknown reasons, the tests showed rather significant increases of endogeneous blood level for day 21.

The in vivo tests by RIA with dexamethasone composites (20% A.I.) show that blood levels of the drug reached an average of 6.8 ng/ml during the first 3 days after injection (Fig. 7), decreased gradually

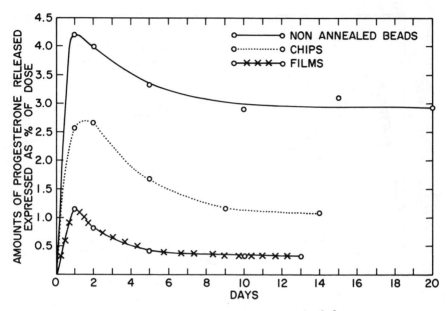

Figure 3. In vitro release of progesterone by dialysis

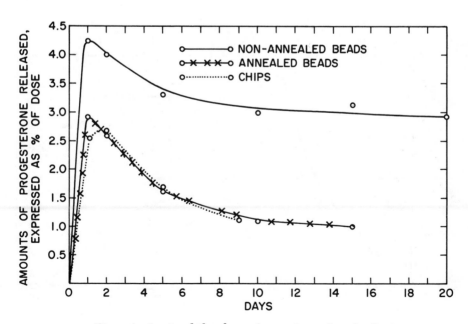

Figure 4. In vitro daily release of progesterone from beads

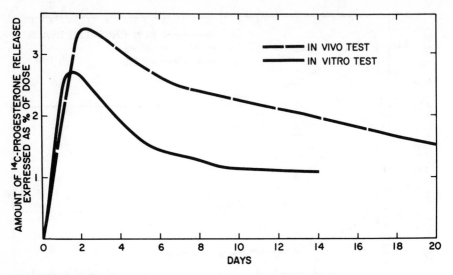

Figure 5.   In vivo vs. in vitro release of progesterone

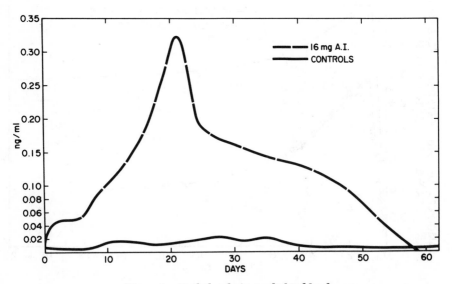

Figure 6.   Daily level of estradiol in blood

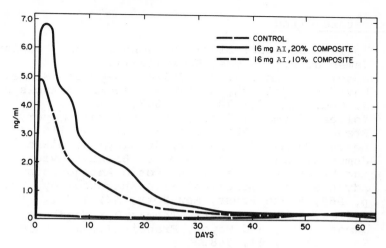

Figure 7.   Daily level of dexamethasone in blood

to about 1 ng/ml during the following 27 days and
then remained constant at about 0.1 ng/ml for the
duration of the test (60 days). Similar profiles
were obtained in tests with composites containing
10% A.I. A maximum blood level of 5 ng/ml was
obtained during the first 2 days. Also in this
case, the higher loading dose showed the higher blood
level.

In a previous paper (2) it was shown that
different profiles for the in vivo rates were
obtained in controlled release of narcotic antagonists from films and chips. Rates for films followed
a first order decay while chips gave a zero order
profile. The difference in behavior may be attributed to the bodies inflammatory processes triggered
by the implant; the one for chips presumably being
more efficient and creating a more effective barrier.
In the blood level work reported in this paper,
lengthy flat profiles are again seen with progesterone and estradiol (Fig. 2 and Fig. 6). However, the
rate curve for dexamethasone is typically first
order (Fig. 7). This behavior supports the hypothesis because dexamethasone is a well-known anti-
flammatory agent.

We gratefully acknowledge the contributions to
this work of Drs. Lloyd Faulkner and Gordon Niswender
of Colorado State University, the guidance of Drs.
E. D. Weiler and M. C. Seidel of Rohm and Haas and
the assistance of Dr. Shayam Hirwe and Robert Allan
Barker of the University of Delaware. This work
was liberally supported by a grant from the Rohm and
Haas Company of Philadelphia, Pennsylvania.

Literature Cited

1. Yolles, Seymour; Eldridge, John E.; and Woodland, James H. R.; Polymer News (1971), 1, 9.
2. Woodland, James H. R.; Yolles, Seymour; Blake, David A.; Helrich, Martin; and Meyer, Francis J.; J. Med. Chem. (1973), 16, 897.
3. Yolles, Seymour; Leafe, Thomas D. and Meyer, Francis J.; J. Pharm Sci. (1975), 64, 115.
4. Leafe, Thomas D.; Sarner, Stanley; Woodland, James H. R.; Yolles, Seymour; Blake, David A.; and Meyer, Francis J.; Narcotic Antagonists - Advances in Biochemical Psycopharmacology, Vol. 8, p. 569, Raven Press, New York, NY, 1973.
5. Yolles, Seymour; Leafe, Thomas D.; Woodland, James H. R.; and Meyer, Francis J.; J. Pharm. Sci. (1975), 64, 348.
6. Yolles, Seymour; Eldridge, John E.; Leafe, Thomas D.; Woodland, James H. R.; Blake, David R.; and Meyer, Francis J.; Controlled Release of Biologically Active Agents - Advances in Experimental Medicine and Biology, Vol. 47, p. 177, Plenum Press, New York, NY, 1973.
7. Niswender, Gordon D.; Steroids (1973), 22, 413.
8. England, B. G.; Niswender, G. D.; and Midgley, A. R.; J. Clin. Endocrinol Metab. (1974), 38, 42.
9. Faulkner, Lloyd C.; Niswender, Gordon D.; Colorado State University, Fort Collins. Private Communication.

Release of Inorganic Fluoride Ion from Rigid Polymer Matrices

B. D. HALPERN, O. SOLOMON, and L. KOPEC

Polysciences, Inc., Warrington, Pa. 18976

E. KOROSTOFF and J. L. ACKERMAN

School of Dentistry, University of Pennsylvania, 40th and Spruce Sts., Phila., Pa. 19104

The objective of this work was the development of a fluoride containing material that will release small amounts of fluoride ion at a constant controllable rate for a period of at least six months. In addition, the material should meet the following requirements:
1. Must be non-toxic, non-allergenic and harmless to oral and gastro-intestinal tissues.
2. Must be able to release fluoride ion at a constant rate ranging from 0.02 mg/day to 1 mg/day through simple modifications of the compound composition.
3. The device based on this material must be capable of easy attachment to the teeth with the possibility of safe removal if the circumstances warrant such removal.

To realize this objective, we have synthesized, developed and evaluated samples and devices of different kinds and shapes, containing fluoride salts and capable of releasing fluoride ions in an aqueous environment at a steady controllable rate. A rate controlling polymer membrane was used to control the release of fluoride ion from a matrix polymer containing the fluoride salt reservoir. The matrix polymers containing fluoride salts are based on recognized biocompatible polymers, frequently used in clinical dentistry and clinical surgery. An intraoral Hawley orthodontic appliance was developed which provides steady-state release of fluoride ion. This device was tested in water over approximately a six month period and it showed steady-state release of fluoride ion. Predetermined rate of fluoride release of up to 1 mg/day was possible by modifying the rate controlling membrane polymer.

Introduction

The efficacy of small doses of fluorides in arresting dental caries is clinically well established. Regardless of the mode of action of fluoride, it is apparent that adequate protection against caries can be obtained by the topical application of fluoride ion on the enamel surfaces. Very little work has been reported on optimum dosage rate of the topical application of fluoride through a sustained long-acting formulation.

An oral release of small amounts of fluoride at a constant rate over a long period of several months to years has several possible advantages. It could provide a means for fluoride treatment for certain segments of the youth population who might otherwise not be treated by available conventional means. Moreover, a constant low dosage sustained oral environment of fluoride ion may have clinical benefits not achieved by episodic topical applications.

The slow release of fluoride can be achieved by the following delivery methods:
1. Diffusion of fluoride ion from a dispersion of the agent in a solid polymer matrix.
2. Diffusion of fluoride ion across a polymeric membrane barrier which encloses the pure or an aqueous dispersion of a fluoride containing agent.
3. Slow release of fluoride from a system which combines system (1) and (2), i.e., dispersion of fluoride salt in a solid polymer matrix (inner core) which is surrounded by an outer rate limiting membrane barrier.

At the outset of our study, we chose to work first with acrylic related polymers because they were already clinically accepted in the dental profession and the means of ready fabrication into dental devices were readily at hand. Preparation of samples of matrixes containing fluoride salt by cold curing redox catalysts is relatively easy. Moreover, the toxicity of this system has never been a problem.

Since the fluoride salt in contact with water provides the ionic species, the diffusion rate from the polymer matrix will be very much dependent on the hydrophilic nature of the polymer and copolymer, the degree of crosslinking, the degree of comminution of the fluoride salt and the solubility of the salt in water. In order to facilitate the fabrication of the final clinical device, we chose a simplified redox polymerization method for incorporation of the fluoride ion in the matrix polymer. The finely divided fluoride salt was dispersed throughout an ultrafine polymethyl methacrylate bead polymer containing residual peroxide and the chosen hydrophilic monomer with dimethyl-p-toluidine was mixed in to allow autopolymerization. This type system is in wide usage in all dental labs and provides an easy way to fabricate a custom dental appliance as would be required for each individual patient.

Experimental: Materials

Different types of liquid monomers selected on the basis of their hydrophilic, hydrophobic or crosslinking ability were used for the preliminary experimental investigations. The monomers

used in this work were: methyl methacrylate (MMA), ethyl
acrylate (EA), 2-hydroxyethyl methacrylate (HEMA), 1,3-butylene
glycol dimethacrylate (BGD), ethylene glycol dimethacrylate (EGD),
and vinyl pyrolidone (VP). Other materials used in the formulation and synthesis of solid polymeric matrices are the following:
- The polymethyl methacrylate (PMMA) had an average MW of
$\sim$ 200,000 with an average bead size of $\sim$22μ.
- The sodium fluoride was of analytical grade and finely
powdered.
A typical procedure for preparation of a polymer matrix
containing a fluoride compound is as follows:
    PMMA powder was mixed thoroughly with $\sim$1% benzoyl peroxide
and the desired amount of fluoride salt was thoroughly dispersed
throughout. The monomer or the mixture of comonomers containing
$\sim$3% w/w N,N-dimethyl-p-toluidine was mixed with the polymer beads
by hand spatulation until a fluid homogeneous paste or a viscous
syrup was formed. The paste or the syrup was poured into a
polyethylene mold and allowed to cure $\sim$10-15 minutes. In this
way cylindrical devices with predetermined dimensions were
obtained. Flat devices were obtained by curing the paste
between two Teflon plates. Discs were obtained by cutting the
flat devices into the necessary dimensions. The Hawley oral
appliances were obtained by curing the paste in an orthodontic
maxillary appliance mold.
    The polymer matrices coated with a thin membrane were
prepared by dipping into a 2% solution of polymer in chloroform,
evaporating the solvent by spinning in the air and vacuum drying.
The membrane thickness was controlled by the number of immersions.

Fluoride Ion Rate Release Measurements:

    Each device containing fluoride salt was subjected to a
general in vitro procedure designed to measure the daily
fluoride release. The extraction of fluoride ion from the
polymer matrices was carried out in polyethylene jars on a
routine basis using 500 ml of distilled water kept at 36-38°C,
mildly agitated with mechanical or magnetic bar stirring.
Periodically the solution was removed and replaced with fresh
distilled water free of fluoride so as not to allow the buildup
of a high concentration of fluoride ion. The determinations
of fluoride ion concentrations in the extract were performed
with a specific fluoride ion electrode in conjunction with a
standard single junction sleeve type reference electrode
connected with an ORION Model 801 digital MV/pH meter. Internal
fluoride standards were made by using ORION reference samples.
Total ionic strength adjustment buffer solution (ORION 94-09-09)
was added to monitor the pH of the samples. In the tested
samples, the Nerns't equation was obeyed over a range of 0.3-3
ppm fluoride ion.

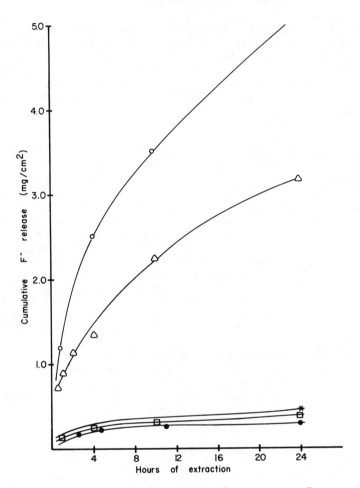

*Figure 1. Release of fluoride ion from polymer matrices. Comono-
mer in the matrix (32–35%): ○, 2-hydroxyethyl methacrylate; △,
ethyl acrylate; *, ethylene glycol dimethacrylate; □, 1,3-butylene
glycol dimethacrylate; ●, methyl methacrylate. Poly(methyl methacrylate) beads: 56–58%. Sodium fluoride: 9.0–10.2%.*

Evaluation Of Fluoride Ion Release Rate From Polymer Matrices:
The Influence Of The Comonomer Nature Of The Rate Of Fluoride
Ion Release From The Polymer Matrices Without Coated Membrane

   The performances of different types of uncoated polymer
matrices containing ∿10% NaF concerning the release of fluoride
ion in an aqueous environment are presented in Figure 1.
   As we can see from the typical release patterns of
different polymer matrices presented in Figure 1, two main groups
can be selected: one group with a fast release and the second

with a slow release. It is obvious that the polymer matrices with a rapid release of fluoride ion are based on hydrophilic polymers such as poly-2-hydroxyethyl methacrylate or polyethyl acrylate. The slow releasing matrices are based on polymers of a more hydrophobic nature or those which yield crosslinked matrices. They can be also characterized as having typical asymptotic type release rate of fluoride ion. Over a long period of time, once the fluoride salt is depleted from the surface of the matrix, the rate of release decays slowly.

An interesting behavior of fluoride ion release is presented by the polymer matrix based on an ethylene-vinyl acetate copolymer shown in Figure 2. The equilibration of the matrix takes a very short time to come to a reasonably steady state of release. Unlike the two component redox system, the NaF has to be incorporated in the ethylene vinyl acetate co-polymer by a milling procedure or by reprecipitation. The matrix must then be formed by heat and pressure or by solvent casting. These fabrication methods are less adapted to the expertise of the average dental laboratory and hence we abandoned this method.

The Influence of the Concentration of the Fluoride Salt in the Matrix on the Rate of Release

As expected, the fluoride ion release from the uncoated polymer matrix increases with the increase of fluoride salt concentration. It can be seen from Figure 3 that the several polymer matrices we studied releases fluoride salt in non-linear fashion as concentration of the fluoride salt increases. Only in the case of a polymer matrix based on a monomer with strong crosslinking ability was a reasonably straight line achieved.

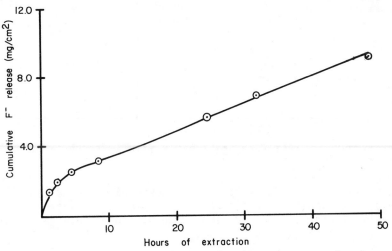

Figure 2. Fluoride ion release from ethylene-vinyl acetate copolymer

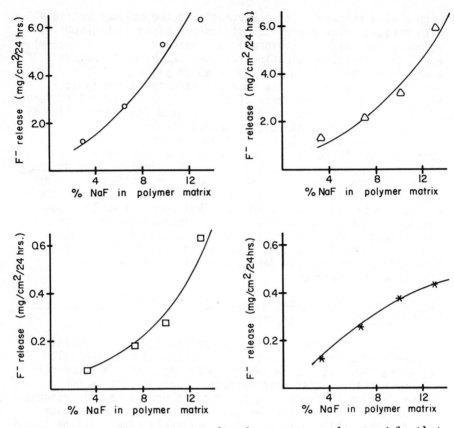

*Figure 3. Influence of NaF content in the polymer matrix on the rate of fluoride ion release in the first 24 hr of water extraction. Comonomer in matrix: ○, 2-hydroxyethyl methacrylate; △, ethyl acrylate, *, 1,3-butylene glycol dimethacrylate; □, methyl methacrylate.*

The Influence of Fluoride Salt Solubility on the Rate of Fluoride Ion Release

Using a fluoride salt with a much greater solubility in water than sodium fluoride would be expected to give a much higher release of fluoride ion. The pertinent data is presented in the following table.

Average Fluoride Ion (Mg/cm²/24 h) Release From Polymer Matrices Based On Hydrophobic Monomers Containing Different Types Of Fluoride Salt At The Same Concentration ∿6%

Time of Sample Extraction	Matrix Containing	
Days	NaF	Na_2PO_3F
10	15.5	82
20	6.5	54
30	4.3	46
60	3.1	31

As we can see from this data, for the same concentration of fluoride salt in the matrix, ∿6%, the matrix containing Na_2PO_3F (which has a solubility in water of 25 g/100 ml instead of 4 g/100 ml for NaF) releases for the same period of time ∿6 to 10 times more fluoride ion. However, the molecular weight of the fluorophosphate is over three times that of the sodium fluoride. This limits the total fluoride salt which can be loaded into the polymer to a level which is less than the reservoir amount needed for a six month period.

Evaluation of Fluoride Ion Release Rate From Polymer Matrices Coated With Membranes

The data discussed thus far shows a non-linear release rate as would be expected from a non-membrane coated matrix. In order to limit the release to a linear release, we found it necessary to use a rate limiting membrane having a lesser degree of hydrophilicity than that of the fluoride reservoir polymer matrix. The membrane coating technique is also very versatile in that it allows easy modification of the rate from 0.02 to 1.0 mg/24 hours and the method is essentially independent of the geometry of the final appliance.

Three prototype designs successfully achieved the desired release characteristics: a cylindrical one, a tablet and an orthodontic Hawley appliance. Data obtained for the daily rate release follows a pseudo zero-order kinetic. (See photograph of Hawley appliance).

Figure 4 graphically demonstrates the restraining effect caused by the membrane on fluoride ion rate release from the polymer matrix. All the membranes including the matrix used in this case are hydrophilic. As we can see from the data presented in Figure 4, the barrier membrane effectively monitored the release rate and made it possible to achieve the desired delivery of fluoride ion. The hydrophilic nature of the membrane influences greatly the slope of the curve and brings it to a straight line.

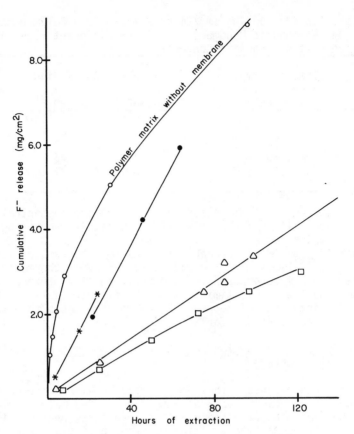

*Figure 4.   Release of fluoride ion from polymer matrix coated with membrane. Comonomer in the matrix: 90 HEMA: 10 MMA; 35%. Poly(methyl methacrylate) beads: 47.6%. Sodium fluoride: 16.7%. Membranes: □, polyethylene vinyl acetate, 20μ; ●, poly(ethoxyethyl methacrylate–2-hydroxyethyl methacrylate), 16μ; *, cellulose acetate, 10μ; △, poly(methyl methacrylate), 15μ.*

From this data, it is seen that all four membranes we studied permit a steady release of fluoride ion, the highest release being achieved when the hydrophilic copolymer of ethoxyethyl methacrylate and 2-hydroxyethyl methacrylate is used for coating.

The same steady state slow release effect can be achieved even in the case of a very hydrophilic matrix such as the one prepared from HEMA:MMA: vinyl pyrrolidone and coated with a polyethylene vinyl acetate membrane as can be seen from Figure 5.

The very strong fluoride ion releasing polymer matrices such as those based on 90 HEMA:10 MMA can be easily moderated by applying a hydrophobic membrane of PMMA. The manner that such a

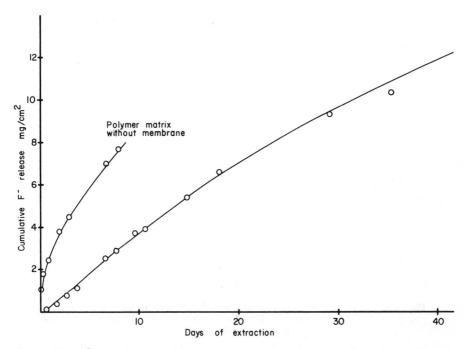

Figure 5. Release rate of fluoride ion from polymer matrices containing N-vinyl pyrrolidone and coated wtih a membrane of polyethylene vinyl acetate. Comonomers in the matrix: 40 HEMA: 30 MMA: 30 N-vinyl pyrrolidone, 35.7%. Poly(methyl methacrylate) beads: 47.6%. Sodium fluoride: 16.7%.

membrane is acting is presented in Figure 6. The tailing in release is starting to occur after 50-60 days because the fluoride salt reservoir was beginning to deplete.

Figure 7 shows the simple dependence between the thickness of the membrane and the release rate of fluoride ion from the device. Increasing the membrane thickness by approximately 50% causes about a 40% decrease in transport of fluoride ion.

We also made a barrier membrane from poly-n-butyl methacrylate so as to allow a flexible coating less subject to failure during flexure or abrasion in a clinical usage of a device. It, too, had straight line release as shown in Figure 8.

The data obtained on long-term, in vitro evaluations of two of the final Hawley devices fabricated into actual shapes similar to that used in clinical situations is shown in Figure 9. Figure 10 represents the Howley Appliance used in this experiment.

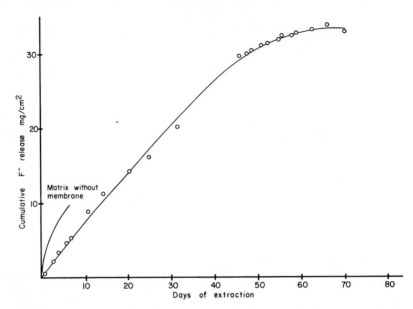

Figure 6. Release of fluoride ion from a polymer matrix. Comonomers in the matrix: 90 HEMA: 10 MMA, 37.5%. Poly(methyl methacrylate) beads: 47.6%. Sodium fluoride: 16.7%.

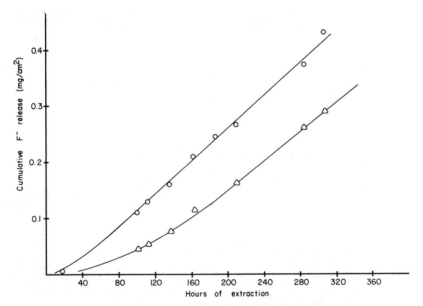

Figure 7. Release of fluoride ion from a polymer matrix. Comonomer in the matrix: 30 HEMA: 70 MMA; 35.7%. Poly(methyl methacrylate) beads: 47.6%. Sodium fluoride: 16.7%. Thickness of poly(methyl methacrylate) membrane: ○, 19μ, △, 26μ.

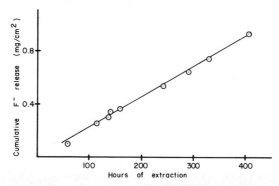

Figure 8. Release of fluoride ion from a polymer matrix coated with poly(n-butyl methacrylate) membrane (49μ). Comonomer in the matrix: 90 HEMA: 10 MMA, 35.7%. Poly(methyl methacrylate) beads: 47.6%. Sodium fluoride: 16.7%.

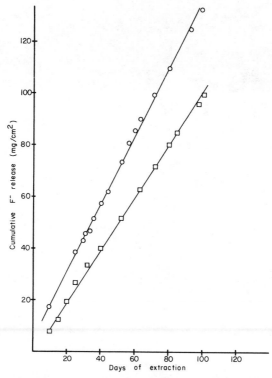

Figure 9. Release of fluoride ion from oral devices. Comonomers in the matrix: 37.5%, ○, 70 HEMA: 30 MMA; □, 90 HEMA: 10 MMA. Poly(methyl methacrylate) beads: 47.6%. Sodium fluoride: 16.7%. Thickness of PMMA membranes: ○, 22μ; □, 19μ.

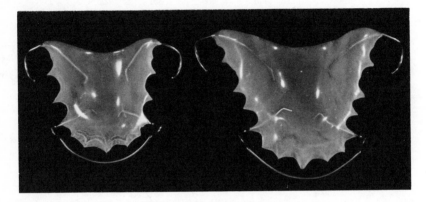

Figure 10. Howley appliance

10

Fallopian Tube Cauterization by Silver Ion–Polymer Gels

HARRY P. GREGOR, H. T. HSIA, and SHEILA PALEVSKY
Department of Chemical Engineering and Applied Chemistry,
Columbia University, New York, N.Y. 10027

R. S. NEUWIRTH
St. Luke's Hospital Center, New York, N.Y. 10025

R. M. RICHART
College of Physicians and Surgeons, Columbia University, New York, N.Y. 10032

The specific stimulus for this study was the observation of Neuwirth and Richart (1) that permanent female sterilization could be effected by Fallopian tube closure in a non-surgical manner by injection of a silver nitrate solution retrograde into the tube. However, solutions were much too fluid and could not be localized effectively. The use of a hydrophilic ointment as the carrier for silver nitrate was studied. Closure with rabbits, monkeys and also a few humans was observed. However, this delivery system was difficult to control although closure did occur with the requisite reliability. In addition, there was the problem of material being introduced into non-desirable parts of the body cavity.

It was then postulated that if one could effect the release of silver ions by a solid, rod-like device which can be inserted into the Fallopian tube with the use of a hysteroscope, a practical solution could result. The hysteroscope is a fiber optic endoscope which allows transuterine delivery of an agent without the necessity of surgery.

The purpose of this study was to examine the employment of various non-toxic polymers which can form a matrix for the release of silver ions at desirable rates. Use was made of alginates and Pluronics, using silver nitrate as the active agent. A model in vitro system was developed and the rate of silver release investigated.

Materials

The Pluronics (BASF Wyandotte) are block copolymers of ethylene oxide and propylene oxide with the
empirical formula

$$HO[CH_2CH_2O]_a[C(CH_3)HCH_2O]_b[CH_2CH_2O]_cH$$

where a and c are approximately equal. Pluronics are
highly resistant to either acid or alkali attack, not
precipitated by most metallic ions and, although most
are soluble in water, they are relatively non-hygro-
scopic. The Pluronic polyols are non-ionic surfactants
with unusually low toxicity. Typical toxicological results which have been reported (2,3) include: intravenous injection of a Pluronic at 0.1 g/kg body weight
into dogs and 1.0 g/kg body weight into rabbits caused
no toxic symptoms; Pluronics are neither metabolized by
the body nor absorbed by it; the acute oral toxicity of
the Pluronic compound used here (F127) was 15 g/kg; the
intravenous acute toxicity was 2.25 g/kg.
Alginic acid is a linear block copolymer of D-
mannuronic (M) acid and L-guluronic (G) acid, with 1,4
linkage resulting in one free carboxylic and two free
hydroxyl groups per uronic acid residue; the aldehydes
are blocked(Fig.1). The distribution of the uronic
acid residues in the polymer molecules and their sequence are not accurately known, and alginic acid is
known to be chemically heterogenous(4). The linear
alginate molecule consists of blocks, in which one or
the other uronate predominates. These have a number
average of 20-30 monomer units and are separated by
regions which contain alternating mannuronic and guluronic acid residues (5,6). The use of IR techniques
gives an indication of the uronate composition (7).
While absorption bands at 10.8 and 12.4 μm were stronger for samples rich in mannuronic residues, the bands
at 10.6 and 12.7 μm were stronger for those with higher
contents of guluronic acid.
The ratio of mannuronic to guluronic monomer units
is dependent upon the exact algae, its age and its location. The dissociation constant of alginic acid is a
function of this ratio. The pK_a values of mannuronic
acid and guluronic acid are 3.38 and 3.65, respectively.

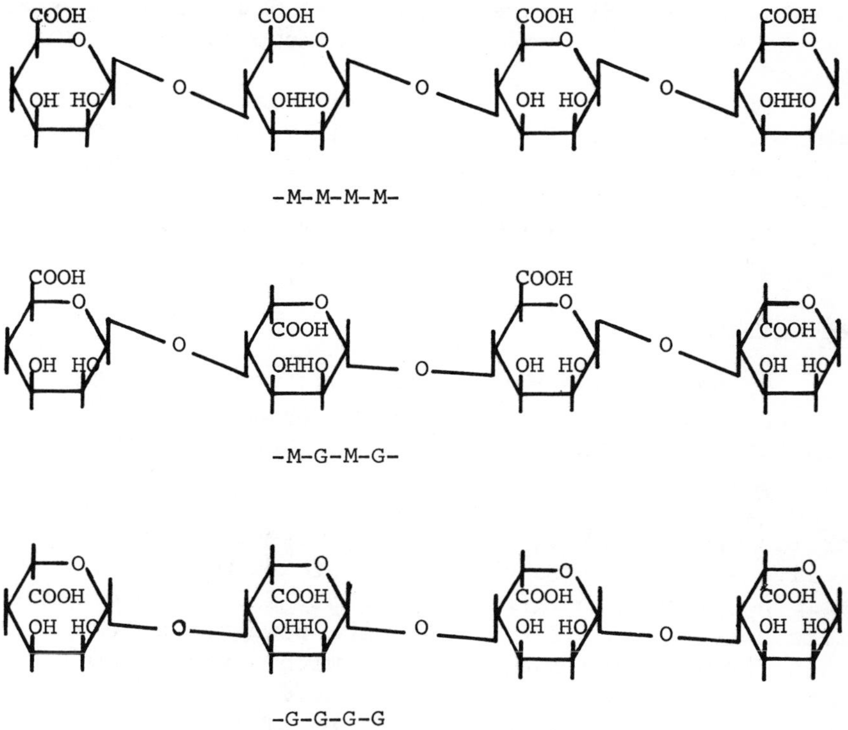

−M−M−M−M−

−M−G−M−G−

−G−G−G−G

Figure 1. Structure of alginic acid

Data obtained from thin-layer chromatography, pH and viscosity measurements indicate that ions are held by alginic acid via ion exchange as well as chelating mechanisms. Mechanisms not involving ion-exchange are due primarily to the presence of the two vincinal hydroxyl groups in each uronic acid residue. Chelation with Ca is strong (8) and cross-linking occurs. Mg does not react or form gel-like complexes as does Ca (9, 10). The intermolecular forces and mechanisms involved in ionic cross-linking are not well understood.

The sodium alginate used in this study was Kelcosol (Kelco Co.), a Na alginate of high molecular weight. The toxicity of the alginates has been investigated extensively over many years. Some of the results obtained are: incorporation of sodium alginate into diet of rats, mice, chicks, cats and guinea pigs for prolonged periods caused no deleterious effects (11,12); the LD_{50} of alginates is above 5 g/kg body weight (13); the im-

plantation of calcium alginate around the femoral shaft
in the guinea pig showed complete absorption within a
period of two weeks (14).

Silver alginate was prepared from a 2% (w/v) solution of Kelgin-Gel LV (low molecular weight sodium form)
which was added to a 3% (w/v) silver nitrate solution.
Vigorous agitation, followed by washing, filtration and
air-drying, then ground to 50-100 microns with a Micro-
Mill gave a tough and hard material.

Experimental

Silver impregnated solid plugs were prepared
either by compressing a powder or by melting a compressed powder mixture in a mold. Excessive exposure
to light caused photodecomposition. Aluminum blocks
were used as molds, with holes having diameters of 0.9
or 1.4 mm drilled and their tops reamed. A piece of
Lucite was bolted to the bottom of the metal mold. The
molding process required repeatedly filling the dish-
like hole on top of the mold with powdered material and
then forcing this into the hole with a steel rod having
the same diameter. Force was exerted by the use of a
small drill press with a lever arm of about 8 inches,
applying the normal pressure that can be exerted manu-
ally by the operators. The limit of pressure used was
determined by the stress failure of the rods. The solid plug was then ejected from the die after removing
the Lucite plate. It could be used "as is" or be subjected to a coating treatment.

When solid Pluronics were used, the mold was
placed on a hot plate after the removal of the Lucite
block. The same powder was placed in the reamed out
cone. When the powders liquified and filled the hole,
the assembly was removed from the heater, cooled to
room temperature and the inserts ejected.

With the sodium alginate-based formulations, a
paste of the mixed powders was prepared by the dropwise
addition of a small quantity of distilled water, followed by rapid mixing, and then the plugs were formed
in the mold. Powdered mixtures that were too dry were
difficult to dislodge from the mold and did not remain
coherent afterwards; those containing too much water
were soft and lacking in mechanical strength.

Some of the inserts were coated by dipping in a 1% high MW sodium alginate solution and then into 10% calcium nitrate solution. The coating immediately hardened with slight shrinkage. With this treatment the suppositories became much stronger and easier to handle. Upon exposure to aqueous media, all treated inserts retained their structural integrity much longer than their uncoated counterparts.

Small tubes of regenerated cellulose were used as model Fallopian tubes. A casting solution of 3% cellulose triacetate (acetyl content 39.4% Eastman Kodak) in acetone was used. Glass tubes having a uniform diameter of 1.4-1.6 mm (melting point capillary tubes) were dipped into this solution, rotated horizontally in ambient air for drying, dipped and dried two more times to form a film of the desired thickness. The last coat was not allowed to dry completely; as soon as it began to become opaque, the tube was placed in a hydrolysis solution of 0.1 M sodium carbonate, 0.1 M sodium bicarbonate at pH 10 for 24 hours at 65° C. These tubelets were then rinsed and stripped off the glass tubes. Depending upon the mode of preparation, these tubes had a wall thickness of 20 $\pm$ 6 microns and had a water content of about 70%.

In vitro rate studies were carried out by placing inserts into the moist cellulose tubelets. After the ends were tied off with thread, each set was placed into a 10 ml beaker and 5 ml of a saline solution was added. The composition of this solution was: 145 mM in $NaNO_3$, 4.6 mM in KNO_3, and 3.5 mM in $Ca(NO_3)_2$, approximating the cationic composition in the Fallopian tube of the rabbit (15,16). At appropriate time intervals, aliquots were removed and analyzed for their silver content by titration.

For the animal experiments, the surgical procedure was as follows: a midline abdominal incision was made and the fimbrial end of the Fallopian tube identified, followed by insertion of the plug. This insert was then squeezed down (toward the interstitial portion) as far as possible, preferably to a point about 4 cm from the proximal end of the tube. Table I lists some of the inserts and their gross composition.

TABLE I
COMPOSITION (WEIGHT %) OF INSERT PREPARATION

Insert No.	AgNO3	NaAlg HMW	CaAlg2 LMW	AgAlg LMW	Pluronic (F127)	CGP***
1*				100		
2*			50	50		
3*			75	25		
7	30	9			60	1
8	30	22			45	3
9	60		40			
11	50		30	15		5
12	60				40	
14	60			30		10
17	50			40		10
18	80			9	10	1
19	70			13	15	2
20	80			18		2
21	10				90	
22**	10				30	
23*	20				80	
24*	30				70	

*   Post-coated with 1% NaAlg (HMW), hardened in 10% $Ca(NO_3)_2 \cdot 2H_2O$.
**   Add 60 parts sucrose.
***   Calcium glycerophosphate.

Results

In in vitro tests, each insert swelled slightly during the course of these studies. At the end of each experiment, the axial expansion was about 15% while radial swelling amounted to 5-10%. Figure 2 shows the cumulative release of silver as a function of time. When Pluronic was the only polymer carrier, most of the silver was released within the first fifteen minutes. This rapid release was observed for all Pluronic polyols. When a sodium alginate was used as the polymer carrier, this rate was slowed down substantially. The same effect was obtained when an additional Ag source was silver acetate suspended in sesame oil.

Histological results are in Table II. The death of a circumscribed tissue or of an organ is termed necrosis. Fibrosis refers to the development in an

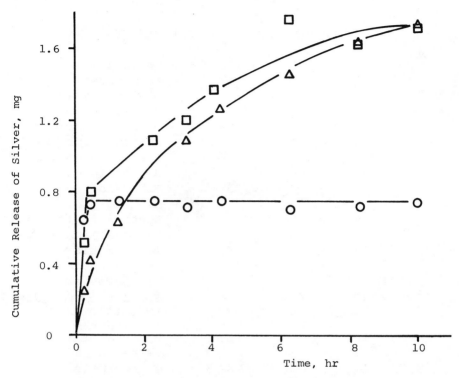

Figure 2. Silver release in vitro. ○ *AgNO₃ 30%, pluronic F127 70%;* □ *AgNO₃ 50%, low MW NaAlg. 50%;* △ *AgNO₃ 30%, silver acetate 10%, low MW NaAlg 60%.*

organ of excess fibrous connective tissues, often in response to necrosis. Fibrosis is a necessary but not sufficient condition leading to tubal blockade. When tubal tissues are severely damaged, the tube may enlarge in diameter and be filled with fluid, a condition known as hydrosalpinx.

It should be noted that bilateral tubal obstruction is difficult to achieve in rabbits, attributed to the morphology of its oviduct. Other investigators have found that formulations and delivery methods which produced closure in primates such as pigtail monkeys did not necessarily effect closure in rabbits. In our study, there was no significant difference in tissue damage when the period between insertion and sacrifice

TABLE II

RESULTS OF ANIMAL EXPERIMENTS

A *	B	C	D **	E
1	1	2	4+	Hydrosalpinx
2	1	4	4+	4+ necrosis
3	2	2		Minimal damage
4	2	4		Minimal damage
5	3	2	2+	Minimal necrosis
6	3	4		Minimal necrosis
7	7	3	2+	Acute inflammation
8	7	6	4+	Hydrosalpinx
9	8	3	3+	Fibrosis
10	8	6	0	Hydrosalpinx
11	9	2	3+	Acute inflammation
12	9	6		Hydrosalpinx
13	11	3	4+	4+ necrosis
14	11	6	1+	Hydrosalpinx, 4+ necrosis
15	12	3	3+	Focal necrosis, deep
16	12	6	3+	Hydrosalpinx, 4+ necrosis
17	14	3	3+	Hydrosalpinx, 4+ necrosis
18	14	6	4+	4+ necrosis, into muscularis
19	17	3	4+	4+ necrosis extending into fat
20	17	6	3+	Hydrosalpinx, necrosis, fibrosis
21	18	2	3+	Necrosis, thru wall
22	18	6		4+ necrosis
23	19	2	3+	Necrosis, thru wall
24	19	6	4+	4+ necrosis, thru wall
25	20	3	3+	Hydrosalpinx, 4+ necrosis
26	20	6	4+	4+ necrosis
27	21	3		No significant
28	22	3		alterations
29,30	23	6	0	Necrosis, epithelium
31,32	24	6	0	regenerated

A-animal no.; B-Insert no.; C-Period to sacrifice(wks);
D-Residuum of insert; E-Observations.
 * 1-28, New Zealand rabbits; 29-32, pigtail monkeys.
** Amt. of insert remaining: 0,1+ to 4+.

was increased from 2-3 weeks to 4-6 weeks. No tubal blockade was achieved either in rabbits or pigtail monkeys.

Discussion

When silver alginate was used, it was so slowly absorbed by the surrounding tissues in the rabbit that it was concluded that, however effective calcium ions were in displacing silver ions from the algin complex, the oviducal environment did not furnish enough calcium for this purpose. Calcium alginate gels were, on the other hand, completely absorbed within 4 weeks even in the presence of silver ions.

The silver nitrate releasing formulations, when placed in the rabbit Fallopian tube, produced necrosis of the epithelium and the wall at higher concentrations, with no observable effect at the lower concentrations. Sections of the oviduct not in contact with the insert were not affected. It was apparent that localized release was obtained, but it was necessary to control the amount of silver nitrate present and its rate of release so as not to produce so much necrosis that peritoneal damage occurred.

It was concluded that failure to obtain closure was due to two factors. First and more important, the highly invaginated nature of the oviduct was such as to prevent silver ions from reacting with the entire epithelial surface over a sufficient length of the tube. Regeneration of the epithelium is known to proceed rapidly, so islands of non-cauterized tissue grow and prevent the slower infiltration of fibroblasts from the cells below the epithelium. Second, the duration of chemical cauterization probably was not long enough. Experiments with other chemical cauterizing agents have shown that a severe but very rapid burn does not necessarily produce closure.

A subsequent study, one still in progress, makes use of paste-like formulations of alginate and silver salts, which distends the tube as it is injected. With this formulation, tubal closure has been observed in the rabbit.

Acknowledgments

This work was supported by NICHD contract Nol-HD-3-2797. The authors express their thanks for the technical assistance of Messrs. George Cottral and Douglas Rosenberg.

Literature Cited

1. Neuwirth, R., Richart, R., and Taylor, H.,Jr.,
    Amer.J.Obstet.Gynec.,(1971),38,51.
2. "The Wonderful World of Pluronic Polyols",
    BASF Wyandotte Co., 1973, p.2.
3. Private Communications from Wyandotte Co.
4. Haug, A., Acta Chem.Scand.,(1959),13,601.
5. _____ , ibid.,(1966), 20, 183.
6. _____ , ibid., (1967), 21, 691.
7. _____ , Colloques Internationaux du Centre
    National de la Recherche Scientifique,(1960),
    No. 103.
8. Cozzi, D., Desideri,P. and Lepri, L., J. Chromatogr.,(1969),40 (1), 130.
9. Wassermann, A. and Cooper, R., Nature, (1957),
    180, 1072.
10. Thiele, H. and Schact, G., Kolloid Z.,(1958),
    161, 120.
11. Nilson, H., and Wagner, J., Pro.Soc.Exp.Bio.
    Med., (1951), 76, 630.
12. Johnston, J., Lobdell, B., and Woodard, G.,
    Woodard Research Corp., unpublished data.
13. Johnston, D., SS-3428 and SS-3429, Woodard
    Research Corp., unpublished data.
14. Blaine, G., Annals of Surgery, (1947),125,102.
15. Mastroianni, L.,Jr., Urzua, M., Avalos, M.,
    and Stambaugh, R., Am.J.Obstet.Gynec., (1969),
    103, 703.
16. David, A., Brackett, B., Garcia, C., and
    Mastroianni, L.,Jr., J.Reprod.Fert., (1969),
    19, 285.

11

Controlled Release of Delmadinone Acetate from Silicone Polymer Tubing: In Vitro-In Vivo Correlations to Diffusion Model

JOHN S. KENT

Institute of Pharmaceutical Sciences, Syntax Research, Palo Alto, Calif. 94304

Introduction

Over the past decade, there has been a great interest in silicone polymers as substances for controlling the release of a drug or chemical substance. The research in this area has been summarized at a Symposium (1). The present report deals with silicone polymer (Silastic®) tubing as a substance for controlling the release of a steroid, delmadinone acetate. It has been discussed (1, p. 103) that silicone polymer tubing packed with drug crystals leads to variable and unpredicably low results. To avoid this it has been suggested in our laboratory and elsewhere (2-5) that the drug be present in the tube in the form of a suspension. This allows a uniform supply of the drug to the tubing inner wall, assuming that the suspending medium provides solubility for the drug and does not rapidly diffusion from the tube. A device such as this was developed and used in the following experiments.

The experiments reported here determine the long term release characteristics of a drug-suspension silicone polymer tube implanted in vivo, determine if the drug release is membrane and/or diffusion layer controlled and examine if there is a correlation between in vivo and in vitro release.

Theoretical

The mathematical relationship for diffusion in a cylinder has been discussed (6). It was of interest to determine if the steroid released from the silicone polymer tubing devices studied here was controlled by the tubing thickness and/or a boundary diffusion layer. The physical model is shown in Figure 1a. The symbols are defined as: C_s = the saturation concentration of drug in the suspension medium; C_1 = concentration of drug in the silicone polymer tubing at the suspension - inner wall interface; C_2 = concentration of drug in the silicone polymer tubing at the outer tubing wall - receptor interface; C_3 =

concentration of drug in the receptor at the outer tubing wall -
receptor interface; A = inner tube radius; B = outer tube radius;
E = outer radius of boundary diffusion layer. Certain
assumptions are necessary in the derivation of the mathematical
model:

     1. Steady state is established such that the flux, J, is
constant through every concentric cylindrical shell;

     2. There is no significant boundary layer within the
cylindrical tubing. The diffusional resistance comprises
the tubing and the external boundary diffusion layer, hence no
interfacial barriers;

     3. There is no significant diffusion through the ends of
the tubing sections;

     4. The diffusion layer is symmetrical over entire tubing
surface.

The derivation of this model has been recently discussed in
detail (7). However, for convenience the derivation is included
here. The general case for diffusion through a cylinder can be
written as:

$$\text{Flux} = J = -2\pi \ rhD \ \frac{\partial C}{\partial r} \qquad\qquad \text{Eq. 1}$$

where r = cylinder radius, h = cylinder length, D = diffusion
coefficient and C = diffusing species concentration. By
rearrangement of this equation and defining D_m as the apparent
diffusion coefficient in the silicone polymer tubing, the
following equation is obtained.

$$\frac{\partial r}{r} = \frac{-2 \ \pi h D_m \ \partial C}{J} \qquad\qquad \text{Eq. 2}$$

By integration between the inner (A) and outer (B) radii and
between C_1 and C_2, equation 2 becomes:

$$J = \frac{-2 \ \pi h D_m \ (C_2 - C_1)}{\ln \ (B/A)} \qquad\qquad \text{Eq. 3}$$

If the same derivation is applied to the cylindrical boundary
diffusion layer, with integration between B and E and concentrations C_3 and C_0 the resulting equation is:

$$J = \frac{-2 \ \pi h D_a \ (C_0 - C_3)}{\ln \ (E/B)} \qquad\qquad \text{Eq. 4}$$

Equations 3 and 4 are combined by using the partition
coefficients defined as follows:

    K_I = Partition coefficient between the core suspending
         medium and the silicone polymer tubing (C_s/C_1).

    K_{II} = Partition coefficient between the silicone polymer
         tubing and the receptor phase ($C_2/C_3 \equiv C_1/C_{sr}$).
         Where C_{sr} = solubility of the drug in the receptor
         phase.

The equation is then:

$$J = \frac{2\pi h D_m D_a C_s}{D_a K_I \ln(B/A) + D_m K_I K_{II} \ln(E/B)}$$ Eq. 5

The product of K_I and K_{II} can be defined as K_{III} which is the partition coefficient between the suspension medium and the receptor phase. Equation 5 defines the flux, J, as being dependent on tubing thickness and the boundary diffusion layer. The equation is simplified if one or the other diffusional resistances predominates. If $D_a K_I \ln(B/A)$ is greater than $D_m K_{III} \ln(E/B)$, the diffusion process is membrane (tubing thickness) controlled. The resulting equation being:

$$J = \frac{2\pi h D_m C_s}{K_I \ln(B/A)} = \frac{2\pi h D_m C_m}{\ln(B/A)}$$ Eq. 6

where $C_1 = C_m$ = saturation solubility of the diffusing species in the silicone polymer.

If the opposite is true, the diffusional process is boundary layer controlled. That equation is then:

$$J = \frac{2\pi h D_a C_s}{K_{III} \ln(E/B)} = \frac{2\pi h D_a C_{sr}}{\ln(E/B)}$$ Eq. 7

Experimental

Materials. Delmadinone acetate (DA; 6-chloro-17α hydroxy-pregna-1,4,6-triene-3,20-dione acetate) was used in the micronized form. For some partitioning and solubility studies tritium labeled delmadinone acetate with a specific activity of 0.152 μCi/mg was used. Deionized water was used in the in vitro diffusion studies. Silicone polymer (Silastic®) tubing and Silastic® Medical Grade Adhesive Type A (Dow Corning, Medical Products Division) was used throughout the experiment. The suspending fluid used in the silicone polymer tube devices was polysorbate 80 (Tween 80, ICI-United States).

Preparation of Filled Silicone Polymer Tubes. Specified lengths of the various sizes of silicone tubing were washed with acetone and dried. One end was then plugged with Silastic® Medical Adhesive Type A and allowed to cure. The tubes for the in vivo study were then weighed and then again after filling with the steroid suspension so the fill weight could be calculated. The steroid suspension was composed of 50% micronized delmadinone acetate and 50% polysorbate 80 except as noted under the in vivo studies. After the tubes were filled with the steroid suspension, they were sealed with the Silastic® Medical Grade Adhesive. A summary of the materials and tubing devices used in the in vivo and in vitro studies is found in Tables I and II.

In Vitro Diffusion Studies. The DA suspension filled silicone polymer tubes (DA tubes) were fastened between an upper

TABLE I

PHYSICAL PARAMETERS OF THE SILICONE POLYMER TUBING DEVICES USED IN THE IN VITRO DIFFUSION STUDY AND CONDITIONS OF THE STUDY.

CONDITIONS

Paddle Rotation - 50 rpm

Temperature - 25°C

Volume - 1 L. Distilled Water

MATERIALS

GROUP	TUBING SIZE, i.d. x o.d., in., (cm)	THICKNESS mil, (cm)	EXTERNAL SURFACE AREA cm²/TUBE	STEROID EXPOSED LENGTH, cm.	NUMBER OF TUBES PER BEAKER	AVERAGE MG. DA PER SEALED TUBE
A	.115 x .125 (.292 x .318)	5(.013)	1.0	1.0	2	42.3
B	.105 x .125 (.267 x .318)	10(.025)	1.0	1.0	4	30.9
C	.132 x .183 (.335 x .465)	25.5(.065)	2.2	1.5	4	74.5
D	.104 x .192 (.264 x .488)	44.0(.112)	3.1	2.0	4	60.6

TABLE II

PHYSICAL PARAMETERS OF SILICONE POLYMER
TUBING DEVICES USED IN THE IN VIVO DIFFUSION STUDY

GROUP	TUBING SIZE, i.d. x o.d., in., (cm)	THICKNESS mil, (cm)	EXTERNAL SURFACE AREA cm²/TUBE	STEROID EXPOSED LENGTH, cm	NUMBER IMPLANTED PER RAT	AVERAGE MG. DA PER SEALED TUBE
A	.115 x .125 (.292 x .318)	5(.013)	1.0	1.0	4	16.6
B	.105 x .125 (.267 x .318)	10(.025)	2.0	2.0	4	25.5
C	.132 x .183 (.335 x .465)	25.5(.065)	1.47	1.0	4	53.3
D	.104 x .192 (.264 x .488)	44.0(.112)	2.33	1.5	4	40.9

and a lower paddle that were on a single stirring shaft (Figure
1b). The shafts were rotated at 50 r.p.m. using a multiple
spindle stirring apparatus (Phipps-Bird, Richmond, Va.). The
receptor was 1.0 liter of deionized water which was changed at
daily intervals to maintain sink conditions. The water bath
holding the receptor beakers was maintained at 25°C. The
receptor phase was assayed for DA by extraction with chloroform,
evaporation to dryness, reconstitution with ethanol, U.S.P. and
absorbance determined at 301 nm. Amount of DA present was
determined by conversion of absorbance to weight by using the
Beer's Law plot for DA in ethanol U.S.P. Each time point
represents the average of three determinations.

   In Vivo Diffusion Studies. The in vivo studies consisted
of two separate experiments. One study consisted of groups A
and B the other C and D. The study with groups A and B used
silicone polymer tubing implants that contained 11% DA, 15%
polysorbate 80 and 75% inert filler. These tubes had shown
equivalent release to the 50% DA formulation described
previously and were tested for release termination characteristics. The experiment with groups C and D used the 50%
suspension formulation. In both experiments four sealed tubes
were implanted subcutaneously on the dorsal side of albino rats.
For groups A and B, two rats were sacrificed and the sealed
tubes removed at one month intervals. The sealed tubes were
then assayed for remaining DA. In the remaining groups, the
animal sacrifice and sealed tube removal was at two month
intervals. The assay of DA remaining in the sealed tubes was
performed by extraction with chloroform. The extract was placed
on a silica gel plate with development by using 70:30,
benzene:ethyl acetate. The spot corresponding to DA was
removed and reacted with 4-aminoantipyrine hydrochloride.
The absorbance of each sample was determined at 420 nm against
the plate blank.

   Solubilities and Partition Coefficients. The aqueous
solubilities of DA were determined at 25°C and 37°C using
tritium labeled DA with a specific activity of 0.152 µCi/mg.
Samples were equilibrated for 4.5 days and then filtered
through a 0.4µ filter (Gelman). Four ml samples were dried,
scintillation fluid (methanol-dioxane) added and counted for
radioactivity.
   The saturated aqueous solutions of DA were then used to
determine the partition coefficients between the silicone
polymer tubing and water. The silicone polymer tubing used was
a) .132" x .183" and b) .104" x .192", i.d. x o.d. A 10 and
5 cm length of each, respectively, were equilibrated with
solutions of DA. After equilibration (2 days) the tubes
were removed, extracted with chloroform, the extract dried and
counted. Aqueous samples were counted as before. The partition

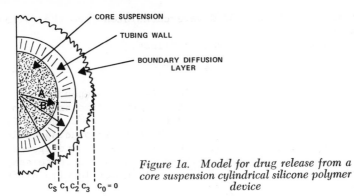

Figure 1a. Model for drug release from a core suspension cylindrical silicone polymer device

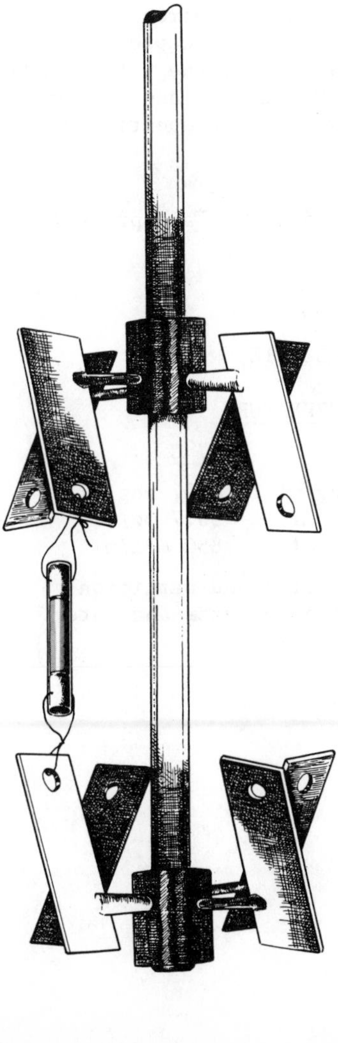

Figure 1b. Paddle assembly for in vitro diffusion experiments

coefficients at 25 and 37°C were calculated from the following expression:

$$K = \frac{DPM_{silastic} \text{ per Volume Silastic}}{DPM_{water} \text{ per Volume Water}}$$

Theoretically, partition coefficients are independent of temperature. As this was essentially true, the partition coefficients reported are from data at both 25°C and 37°C.

The solubility in the polysorbate 80 suspending medium was determined by equilibration of DA with the suspending medium, centrifugation of the samples, removal of a supernate sample and analysis of DA as described previously under in vivo diffusion studies.

Data Analysis. The computation of D_m and the diffusion layer, ℓ, as well as the goodness of fit of the data to equation 5 was accomplished through non-linear regression analysis using NONLIN (8). The values for the receptor diffusion coefficient (D_a) were calculated from the Sutherland-Einstein equation (9). The values for D_a at 25°C and 37°C were 4.90 x 10^{-6} cm^{2}sec^{-1} and 5.10 x 10^{-6} cm^{2}sec^{-1}, respectively.

Results

The solubilities and partition coefficients are presented in Tables III and IV respectively.

TABLE III

SOLUBILITIES OF DELMADINONE ACETATE

MEDIUM	TEMPERATURE	
	25°C	37°C
Water	4.57 mcg/ml	6.07 mcg/ml
Polysorbate 80	28.5 mg/ml	36.7 mg/ml
Silicone Polymer*	640 mcg/ml	850 mcg/ml

*Calculated from water solubilities and partition coefficients between the silicone polymer and water.

TABLE IV

PARTITION COEFFICIENTS OF DELMADINONE ACETATE
(The partition coefficients are essentially equivalent
at both 25° and 37°. Therefore data from both temperatures was used in calculating the K values reported here.)

MEDIUM	K
Silicone Polymer/Water	K_{II} = 140
*Polysorbate 80/ Silicone Polymer	K_I = 43.9
*Polysorbate 80/Water	K_{III} = 6.15 x 10^3

*Calculated from solubilities

Figures 2 and 3 exhibit the cumulative amounts of DA released per cm length of tubing. The solid line in each case
represents the least squares fit of the data. The slope
of each line which is the flux per cm length of tubing, J_h, is
found in Table V. Also the inverse of the natural logarithm
of the ratio of the outer diameter over the inner diameter of the
silicone polymer tubings is listed as well.

TABLE V

IN VITRO DIFFUSION STUDY OF DELMADINONE
ACETATE FROM SEALED SILICONE POLYMER TUBES

GROUP	J_h(mcg day^{-1}cm^{-1})	$[\ln\frac{(o.d.)}{(i.d.)}]^{-1}$
A	126.0	12.0
B	68.7	5.74
C	39.7	3.06
D	21.1	1.63

If the in vitro data is plotted according to equation 5
and then fit to that equation using non-linear regression
analysis, the result is that shown in Figure 4. The calculation
for D_m and ℓ, the diffuion layer from this analysis are in
Table VI.

The results of the in vivo diffusion experiments are
plotted in Figure 5. The solid line is the least squares fit
of the data, the slope of which is the flux, J. The values for
the flux per cm length of tubing, J_h, and the inverse of the
natural logarithm of the ratio of the outer diameter over the
inner diameter of the silicone polymer tubing are listed in
Table VII. The plot of the data according to equation 5 is
depicted in Figure 6. The dashed line is the fit of the data
to equation 5 using non-linear regression analysis. The values
for D_m and ℓ from this analysis are presented in Table VI.

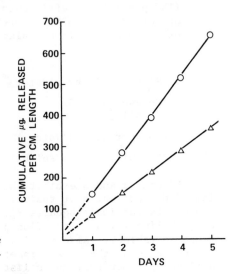

Figure 2. In vitro diffusion of delmadinone acetate from sealed silicone polymer tubes. Key: ○ *Group A,* △ *Group B.*

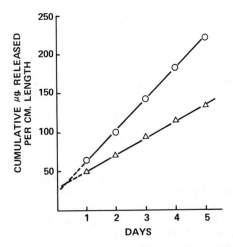

Figure 3. In vitro diffusion of delmadinone acetate from sealed silicone polymer tubes. Key: ○ *Group C,* △ *Group D.*

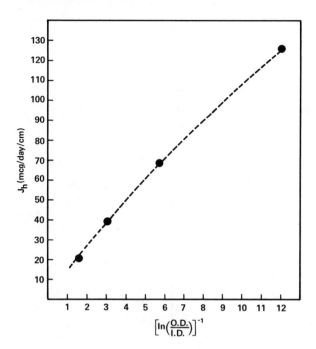

Figure 4. In vitro diffusion data. Key: ——— data fit to diffusion. C.C. = 1.000.

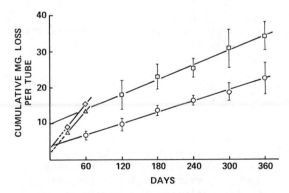

Figure 5. Diffusion of delmadinone acetate from silicone polymer tubes implanted in rats. Key: △ Group A, ◇ Group B, □ Group C, ○ Group D.

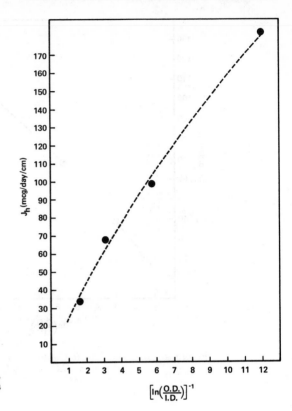

Figure 6.   In vivo diffusion data.
Key: – – – data fit to diffusion
*   model. C.C. = 0.997.*

$$\left[\ln\left(\frac{O.D.}{I.D.}\right)\right]^{-1}$$

Discussion

The in vivo and in vitro diffusion data correlate well with
the diffusion model (Eq. 5). As indicated in Figures 4 and 6,
the correlation coefficients to this model (Eq. 5) for the in
vitro and in vivo diffusion data are 1.000 and 0.997, respectively. Also, the in vivo data (Figure 6) demonstrates the
utility of a drug-suspension within a silicone polymer tube as
a device for uniform delivery of drug over a period of at least
one year.

The activation energy (ΔEa) for diffusion of DA in silicone
polymer can be calculated using the Arrhenius expression (10)
which describes the relationship between the diffusion coefficient in a polymer and temperature. The apparent diffusion
coefficients (D_m, Table VI) for DA in the silicone polymer have
been calculated as the result of the data fit to the theoretical
expression (Eq. 5) for drug diffusion. Since the values for D_m
are at 25°C and 37°C, an estimate of ΔEa was calculated as 3.3
kcal mole^{-1}. This is consistant for values of ΔEa which have
been reported (11–13) as 3.6 to 18.2 kcal/mole for various
compounds in silicone polymer. This result indicates that the

TABLE VI

IN VITRO AND IN VIVO VALUES FOR D_m AND ℓ BY DATA FIT TO
DIFFUSION MODEL BY NON-LINEAR REGRESSION ANALYSIS

	D_m	ℓ (microns)
IN VITRO	$3.27 \times 10^{-3} cm^2/day$	30.2
	$3.78 \times 10^{-8} cm^2/sec$	
IN VIVO	$4.12 \times 10^{-3} cm^2/day$	41.6
	$4.77 \times 10^{-8} cm^2/sec$	

TABLE VII

IN VIVO DIFFUSION STUDY OF DELMADINONE
ACETATE FROM SEALED SILICONE POLYMER TUBES

GROUP	J_h (mcg day^{-1}cm^{-1})	$[\ln \frac{(o.d.)}{(i.d.)}]^{-1}$
A	183	12.0
B	99	5.74
C	68	3.06
D	34	1.63

values for D_m are reasonable and the diffusion process in the
polymer has a low energy requirement.

The values for the diffusion layer (Table VI) for the
in vivo and in vitro experiments can be explained. The results
suggest that a decrease in the stirring or hydrodynamics of the
in vitro system would increase the diffusion layer (ℓ) to the
value of that observed in the in vivo experiment. Then, providing equivalence of the experimental temperatures, a direct
correlation could be obtained between in vivo and in vitro drug
diffusion from the tubing devices. The in vitro value for ℓ was
slightly less than the value of 66.8 microns reported in an
earlier in vitro study (14) with a matrix-drug system. However,
differences in the mixing or hydrodynamics in the receptor of
these two experiments could easily account for the observed
difference in diffusion layer thickness.

The reduction of equation 5 to that for membrane controlled
drug release (Eq. 6) is dependent on the value of K_{III} and the
tubing thickness. In the present experiment, the value of K_{III}
is very large so reduction to membrane controlled drug release
occurs at values for the tubing thickness much larger than
otherwise might be observed.

A direct correlation between in vivo and in vitro drug
diffusion in this system is suggested if a) the hydrodynamics
of the in vitro system are controlled such that the diffusion
layer values are equal (also, temperatures of the systems must be

equivalent); or b) the tubing wall thickness is large enough such that the value for the diffusion layer thickness becomes negligible and the diffusion process becomes membrane (tubing) controlled (Eq. 6).

In summary, it has been observed that: 1) drug suspension filled silicone polymer tubes allow uniform release of drug over periods of at least one year. 2) In the _in vivo_ and _in vitro_ situation, diffusion of delmadinone acetate from this silicone polymer device is a membrane and diffusion layer controlled process which is described theoretically (Eq. 5). 3) The correlation between _in vitro_ and _in vivo_ results is dependent on _in vitro_ hydrodynamics (stirring) that will provide a diffusion layer thickness equivalent to the _in vivo_ value. 4) The drug diffusion model (Eq. 5) reduces to a membrane controlled process provided the tubing thickness increases such that the contribution by the boundary diffusion layer is not significant and/or the conditions are changed such that K_{III} decreases in value.

Acknowledgements: Mr. Dale Herriott, Mr. Mark Yost, Miss Nicola Nanevicz, the Dept. of Pharmaceutical Analysis and the Dept. of Toxicology for their technical assistance. Drs. R. E. Jones and G. L. Flynn for their helpful discussions and Dr. B. Poulsen for his support and encouragement.

Literature Cited

(1) Tanquary, A.C. and Lacey, R.E., "Controlled Release of Biological Active Agents", Advances in Experimental Medicine and Biology, Vol. 47, Plenum Press, New York (1974).
(2) Kincl, F.A. and Rudel, H.W., _Acta. Endocrinological_, Suppl. __151__, 5 (1971)
(3) Zaffaroni, A., U.S. Patent 3,845,761 (1974).
(4) Zaffaroni, A., U.S. Patent 3,895,103 (1975).
(5) Zaffaroni, A., U.S. Patent 3,896,819 (1975).
(6) Crank, J., "The Mathematics of Diffusion", Oxford University Press, London, England, (1964), p. 62.
(7) Flynn, G.L., _et al_, _J. Pharm. Sci._, __65__, 154 (1976).
(8) Metzler, C.M., "A User's Manual for NONLIN", Tech. Rep. 7297/69/7297/005, The Upjohn Co., Kalamazoo, Mich., 1969, as modified.
(9) Martin, A.N., Swarbrick, J., and Cammarata, A., "Physical Pharmacy", 2nd Ed., Lea &Febiger, Philadelphia, PA., (1970), p. 452.
(10) Meares, P., "Polymers: Structure and Bulk Properties" D. Van Nostrand Company Ltd., London, England, 1965, p. 324.
(11) Garrett, E.R. and Chemburkar, P.B., _J. Pharm. Sci._, __57__, 949 (1968)
(12) Garrett, E.R. and Chemburkar, P.B., _J. Pharm. Sci._, __57__, 1401 (1968)
(13) Hwang, S.T. _et al_, _Invest. Urology_, __8__, 245 (1970)
(14) Roseman, T.J. and Higuchi, W.I., _J. Pharm. Sci._, __59__, 353 (1970)

Steroid Release via Cellulose Acetate Butyrate Microcapsules

DAVID L. GARDNER, DAVID J. FINK, ALBERT J. PATANUS,
WILLIAM C. BAYTOS, and CRAIG R. HASSLER

Battelle, Columbus Laboratories, 505 King Ave., Columbus, Ohio 43201

Many novel systems for a controlled drug delivery are now being developed. For instance, during the last few years, several investigators have explored the possibility of preventing conception through the use of intrauterine or intravaginal administration of drugs released from reservoirs such as Silastic vaginal rings and tubes (1-5). These devices are impregnated with progestational steroids, such as medroxyprogesterone acetate (MPA), Norgestral, etc., and then inserted in the uterus or vagina. Once inserted within the uterus or vagina, the device slowly releases the steroid, sometimes over prolonged periods of time, and is effective in preventing conception.

An alternative controlled drug delivery system might be a system based upon transcervical or intrauterine migration of particles for either contraceptive or medicative purposes. Egli and Newton (6) discovered that inert carbon particles, placed in the posterior fornix of the vagina in three women about to undergo an abdominal hysterectomy, migrated within 35 minutes into the fallopian tubes in 2 out of the 3 cases. deBoer (7) found that when a quantity of India ink (a colloidal suspension of carbon) was placed in the uterine cavity of patients about to undergo an abdominal surgical procedure (hysterectomy, oophorectomy, or tubal ligation), the ink particles had been transported to the fallopian tube in more than 50 percent of the observed patients and migration of the particles from the cervical canal had occurred in nearly 30 percent of the patients. Both of these studies indicate that inert particles can migrate from the vaginal tract or uterine cavity into the fallopian tube.

A drug delivery system based upon the transcervical migration of particles might make use of microcapsules. Microcapsules are spherical membranes ("synthetic cells") which can vary in diameter from a few microns to several millimeters and which can contain either a drug solution, suspension, or emulsion. This paper describes preliminary results of steroid release from cellulose acetate butyrate microcapsules.

Materials and Methods

Cellulose acetate butyrate (CAB) microcapsules containing two core preparations for drug delivery were prepared by a phase-separation technique. The first core consisted of tritiated progesterone dissolved in a high molecular weight oil (olive) and emulsified in a phosphate-saline buffer solution (pH 7.3). In the second core solution, tritiated progesterone or estrone was suspended directly in the aqueous medium (phosphate-saline buffer). Microcapsules were prepared in which the core solution contained 100 μCi of tritiated progesterone (specific activity of 50.3 Ci/mmole plus 20 mg of unlabeled progesterone) or 50 μCi of tritiated estrone (specific activity of 48 Ci/mmole plus 20 mg of unlabeled estrone).

In vitro release rate studies were performed on several different preparations of progesterone and estrone microcapsules by two procedures. In the first procedure, a known weight of capsules was placed in a volume of phosphate-saline buffer (pH 7.3) with the addition of Triton X-100 surfactant. The flask containing the capsules and buffer solution was then placed in a constant-temperature bath at 37 C and agitated. Samples of the suspension were periodically removed and filtered, and the concentration of drug in the supernatant determined by liquid scintillation spectrometry. In this procedure, there was a continual increase of the drug in the supernatant solution since the supernatant solution was not changed during the period of study.

The second procedure involved exchanging the test solution daily. Drug-containing capsules and buffer were placed in a test tube with a specially fitted rubber stopper. The test tube was agitated in a thermostatically controlled water bath (37 C). A plastic screen at the base of the stopper permitted removal of the supernatant solution while the capsules were retained in the tube. The supernatant was withdrawn daily from the capsules and the drug concentration determined as above. Fresh test solution was added back to the tube to restart the test.

Results

In Vitro Progesterone Release Studies. The first study involved 200-300-μ-diameter capsules which contained three different concentrations of progesterone in an oil-in-water emulsion. The progesterone concentrations for each capsule preparation were: Preparation 1 - 440 ng/100 mg capsules, Preparation 2 - 155 ng/100 mg, and Preparation 3 - 83 ng/100 mg.

Release rates from 100 mg of each of these capsule preparations were measured into the following solutions (200 ml).

Solution A: Phosphate-saline buffer, pH 7.35
Solution B: Phosphate-saline buffer, pH 7.35, plus
             2 drops of surfactant (Triton X-100)

The presence of surfactant greatly enhanced the rate of progesterone transport from the capsules as shown in Table I. The release rates in the presence of surfactant (Figure 1) indicate a rapid initial release of progesterone from the capsules followed by a more constant release rate. We attribute the high initial rate either to rupturing of incompletely formed capsules or the release of surface-adsorbed progesterone into the test solution.

TABLE I. RELEASE OF PROGESTERONE FROM CAPSULES CONTAINING DIFFERENT CONCENTRATIONS OF PROGESTERONE IN AN OIL/WATER EMULSION

	Cumulative Nanograms of Progesterone Released/100 mg of Capsules					
	Prep. 1 Solution		Prep. 2 Solution		Prep. 3 Solution	
Times, hr	A	B	A	B	A	B
1	23	56	5	20	7	15
3	24	109	18	41	13	16
6	24	122	18	46	1	36
24	30	159	23	52	9	39
48	40	170	18	70	18	41
72	53	190	28	72	21	48
144	88	210	38	91	30	63

The "constant" release rates from 24 hours to 144 hours for each batch of capsules were: Preparation 1 - 10.2 ng/day, Preparation 2 - 7.8 ng/day, and Preparation 3 - 4.8 ng/day. The long-term release rate of Preparation 1 was roughly twice the release rate of Preparation 3, although the initial progesterone concentration was approximately 5 times greater. This indicates that the progesterone concentration may be increased in the capsule without a corresponding linear increase in release rate. Thus, a combination of factors such as drug solubility, partitioning rate, and membrane transport rate may contribute to the control of the drug release rate.

The second release rate study involved the release of progesterone from CAB microcapsules containing progesterone particles suspended in phosphate-saline buffer containing bovine serum albumin. In this study, 500 mg of 420–500-μ capsules and 2 g of 510–700-μ capsules were placed in 5 ml of a phosphate-saline buffer solution containing 1 drop of Triton X-100 surfactant. The 5-ml test solution was separated daily from the capsules as described earlier and fresh test solution (phosphate-saline buffer plus surfactant) was added back to the capsules. Duplicate aliquots of the filtered test solution were then counted to determine the progesterone release rate.

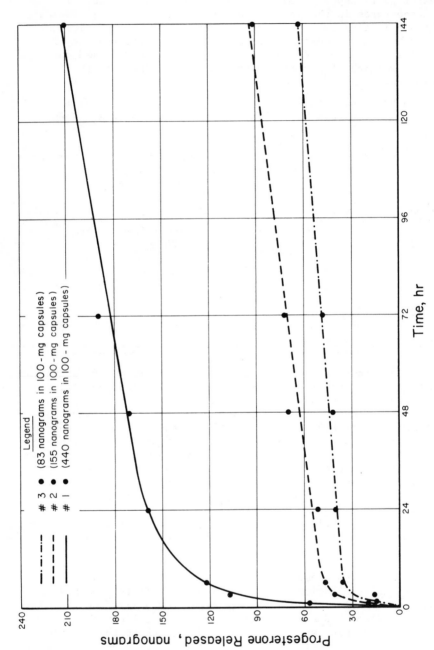

Figure 1. Effect of progesterone concentration within microcapsules on release rate

The results of this study (Table II) indicate that the progesterone release rate was considerably greater and more constant over the four test days than the release rates seen with the smaller capsules (200–300 μ) in the first test (Table I). We believe that the increased transport reflects the different core preparations, i.e., emulsion (Table I) and suspension plus albumin (Table II). The micrograms of progesterone released per day approximated 2.4 μg/g for the 420–500-μ capsules and 1.6 μg/g for the 510–700-μ capsules.

TABLE II. IN VITRO RELEASE RATE OF PROGESTERONE FROM MICROCAPSULES CONTAINING SOLID PROGESTERONE SUSPENDED IN A PHOSPHATE–SALINE–ALBUMIN CORE

Time, days	420–500 μ Net CPM Released/ Day/g Capsule	Time, days	510–700 μ Net CPM Released/ Day/g Capsule
1	18,400	1	8,275
2	13,700	2	8,350
3	12,500	3	8,225
4	12,700	4	8,200

In Vivo Progesterone Release Rate. To determine the in vivo release rate of progesterone from the above 420–500-μ–diameter capsules, 100 mg of moist capsules were placed in the uteri of each of two rabbits via a simple laparotomy. 100 mg of moist capsules is equivalent to 3.21 mg on a dry weight basis and contained 4049 CPM/mg dry capsules. Dry weight was determined after air drying for 24 hours. The rabbits were sacrificed 4 and 6 hours after insertion of the microcapsules, and the uteri were removed and flushed with a phosphate–saline buffer solution to recover the remaining capsules. The flushed solution was passed over a screen designed to retain this particular sized capsule. The recovered capsules were then air dried for 24 hours. The progesterone remaining in the dried capsules is shown in Table III and a comparison between the release rate obtained in vitro and in vivo is shown in Figure 2.

The in vivo progesterone release rate from these capsules is at least 17 times greater than the in vitro rate determined in the preceding release rate study (Table II) using identical capsules. We believe this increased rate is due to the highly lipophilic uterine environment. Lipophilic materials which penetrate the capsule wall would probably lead to increased progesterone solubilization and perhaps also to higher membrane transport rates. This experiment again points out the necessity for correlation of in vivo and in vitro transport rates when devising in vitro testing procedures.

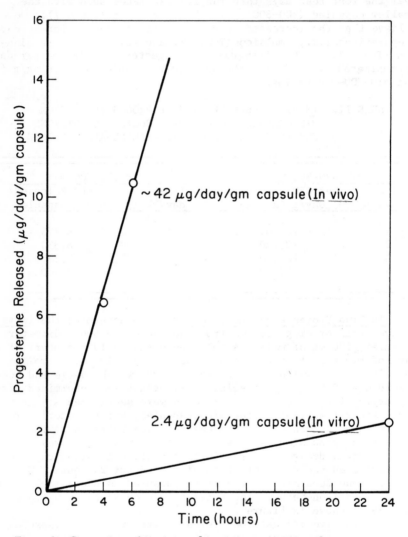

Figure 2.   *Comparison of in vitro and in vivo progesterone release rates from 420–500-μ-diameter microcapsules*

TABLE III. PROGESTERONE–LOADED CAPSULES RECOVERED
FROM RABBIT UTERI AT 4 AND 6 HOURS

Rabbit No.	Uterine Horn	Dry Weight of Recovered Capsules, mg	Net CPM	CPM/mg Dried Capsule	Average CPM/mg Dried Capsule
104	Rt side	0.30	890	2967	2935
(4 hr)	Lf side	0.54	1568	2904	
113	Rt side	0.35	689	1968	2238
(6 hr)	Lf side	0.56	1401	2502	

In Vitro Estrone Release Rate. The first estrone release
rate study involved two different microcapsule sizes from the
same microcapsule preparation, i.e., 297–420 μ and 420–500 μ
diameter. The test solution consisted of 5 ml of phosphate-
saline buffer (pH 7.3) plus 1 drop of surfactant (Triton X-100).
Two hundred mg of capsules were added to the test solution and
the tubes were agitated in a thermostatically controlled water
bath (37 C). Two hundred mg of capsules contained approximately
90 μg of estrone. The results of this study are presented in
Table IV.

TABLE IV. ESTRONE RELEASE FROM TWO DIFFERENT
MICROCAPSULE SIZES

Sampling Time, hr	297–420 μ μg Released/ 200 mg Capsules	420–500 μ μg Released/ 200 mg Capsules
24	4.6	6.0
48	4.4	4.5
72	3.5	2.7
96	2.9	1.1

The results suggested that the release rate was nonlinear
over the time of release monitored. To determine if a zero-order
release rate could be obtained over a longer time period, duplicate 500-mg capsule samples (A and B) were placed in 5 ml of
phosphate-saline buffer solution containing a surfactant (5 drops
of Triton X-100/1000 ml). These capsules (297–420 μ), however,
were of a different microcapsule preparation than those used in
Table IV and contained 290 μg estrone/500 mg capsules. The
results of the release rate study are presented in Figure 3 and
the single point represents the average between duplicate samples.

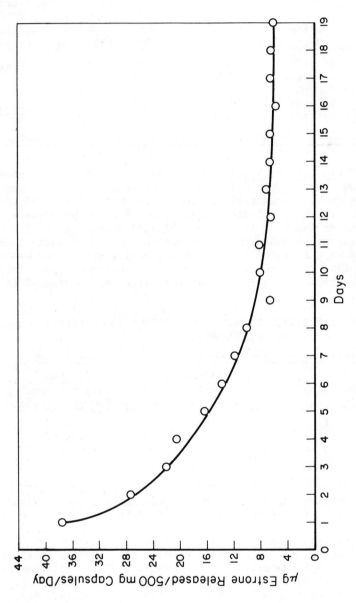

Figure 3. Long-term estrone release from 297–420-μ-diameter microcapsules

It is clearly evident from this study that a near zero-order release rate may be obtained from cellulose acetate butyrate microcapsules. The reason for the nonlinear release rate over the first 8 days is believed to be due either to estrone entrapped in the membrane wall or the rupturing of imperfect microcapsule walls. After the initial period, a zero-order release rate is observed during which the drug inside the capsule is maintained at a fixed concentration, i.e., at its solubility limit.

Discussion

The encapsulation of the oil-in-water emulsion is signifi-cant since this approach permits encapsulation of hydrophobic steroids by the nonaqueous phase-separation method. Prior to this, the nonaqueous phase-separation method had been limited to hydrophilic materials.

The in vitro release of progesterone was significantly slower than that observed in the single in vivo study. This difference in release rates is not surprising in view of the highly lipo-philic milieu which exists in the rabbit uterus. If some lipo-philic substances penetrate the capsule wall, the solubility and membrane transport rate for progesterone should be increased.

The penetration of lipophilic materials through the capsule membrane should not prevent the realization of a zero-order release rate since the primary requirement governing zero-order release from a reservoir device is the maintenance of saturation concentrations within the device. This was accomplished in these studies since the solubility of progesterone or estrone is much lower in an aqueous environment (9 µg/ml for progesterone and 30 µg/ml for estrone) (8) than the total amount of steroid encap-sulated. Theoretically, we could maintain the saturated concen-tration level within the capsule until the drug is almost com-pletely voided. Thus, in a reservoir device such as a microcap-sule, a zero-order release rate should be feasible but other parameters may affect the release rate. These parameters might include the total number and size distribution of the microcap-sule, the microcapsule wall thickness, the type of polymer used for the microcapsule membrane, the rate of drug solubilization within the microcapsule, and the in vivo rate of drug removed from the drug interface area surrounding the microcapsule.

Table V was constructed to determine if the preliminary release rates from cellulose acetate butyrate microcapsules might be satisfactory for use as a transcervical drug delivery device. This table depicts release rates required of microcapsules and assumes different percentages of transcervical migration and possible effective localized drug dosages. In addition, we have examined three different drug delivery rates which might be required at a localized site.

The amount of drug which will be required at a localized site of action is relatively unknown. However, estimates of the

TABLE V.   RELEASE RATES REQUIRED OF MICROCAPSULES WHEN COMPARING DIFFERENT PERCENTAGES
OF TRANSCERVICAL MIGRATION AND EFFECTIVE LOCALIZED DRUG DOSAGES

Capsule Diam., μ	Capsules Placed in Vagina, g	Assumed Transcervical Migration, percent	Volume of Capsules Migrating, ml	Weight of Capsules Migrating, mg	Number of Capsules Migrating	Assumed Drug Delivery Rate Required at Localized Site, μg/day	Release Rate Required from Migrating Capsules, μg/day
50	10	1.0	0.09	100	1,386,962	50	50
150	10	1.0	0.09	100	51,282	50	50
250	10	1.0	0.09	100	11,099	50	50
150	10	1.0	0.09	100	51,282	10	10
		3.0	0.27	300	153,840	10	3.3
		5.0	0.45	500	256,410	10	2.0
150	10	0.25	0.02	25	12,820	1	4.0
		0.50	0.04	50	25,641	1	2.0
		1.00	0.09	100	51,282	1	1.0

amount of progesterone required per day to prevent conception
indicate that only micrograms or even nanograms of a more potent
drug might be sufficient. Roland (9) has shown that 75 µg of
Norgestral orally administered per day to humans effectively prevented pregnancy by altering the cervical mucosa, thus preventing sperm migration into the uterine cavity. In addition,
Silastic rubber implants attached to a modified Lippes intrauterine loop released 31 µg progesterone/mm capsule/day in
studies conducted by Lifchez and Scommegna (3). At a recent
symposium, an IUD developed by the Alza Corporation was described
which released 50 µg progesterone/day (10).

The first three capsule diameters in Table V would require
a release rate of 50 µg/day/100 mg of capsules. At the 10 µg/
day level, the rate of release required would be 10 µg/100 mg for
1 percent migration, 3.3 µg/100 mg if there was 3 percent migration, or 2 µg/100 mg if 5 percent migration occurred. Even
smaller release rates would be required if only 1 µg/day were
required at a localized site.

In our single in vivo study, we obtained a progesterone
release rate of about 4 µg/day/100 mg of capsules and at this
release rate, we would need approximately 3 percent transcervical migration if 10 µg/day would suffice as an effective localized dosage. An important point to be brought out is that if a
drug were 10 times more effective than progesterone, the release
rates seen in these studies might be adequate if the assumed
transcervical migration occurred.

Thus, from these estimations, a self-administered delivery
system based upon microcapsules and transcervical migration
appears feasible if one considers the small amount of drug which
might be needed at a localized site.

Literature Cited

(1) Mishell, D. R. and Lunkin, M. E., Fertil. & Steril., (1970),
     21, 99.
(2) Scommegna, A., et al., Fertil. & Steril., (1970), 21, 201.
(3) Lifchez, A. S. and Scommegna, A., Fertil. & Steril., (1970),
     21, 426.
(4) Chang, C. C. and Kincl, F. A., Steroids, (1968), 12, 689.
(5) Chang, C. C. and Kincl, F. A., Fertil. & Steril., (1970),
     21, 134.
(6) Egli, G. E. and Newton, M., Fertil. & Steril., (1961), 12,
     151.
(7) deBoer, D. H., J. Reprod. Fert., (1972), 28, 295.
(8) Kabasakalian, P., J. Pharm. Sci., (1966), 55 (6), 642.
(9) Roland, M., Fertil. & Steril., (1970), 21 (3), 211.
(10) Symposium on Drug Therapy and Novel Delivery Systems -
     Challenges and Responses (1974), Battelle Seattle Research
     Center, Seattle, Washington.

13

Controlled Release of Quinidine Sulfate Microcapsules

GEORGE R. SOMERVILLE, JOHN T. GOODWIN, and DONALD E. JOHNSON

Southwest Research Institute, San Antonio, Tex. 78284

Introduction

Controlled release formulations are being utilized in several types of products, including pharmaceuticals, veterinary medical products, pesticides, fertilizers, flavors, aromas and corrosion inhibitors. This paper describes a study to develop a controlled release formulation for quinidine sulfate, a pharmaceutical product which is used primarily in the treatment of cardiac arrhythmia.

In general, the objective of developing the controlled release drug formulation is to be able to deliver the drug at the optimum level over a period of time ranging up to 12 hours or sometimes longer. This does not necessarily mean a completely flat response curve, but the desired response may have an initially elevated level followed by a sufficiently extended response until the next dose is administered.

Experimental

Microencapsulation. Quinidine sulfate was microencapsulated by the multiorifice centrifugal extrusion process. The shell formulation is a liquid during the encapsulation and is hardened after the microcapsule is formed. Any of several types of shell formulations may be utilized, depending upon the material to be encapsulated and the desired properties of the end product. These types include hot melts, solutions and latexes. Hardening mechanisms include cooling--in the case of hot melts--, chemical reaction in an appropriate hardening bath, and solvent extraction or evaporation. Combinations of these general mechanisms may be used in some instances. From an operational standpoint, hot melt systems are the simplest to use, as there is no need for solvent recovery, chemical makeup or capsule drying.

Figure 1 is a schematic representation of the device used in the multiorifice centrifugal extrusion process. The liquid phase to be encapsulated enters the rotating head through the inner of two concentric feed tubes, passing through a seal arrangement to a central chamber. It then passes through tubes which radiate outward from the central chamber and penetrate orifices located about the periphery of the rotating head.

The liquid shell material enters the outer of the two concentric feed tubes, passing through a seal arrangement into the outer chamber of the head. The shell material is then extruded through the annuli created by these sets of tubes and orifices to form fluid sheaths about the fluid "rods" of core material which are discharged from the tubes. Nodes begin to form on these compound fluid "rods", and at some point beyond the periphery of the rotating head, the nodes become more pronounced and individual fluid capsules are formed. Hot melt capsules are cooled in flight, and the resultant capsules are collected. Chemically hardened shells and those from which solvent is extracted are typically caught in a liquid hardening medium. Those systems involving solvent evaporation are generally hardened in flight.

In this encapsulation process, the principal factors influencing capsule size are feed rate, rotational speed and--to a lesser extent--orifice size. Increased feed rate tends to increase the capsule size, whereas increased rotational speed decreases the size. In preparing the quinidine sulfate formulations in this study, the operating parameters were adjusted so as to produce microcapsules in the size range of 420-841 microns.

Capsule formation in the multiorifice centrifugal extrusion process is quite rapid. In a typical operation producing 350-micron capsules, a production rate in excess of 300,000 capsules per second per orifice has been observed. This process has been taken beyond bench-scale, and a pilot plant is in operation with a demonstrated capacity in excess of 90,000 pounds per month.

In the encapsulation of quinidine sulfate, it was necessary to slurry the finely divided drug in a liquid so that it could be pumped and extruded. Several materials were investigated as slurry vehicles, including molten hydrogenated triglycerides, mono-diglycerides and several types of natural and synthetic waxes. The shell components comprised similar molten

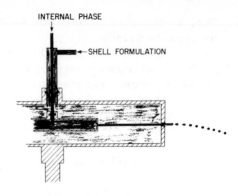

*Figure 1. Multiorifice centrifugal extru-
sion head*

materials, except that no mono-diglycerides were used. Shell
and core hardening, of course, is accomplished by cooling the
capsules as they are projected from the rotating head. Thus,
the resultant product is a continuous shell enclosing a dispersion
of quinidine sulfate particles in a solid matrix.

Analytical Methods. Gas-liquid chromatography was used
for assay purposes, for analysis of in vivo samples, and for
analysis of in vitro samples involving simulated gastric and
intestinal fluids.

The blood samples of the in vivo tests were analyzed by
centrifuging the whole blood and separating the plasma. The
plasma was treated with sodium hydroxide, extracted with chloroform and evaporated to dryness under nitrogen. The dried
samples were reconstituted with chloroform containing an internal standard of cholesterol acetate and analyzed by gas
chromatography with a flame ionization detector. Similar work-
up procedures were used in the in vitro analyses and in the
microcapsule assays. The extraction efficiency of this method
was found to be 88. 6% with a standard deviation of 4. 2.

Standard response curves were developed using the internal
standard of cholesterol acetate spiked with varying amounts of
quinidine and were plotted as quinidine concentration versus the
ratio of the quinidine and cholesterol acetate peak areas. The
quinidine concentrations of unknowns were then converted to
equivalent quinidine sulfate.

Bioavailability Study. Fifteen normal, healthy subjects
were used in the study. Those subjects were selected which had
no history of any physiological problems which would cause concern in administration of quinidine sulfate. In addition, each

subject was given a thorough examination including medical
history, physical examination, blood count and electrocardio-
gram. Each individual bioavailability study involved five individuals. The participants were randomly selected from the total
pool of fifteen subjects. Dosages of 300 mg of both unsustained
and sustained release formulations were orally administered,
and blood samples were taken at 1-, 2-, 4-, 6-, 8- and 12-hour
intervals.

Results and Discussion

Table I presents the compositions of some of the many
formulations which were prepared and evaluated during this
study. It was discovered in the early stages that, with the types
of coating materials under investigation, the slurry vehicles for
the quinidine sulfate affected the release rate to a greater degree
than did the shell components. Other considerations, particularly storage stability, led to changes in the shell components as
the investigation progressed.

TABLE I.
FORMULATIONS OF MICROENCAPSULATED
QUINIDINE SULFATE (Core Material)

| Ingredient | Control | Formulation (parts) | | | | |
		1	2	3	4	5
Quinidine Sulfate	100	59	59	59	59	59
Beeswax		15		10		
Hydrogenated Triglycerides		14	10	10		
Mono-Diglycerides		12	31	21	1	10
Paraffin Wax					40	31
Payload (%)	100	53	53	53	53	53

Note: Formulations 1-3 had a shell of 65 parts beeswax and 35
parts hydrogenated triglycerides. Formulations 4 and 5
had shells of paraffin wax.

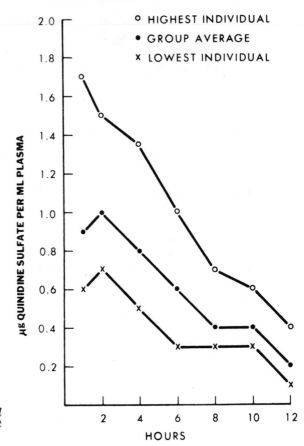

Figure 2.   In vivo blood level variations within subject groups—quinidine sulfate

Figure 2 shows the in vivo results for unencapsulated quinidine sulfate. As indicated, the dark circles represent the group average, and the open circles and crosses represent the results for the highest and lowest individual assays within the group. A threefold difference between extreme values is indicated.

Figure 3 shows corresponding results for one of the slower releasing microencapsulated formulations. The blood levels were initially lower but after six hours were substantially higher than for the uncoated quinidine sulfate; i. e. , about 30% higher at six hours and twice as high at twelve hours.

Comparisons between a relatively slow release formulation, a relatively fast but sustained release formulation and the uncoated drug are presented in Figure 4.

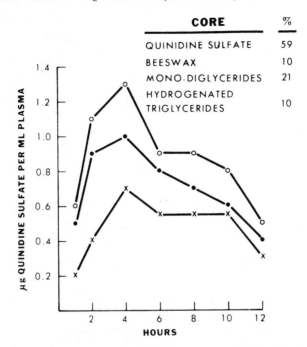

CORE	%
QUINIDINE SULFATE	59
BEESWAX	10
MONO-DIGLYCERIDES	21
HYDROGENATED TRIGLYCERIDES	10

Figure 3. In vivo blood level variations within subject groups—formulation (3)

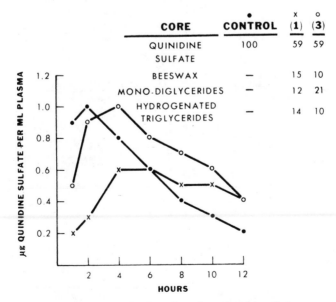

CORE	CONTROL ●	X (1)	o (3)
QUINIDINE SULFATE	100	59	59
BEESWAX	—	15	10
MONO-DIGLYCERIDES	—	12	21
HYDROGENATED TRIGLYCERIDES	—	14	10

Figure 4. In vivo blood levels with various formulations

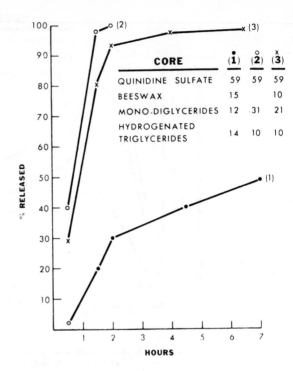

CORE	(1)	(2)	(3)
QUINIDINE SULFATE	59	59	59
BEESWAX	15		10
MONO-DIGLYCERIDES	12	31	21
HYDROGENATED TRIGLYCERIDES	14	10	10

Figure 5. Percent release after storage at ambient conditions for two months in vitro

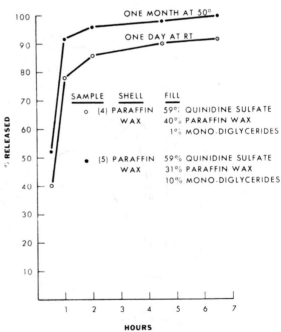

SAMPLE	SHELL	FILL
○ (4)	PARAFFIN WAX	59% QUINIDINE SULFATE 40% PARAFFIN WAX 1% MONO-DIGLYCERIDES
● (5)	PARAFFIN WAX	59% QUINIDINE SULFATE 31% PARAFFIN WAX 10% MONO-DIGLYCERIDES

Figure 6. Percent release after storage in vitro

The in vitro availability of three separate formulations after aging for two months at ambient conditions is shown in Figure 5. Each of these formulations released most of the quinidine sulfate when tested within a day or two after preparation. It is noted that the formulation containing the highest level·of beeswax and the lowest level of mono-diglycerides released the drug quite slowly in this in vitro test.   All three capsules had the same shell formulation, i. e. 65% beeswax and 35% hydrogenated triglycerides, and contained the same amount of drug. Thus, aging had a pronounced effect on the high beeswax formulation.

Figure 6 shows the stability of other formulations in which the beeswax and hydrogenated triglycerides were replaced with paraffin wax, both in the core and in the shell. Although not directly comparable because of differences in aging time and temperature, the formulation containing the greater concentration of mono-diglycerides in the core exhibits greater in vitro availability--and stability--on aging.

Conclusions

This study has indicated that it is possible to prepare controlled release formulations of quinidine sulfate by means of microencapsulation. Shell materials such as waxes and hydrogenated triglycerides were used successfully. The composition of the quinidine sulfate slurry vehicle, which ends up as the core matrix, had a large influence on the release rate of the drug. The presence and proportion of mono-diglycerides in the core had a major effect on the release rate.

It was found that release patterns of the formulations containing beeswax and hydrogenated triglycerides changed significantly during aging. The substitution of paraffin wax in the formulations improved the stability markedly.

Acknowledgment

Southwest Research Institute gratefully acknowledges financial support of Beecham Laboratories in the conduct of the study reported herein.

14

Characterization of Microcapsules Containing Naltrexone or Naltrexone Pamoate

CURT THIES

Department of Chemical Engineering, Washington University, St. Louis, Mo. 63130

Introduction

The concept of long-acting injectable drug formulations has intrigued pharmaceutical scientists for some time. One way to prepare the desired formulations is to synthesize drug-filled microcapsules that can be injected. The coating material used to form such capsules must not only provide controlled drug release, but also be biocompatible and bioabsorbable. These requirements severely restrict the number of acceptable coating materials. However, one promising material is dl-poly(lactic acid)(dl-PLA). Initial results of efforts to develop injectable microcapsules with dl-PLA as the coating material focused on cyclazocine, a narcotic antagonist (1). More recent work has focused upon the use of dl-PLA to encapsulate naltrexone free base (NFB), also a narcotic antagonist, and naltrexone pamoate (NP), the pamoate salt of naltrexone free base. This paper describes some of the properties of selected NFB and NP microcapsule samples.

Experimental

Microcapsules containing NFB or NP were prepared with dl-poly(lactic acid) supplied by Dr. Donald Wise of Dynatech R/D Co., Cambridge, Mass. The capsules contained 33 wt. % NFB or 50 wt.% NP. Several capsule fractions were isolated from each capsule batch by sieving. For each capsule fraction, the smaller number given represents the size of the rectangular screen opening which retained the microcapsule, whereas the larger number represents the size of the rectangular screen opening through which the capsules passed.

In vitro release properties of the capsules were evaluated at 37°C in pH 7.4 phosphate buffer. All evaluations were carried out in a rotating bottle apparatus (40 rpm) manufactured by Ernest Menold, Lester, Pa. The test samples consisted of 15 mg of capsules suspended in 75 ml of buffer. Concentration of

naltrexone in the extracting solution was established spectrophotometrically by using the 282 nm band characteristic of
naltrexone.

Evaluation of microcapsules containing NP was complicated
by non-stoichiometric diffusion of naltrexone and pamoic acid
from such capsules. Pamoic acid has an absorbance maximum at
288 nm. NP release curves based on changes in magnitude of this
peak were constructed. However, NP capsules which released their
payload over a prolonged period did not release naltrexone free
base and pamoic acid in a 1:1 molecular ratio. For this reason,
extracts from such NP capsules were acidified to pH 2.0 with HCl.
This precipitated nearly all of the pamoic acid, so the concentration of naltrexone left in solution could be established
from its absorption maximum at 282 nm. Controls containing only
pamoic acid were treated similarly in order to determine the
amount of pamoic acid remaining in solution at pH 2.0. This contribution to the 282 nm maximum of naltrexone was then sub-
tracted from all actual test runs in order to give corrected
values of the amount of naltrexone released by the capsules.
Release data have been plotted as mg NFB or mg NP released by 15
mg capsules as a function of extraction time.

Results and Discussion
_____

Figures 1 and 2 contain in vitro release data for capsules
isolated from representative NFB and NP encapsulation runs.
Figure 1 shows that the NFB capsules being evaluated release
~50% of their payload within the first few hours of extraction;
the remaining NFB is leached out over a three week period. After
the first surge of NFB release, NFB extraction from the capsules
is essentially zero order.

The relatively large amount of NFB released by the capsules
initially is attributed to rapid and essentially complete release of NFB from capsules that have gross defects in their
walls. The solubility of NFB in pH 7.4 buffer at 37°C is
~450 mg/100 ml. This does not suffice to classify NFB as a
highly water-soluble drug. Nevertheless, the solubility is
sufficiently great to ensure rapid and complete removal of NFB
from defective <106µ capsules. For this NFB capsule sample,
nearly 50% of the capsules appear to be defective.

Why the coatings of certain NFB capsules contain gross defects is unresolved at the moment. However, scanning electron
micrographs of such capsule surfaces reveal that many have
macroscopic craters and pores. Although much of a capsule surface may be free of these gross defects, they presumably are the
points at which drug is transferred rapidly from defective
capsules to the extracting medium. Not all capsules contain
such defects. If the surfaces of a sufficiently large number of
capsules are examined, many capsules free of defects are found.

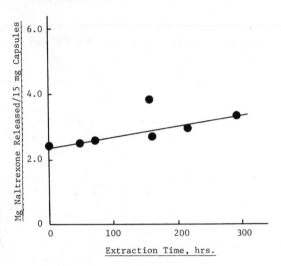

Figure 1. Extraction of naltrexone-free base at 37°C and pH 7.4 from < 106-μ dl-poly(lactic acid) capsules containing initially 33 wt % drug

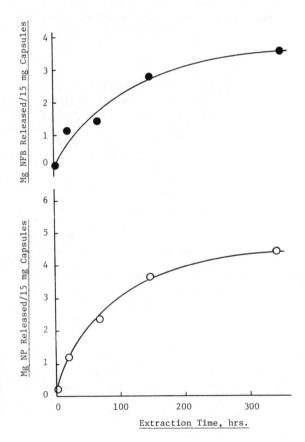

Figure 2. Extraction of naltrexone-free base and apparent extraction of naltrexone pamoate at 37°C and pH 7.4 from 106–180-μ dl-poly(lactic acid) capsules containing initially 50 wt % drug

This is particularly true of NP capsules. Figure 3 is a scanning electron micrograph of such a capsule containing 50 wt. % NP. At present, efforts are being made to produce NFB capsules that appear as free of defects as this NP capsule.

Significantly, the capsules used to obtain the release data in Figure 1 were <106µ in diameter. Such capsules are sufficiently small to pass freely through a 20 gauge needle. Another important practical consideration is that the total

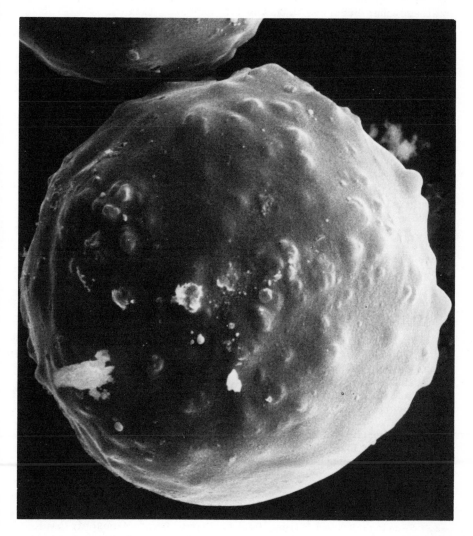

Figure 3.   Scanning electron micrograph of the surface of a 106–108-µ capsule containing 50 wt % naltrexone pamoate

weight of <106µ capsules isolated represents 64% of the total theoretical yield of capsules. That is, small capsules suitable for injection have been synthesized in relatively high yield.

Because the solubility of NP in phosphate buffer is markedly lower than that of NFB, it was hypothesized that the reduction in solubility should reduce the driving force for drug extraction from NP microcapsules thereby enhancing in vitro lifetime. The release data in Figure 2 indicate that this has happened. The NP capsules do not experience the immediate large burst of drug release that occurred with the NFB capsules (Figure 1). After 500 hrs. of extraction, the NP capsules release significantly less drug than the theoretical payload of 7.5 mg NP or 4.5 mg NFB per 15 mg capsules. The release curves shown appear to level off after 300 to 500 hrs. of extraction. However, longer extractions of similar NP capsules have been carried out and results obtained indicate that slow release of NFB continues until the theoretical NFB payload of the NP capsules is reached (2). In contrast, the amount of pamoic acid released does not increase significantly. A substantial fraction of the pamoic acid portion of NP appears to be effectively trapped within the capsule. Thus, the pamoic acid and NFB portions of NP do not diffuse from the capsules in a 1:1 stoichiometric ratio. Analyses based on the 288 nm band characteristic of pamoic acid give misleading results, and the amount of NFB released by the capsules must be monitored directly.

From Figures 1 and 2 it is clear that neither of the two capsule samples being evaluated releases drug at a constant or zero order rate over the entire time the capsules are extracted in vitro. The initial rate of drug release always is higher than the rate observed in the latter stages of the capsule extraction process. Nevertheless, it is becoming apparent that as the poly(lactic acid) encapsulation technology develops, capsules with fewer macroscopic coating defects are being isolated. Although the release of drug from such capsules is not zero order, the better the capsules become, the closer their release behavior approaches the desired zero order goal. Current capsules are capable of providing multi-week drug release in vivo (2); how much additional improvement in capsule quality can be achieved remains to be seen.

Acknowledgements: This work was sponsored by the National Institute on Drug Abuse, Contract No. HSM-42-73-265. The technical assistance of G. Lapka is gratefully appreciated.

Literature Cited

1. Cicero, T., Mason, N., and Thies, C, J. Pharm. Sci., In press
2. Reuning, R. and Thies, C., J. Pharm. Sci., Manuscript in preparation

Effect of Cross-Linking Agents on the Release of Sodium Pentobarbital from Nylon Microcapsules

M. D. DeGENNARO
College of Pharmacy and Allied Health Professions, Northeast Louisiana University, Monroe, La. 71201

B. B. THOMPSON
School of Pharmacy, University of Georgia, Athens, Ga. 30602

L. A. LUZZI
School of Pharmacy, West Virginia University, Morgantown, W.Va. 26506

The process of microencapsulation is currently one of the most extensively investigated means for the storage, protection, taste-masking, and prolongation of release for many pharmaceuticals. This is attested to by the rapid accumulation of scientific articles and patents in the literature in this and other countries. An extensive listing of pharmaceuticals which have been encapsulated has been published by Bakan and Sloan (1). Methods available for encapsulation are numerous and an overview of many of them may be found in a review of the subject by Ranney (2). Herbig (3) has enumerated some of the many materials which may be used as encapsulating membranes or as an adjunct to the encapsulating agent.

Microencapsulation is not a new process. In preparing "carbonless carbon paper," Green and Schleicher (4, 5) made use of the first patented application of microencapsulation. In that process, oil soluble dyes were encapsulated in a gelatin-acacia membrane by the use of complex coacervation (6). Luzzi and Gerraughty (7-9) investigated some of the variables involved in the coacervation of oils and solids and in addition Nixon et al. (10, 11) have extensively studied the preparation and release of gelatin coacervate microcapsules.

It is evident from the literature that most of the published material on microencapsulation pertains mainly to applications of the coacervate system and that very little has been reported, especially using nylon as the encapsulating material for pharmaceuticals. Chang et al. (12) prepared semipermeable collodion and nylon microcapsules containing enzymes which can be used to treat enzyme deficiencies and also reported the use of semipermeable microcapsules in an extracorporeal shunt system (13, 14). Kondo et al. (15-18) prepared microcapsules via interfacial polymerization using a variety of encapsulating membranes. The same authors also reported some of the characteristics of the formed microcapsules.

The only reference to the microencapsulation of a pharmaceutical agent, using a nylon membrane as the encapsulating material, has apparently been made by Luzzi et al. (19). Due to the potential which exists for the encapsulation of pharmaceuticals via interfacial polymerization, this work was undertaken to determine what effect the incorporation of cross-linking agents into the membrane might have upon the release of sodium pentobarbital from nylon 6-10 microcapsules.

Experimental

Materials. The materials used in this study were sodium pentobarbital,[1] carbon tetrachloride[2] (reagent grade), 1,6-hexanediamine[3] (Eastman grade), sebacyl chloride[3] (Eastman grade), diethylenetriamine[4] (95%), triethylenetetramine[4] (technical grade), and Glycerin U.S.P.[5] All materials were used as supplied by the manufacturers without further purification.

Preparation of Drug-Containing Microcapsules. The method utilized for the preparation of the nylon microcapsules containing sodium pentobarbital in this experimentation was a modification of the methods previously reported by Chang et al. (12) and by Luzzi et al. (19). The modified method consisted of adding 100 ml. of an aqueous solution containing the drug to be encapsulated, 1,6-hexanediamine and glycerin to 500 ml. of carbon tetrachloride contained in a 2000 ml. beaker. The mixture was then stirred at a speed setting of 60 using a counter-rotating stirrer[6] for 15 seconds to form a water-in-oil emulsion. Then, 500 ml. of the same organic solvent containing sebacyl chloride was added and the stirring was continued at

---

[1]Abbott Laboratories, N. Chicago, Ill.

[2]J. T. Baker Chemical Co., Phillipsburg, N.J.

[3]Eastman Kodak Co., Rochester, N.Y.

[4]Aldrich Chemical Co., Milwaukee, Wis.

[5]Fisher Scientific Co., Fairlawn, N.J.

[6]Model L2994, Brookfield Engineering Laboratories, Stoughton, Mass.

the stirrer's maximum speed for a total of 10 minutes. The microcapsules thus formed were collected by filtration.

While still damp, the filtered microcapsules were passed through a standard 12 mesh sieve. The microcapsules were then placed in an oven at 37° for 10-12 hours and were then placed in a vacuum desiccator over phosphorous pentoxide for an additional 10-12 hours. This procedure insured removal of residual solvent and moisture.

Effect of Cross-Linking Agents. The effect of the cross-linking agents used in this study, diethylenetriamine and triethylenetetramine, on the release of core material was determined by progressively incorporating them into the aqueous phase in exchange for the 1, 6-hexanediamine. This was done on both active site and molar bases. When the active sites were the criteria, a given quantity of 1, 6-hexanediamine was removed and replaced with two-thirds the number of moles of diethylenetriamine and one-half the number of moles of triethylenetetramine.

Assay Procedure. Ultraviolet spectra for sample solutions of sodium pentobarbital in 0. 1N ammonium hydroxide were recorded using a Perkin-Elmer recording spectrophotometer[7] with 0. 1N ammonium hydroxide solution as a blank. The wavelength of maximum absorbance was found at 240 nm, and all measurements were made at this wavelength while employing appropriate blanks. Samples of empty nylon microcapsules treated in the same manner failed to exhibit absorbance at 240 nm.

Absorbances of the solutions were obtained using a Beckman DU spectrophotometer.[8] These data were then used to prepare a Beer's law plot which was used for comparison to determine the amount of sodium pentobarbital released from the microcapsules.

Assay Procedure for Total Sodium Pentobarbital Content of Microcapsules. Triplicate samples of approximately 100 mg. of the microcapsules were accurately weighed and placed in a 150 ml. homogenizing flask containing 50 ml. of 0. 1N ammonium hydroxide solution. The samples were then completely

---

[7]Model 202, The Perkin-Elmer Corp., Norwalk, Conn.

[8]Model DU-2, Beckman Instrument Inc., Fullerton, Calif.

Table I. Cross-Linking Replacements Carried Out On An
          Active Site Basis[*]

Percent Diamine Replaced	0	6	9	12
Moles of Diamine Used	0.032	0.031	0.03	0.029
Moles of Diethyl- enetriamine Used	0	0.0012	0.0019	0.0025
Moles of Triethyl- enetetramine Used	0		0.0015	

[*]Diethylenetriamine and triethylenetriamine replacements
were not carried out simultaneously.

15	18	24	60	90	100
0.028	0.027	0.025	0.013	0.0032	0
0.0032	0.0038	0.0051	0.013	0.02	0.022
		0.0039	0.0097	0.015	0.016

ruptured using a Virtis blender[9] at its maximum speed. In
each case, two samples were blended for 10 minutes and complete rupture was assured by blending the third for 15 minutes
with no observed increase in drug content. Complete collection
from the flask assembly was insured by washing with 50 ml. of
0.1N ammonium hydroxide solution. Aliquots were taken and
diluted to an appropriate volume for spectrophotometric assay.

In-Vitro Dissolution Studies.   Dissolution was followed by
examining triplicate samples containing approximately 30 mg.
of drug using the flask method as previously described (20).   In
each case, microcapsules were placed on the surface of
300 ml. of 0.1N hydrochloric acid in a 500 ml. round bottom
flask the temperature of which had been brought to equilibrium
at $37 \pm 0.5^{\circ}$.
     The mixture was stirred at 50 r.p.m. and samples were
withdrawn at appropriate time intervals using a pipet fitted
with a cotton plug. A constant volume of dissolution medium
was maintained by the addition of an equal volume of medium
after each 2 ml. sample withdrawal. In each case, the cotton
plug which had been used as a filter, was added to the dissolution mixture. Appropriate dilutions were made, ultraviolet
absorbances recorded, and comparisons to a Beer's law plot
were made.

Results and Discussion

     Preliminary investigations showed that stable micro-
capsules could be prepared using an aqueous phase consisting
of 10% sodium pentobarbital, 4.5% 1,6-hexanediamine, and 1%
glycerin. After the initial emulsification period, 500 ml. of
carbon tetrachloride containing 3.38% sebacyl chloride was
added to produce capsule formation. The effect of the cross-
linking agents was determined by replacing preselected portions of 1,6-hexanediamine with the two cross-linking agents
on both an active site and molar basis. Table I shows the
quantities of cross-linking agents, diethylenetriamine and triethylenetetramine, on an active site basis used to replace the
indicated percentages of 1,6-hexanediamine. Table II shows
the replacements made using diethylenetriamine on a molar
basis. The amount of sebacyl chloride used was held constant

---

[9]Model 45, Virtis Research Equipment, Gardner, N.Y.

Table II.   Cross-Linking Replacements Carried Out On a Molar Basis

Percent Diamine Replaced	6	9	12	15	18
Moles of Diamine Used	0.031	0.03	0.029	0.028	0.027
Moles of Diethylene-triamine Used	0.0019	0.0029	0.0038	0.0048	0.0058

in all cases.

Figure 1 is a plot of percent sodium pentobarbital released at selected times for the replacement of 1,6-hexanediamine with the indicated quantities of diethylenetriamine on an active site basis. This figure shows that when diethylenetriamine was used to replace the diamine, the percent sodium pentobarbital released at all sampling intervals showed an irregularly increased release with increasing amounts of diethylenetriamine.

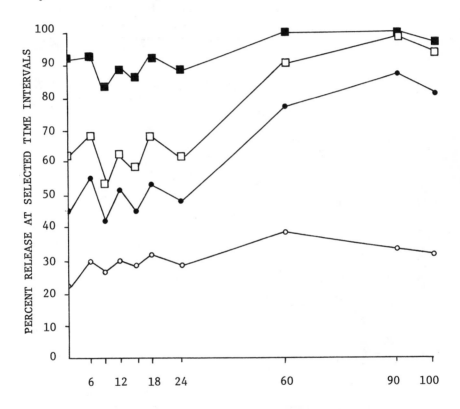

PERCENT DIAMINE REPLACED WITH DIETHYLENETRIAMINE – ACTIVE SITE BASIS

Figure 1. Percent sodium pentobarbital released at selected time intervals vs. diamine replacements with diethylenetriamine on an active site basis. Each value represents the average of at least three determinations on a minimum of two, and in most cases three or four, batches of microcapsules prepared at different times.
○ *5 min;* ● *20 min;* □ *40 min;* ■ *120 min.*

It may be seen from Figure 2 that there was little significant change in the amount of sodium pentobarbital released when between 6 and 24% of the diamine were replaced. However, when 60-100% replacements were carried out, the amount of drug released became significantly greater.

Figure 3 indicates that when triethylenetetramine was used to replace the diamine on an active site basis, the trend was also an increased release with increasing amounts of cross-linking agent. The one exception was at the 9% replacement level. This level of replacement yielded only slightly slower release than did that which had no cross-linking agent.

From Figure 4 it may be seen that when diethylenetria-

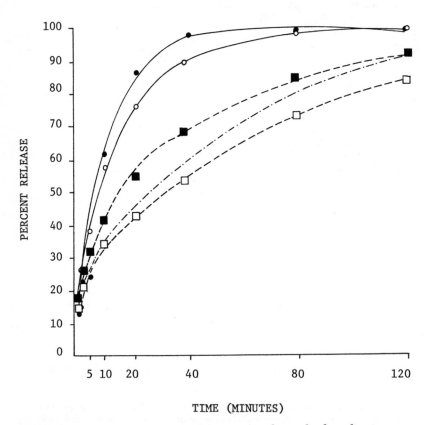

TIME (MINUTES)

Figure 2. Extremes of the two release ranges observed when diamine was replaced with diethylenetriamine on an active site basis. Each value represents the average of at least three determinations on a minimum of two, and in most cases three or four, batches of microcapsules prepared at different times. — higher limits: ● 90% replaced, ○ 60% replaced; – – – – lower limits: ■ 6% replaced, □ 9% replaced; – · – 0% cross-linking.

mine was used to replace 1,6-hexanediamine on a molar basis, there was a general trend towards faster release rates as the amount of cross-linking agent was increased. Here again, as when replacements were carried out on an active site basis, the increase in release was not always directly related to the percentage of diamine replaced by diethylenetriamine.

Since nylon 6-10 is a linear polymer, it was desired to add cross-linking agents to the aqueous phase in order to produce a non-linear polymer, and it was thought that the addition of cross-linking agents would have a profound effect upon both the porosity and strength of the nylon membrane. However, it appears that the addition of cross-linking agents is not a suit-

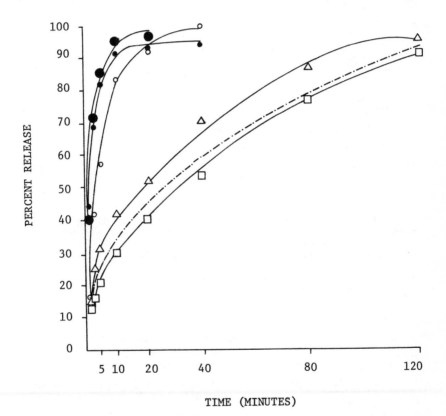

TIME (MINUTES)

Figure 3. Percent sodium pentobarbital released when diamine was replaced with triethylenetetramine on an active site basis. Each value represents the average of at least three determinations on at least two, and in some cases three or four, batches of microcapsules prepared at different times. □ *9%;* △ *24%;* ○ *60%;* ● *90%;* ● *100%;* − · − *0% cross-linking.*

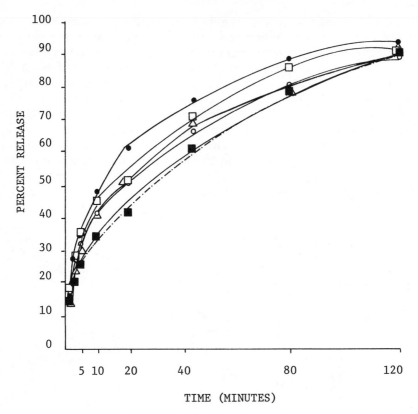

Figure 4. Percent sodium pentobarbital released when diamine was replaced with diethylenetriamine on molar basis. Each value represents the average of at least three determinations on at least two, and in most cases three or four, batches of microcapsules prepared at different times. ■ *6%;* □ *9%;* ○ *12%;* △ *15%;* ● *18%; – · – 0% cross-linking.*

able means for prolonging drug release from nylon 6-10 microcapsules. This may be due to any one of a combination of factors.

Kondo (18) revealed that microcapsules prepared using different monomer combinations were of different sizes. In the present report, the addition of diethylenetriamine and triethylenetetramine to the aqueous phase could possibly have caused changes in the release rates by bringing about changes in porosity or in membrane thickness. Changes in both of these factors may have been due to the different polymerization characteristics of each combination of monomers.

The addition of cross-linking agents to the aqueous phase also produces other changes which are not as obvious. Small additions of cross-linking agents to the aqueous phase produce changes in reactant concentrations as well as in the ratio of reactants to each other, and since the diamine concentration would be reduced, the cross-linking agents also serve as diluting agents. It has been reported (21) that while reactant concentrations determine membrane thickness, there exists an optimum proportion of diamine to acid halide for each pair of reactants in a given system (16, 22). Each addition of cross-linking agent produces new ratios of reactants for which optimum concentrations must be determined. Changes in the ratio of reactants may produce an excess or may alter the availability of the amines in such a way that products with rapid release rates are produced.

The most plausible rationale which seems to explain the more rapid release rates observed in each case where diamine was replaced by diethylenetriamine or triethyltenetetramine involves the individual diffusion rate of the amines and the effects of the presence of diethylenetriamine and triethylenetetramine on the diffusion rate of the diamine. Although an orientation argument would be plausible, it would appear that on a functional group basis, the diamine would be more freely soluble in nonaqueous systems than either of the cross-linking agents investigated (23). It follows that diffusion into the nonaqueous phase for a mixture of these amines would allow a gradation of transfer, thus limiting the concentration of amine available for "nylon" formation at, or near, an aqueous/nonaqueous interface. This rationale is strengthened if there is a competition for available water molecules among the mixture of amines, the drug, and the glycerin, all of which are found in the aqueous phase.

The result may be that a lower molecular weight nylon is initially formed by the early migration of the diamine. This is followed by the formation of higher molecular weight polymer brought about by the subsequent diffusion of the diethylenetriamine or triethylenetetramine. The higher molecular weight polymer may be less compact due to several factors including a possible predisposition to a combination of vertical and tangential polymer backbones.

It is evident that the effects produced by the addition of cross-linking agents show definite trends towards increased rates of release. However, these trends are produced on an irregular basis, regardless of whether the cross-linking agent is added on an active site or molar basis. It is apparent that the addition of cross-linking agents alters several factors, one or more of which might account for the changes in release rates observed. In order to determine which of these factors is primarily responsible for the observed results, additional studies must be carried out.

Conclusions

The objective of this study was to determine the effect that the addition of cross-linking agents to the aqueous phase during microcapsule formation via interfacial polymerization might have upon the release of core material from the microcapsules. In this study, two cross-linking agents, diethylenetriamine and triethylenetetramine, were investigated. Substitution of the cross-linking agents was carried out on an active site as well as molar basis.

The conclusions resulting from this investigation are:

1. The progressive addition of diethylenetriamine or triethylenetetramine to the aqueous phase as cross-linking agents, on an active site basis, produced microcapsules having increased rates of release. The increase observed followed no discernible pattern.

2. The addition of diethylenetriamine to the aqueous phase, on a molar basis, also produced microcapsules with increased release rates as more diethylenetriamine was added. Again, the increase followed no discernible pattern.

3. Progressive addition of cross-linking agents into the aqueous phase probably produced encapsulating shells with increased porosity.

Literature Cited

1. Bakan, J. A. and Sloan, F. D., Drug and Cosmetic Ind., (1972), 110, p. 34.
2. Ranney, M. W., "Microencapsulation Technology," Noyer Development Corp., Park Ridge, 1969.
3. Herbig, J. A., "Encyclopedia of Chemical Technology," 2nd ed., vol. 13, p. 441, Interscience, New York, 1967.
4. Green, B. K. and Schleicher, L., U.S. Pat. 2,730,456 (1956).
5. Green, B. K. and Schleicher, L., U.S. Pat. 2,730,457 (1956).
6. Bungenberg de Jong, H. G., "Colloid Science," Ed. by H. R. Kruyt, Vol. II, Elsevier, New York, 1949.
7. Luzzi, L. A. and Gerraughty, R. J., J. Pharm. Sci., (1964), 53, 429.
8. Ibid., (1967), 56, 634.
9. Ibid., (1967), 56, 1174.
10. Khalil, S.A.H., Nixon, J. R. and Carless, J. E., J. Pharm. Pharmacol., (1968), 20, 215.
11. Nixon, J. R. and Walker, S. E., Ibid., (1971), 23, 1475.
12. Chang, T. M. S., MacIntosh, F. C. and Mason, S. G., Can. J. Physiol. Pharmacol., (1966), 44, 115.
13. Chang, T. M. S., Trans. Amer. Soc. Artif. Int. Organs., (1966), 12, 13.
14. Chang, T.M.S., Pont, A., Johnson, L. J., and Malave, N., Ibid., (1968), 14, 163.
15. Suzuki, S., Kondo, T. and Mason, S. G., Chem. Pharm. Bull., (1968), 16, 1629.
16. Koishi, M., Fukuhara, N. and Kondo, T., Ibid., (1969), 17, 804.
17. Shigeri, Y. and Kondo, T., Ibid., (1969), 17, 1073.
18. Shigeri, Y., Koishi, M., Kondo, T., Shiba, M. and Tomioka, S., Can. J. Chem., (1970), 48, 2047.
19. Luzzi, L. A., Zoglio, M. A., and Maulding, H. V., J. Pharm. Sci., (1970), 59, 338.
20. Underwood, T. W. and Cadwallader, D. E., J. Pharm. Sci., (1972), 61, 239.
21. Chang, T.M.S., Science, (1964), 146, 524.
22. Morgan, P. W. and Kwokek, S. L., J. Polym. Sci., (1959), 40, 299.
23. Weast, R. C., Ed., "Handbook of Chemistry and Physics," 51st ed., Chemical Rubber Co., Cleveland, Ohio, 1970.

16

New Concepts in the Application of Controlled Release Systems to Agriculture

NATHAN F. CARDARELLI

Engineering and Science Division, University of Akron, Akron, Ohio 44325

As worldwide population growth outdistances the annual increase in agricultural yield a global imperative to increase food production has resulted. Food shortages lead not only to starvation and malnutrition, but also to social, political and economic instability. The recent increases in U.S. food exports emphasizes the growing inability of nations, especially in the third world and the underdeveloped soviet sphere, to feed themselves. Agricultural surplus in the United States seldom exceeds 6% of the annual harvest and considering our own demographic increase it is likely that we will experience difficulty in meeting our own needs in future years.[1]

Two viable alternatives exist to meet the foreseeable crises in agriculture; increased tilled acreage and pasturelands and/or increase crop yield per acre. Certainly both routes will be followed - and both will lead to serious, perhaps grave, environmental consequences. Considering the present methods of growing foodstuffs we cannot achieve both increased farm output and assure a quality environment. The need for fertilizers, herbicides, insecticides, fungicides, rodenticides, nematicides and predator control is absolute. It is well recognized that the chemical agents used create a negative environmental impact. Through soil, air and water contamination, and biomagnification nontarget members of the biota including man, can be drastically effected.

Agricultural pesticides and fertilizers are responsible for perhaps 60% of the total U.S. food production. Contamination arising from such usage cannot be checked without grave national consequences. It is noted that economic and social dislocations arising from the reduction of industrial contamination pale to insignificance compared to the consequences of decreasing the use of agricultural chemicals.

Present levels of contamination from agricultural chemicals do not pose any serious threat to human life or its quality <u>at this time</u>. A great increase in the quantities of pesticides and other agents used - as will be necessary for any substantial increase in farm production, could result in a major alteration in biospheric interactions with perhaps grave consequences for humanity. Thousands of articles have been written pro and con on this issue and whereas the possibility is remote; so is the demise of the human race as a consequent of nuclear war remote - however in neither case do we wish to initiate the experimentation necessary to deny the hypothesis!

Crops and livestock are produced in a hostile environment shared by 50,000 species of fungi, 30,000 species of competing weeds, 1,500 species of economically important nematodes, over 10,000 species of insects; grain devouring birds and rodents; predators such as the coyote and vampire bat that destroy sheep and cattle, and a host of parasites and pathogenic microbes. Crops and cattle remove nutrients from the soil which must be replaced if yield is not to drastically decline. Without chemical assistance man would be, and has been through most of history, hard put to feed only himself and his immediate family.

It is hypothesized that Controlled Release Methodology, if applied to the use of agricultural chemicals, will allow the increased production of foodstuffs while simultaneously decreasing the amount (and type) of agents used.

Past experience with controlled release techniques have demonstrated that one can reduce the use of antifouling agents by a factor of 12; a thirty-fold or greater decrease in molluscicide usage has been demonstrated, and an unknown, but substantial, decrease in the amount of various aquatic herbicides necessary to control specific water weeds and algae is promised (2, 3). This emerging technology is now providing indirect benefits to agriculture through mere efficient human disease control - an important element in many nations where the productivity of the farmer and herder is greatly dependent on his state of health. Individuals suffering from debilitating parasitic infections, such as Schistosomiasis and malaria, are not physically capable of the labor necessary to create agricultural surpluses. Indeed many cannot adequately feed themselves. Where 60 to 80% of the rural population are victims of Schistosomiasis, a not unusual condition in vast areas of

Africa, the eradication of this one malady should
result in a significant rise in crop yield. Controlled
release molluscicide may well be the key to intervention of the Schistosomiasis transmission cycle.
Also controlled release technology will assist in
improving protection for stored grains against insect
and rodent pests. In India and other nations rodents
alone consume 10% or more of the harvested and stored
crops. Encapsulated rodenticides in bait formulations
are better accepted by rodents (4). Insecticides and
insect repellents released from various polymeric
based dispensing mechanisms such as the HERCON^{tm} or
CONREL^{tm} dispensers promise more efficient pest control
while using less chemical (5, 6).

The above mentioned technology, once widespread,
should substantially increase available foodstuffs;
however, the really dramatic (and necessary) rise in
agricultural productivity will be in the field. To
date little has been done in the application of this
new technology to both the protection and nutrition of
growing crops, and the decrease in the quantity of
chemical agents utilized. Pioneering efforts are
presently underway in the controlled release of sex
attractant pheromones from a plastic or elastomer
dispensing system. Pheromones have been used as
confusants (gypsy moth) (7) to prevent location of one
sex by another; in mechanical trapping devices (Boll
Weevil (8), Cabbage Looper (9), etc.) or in contact
baits (10, 11). Varying degrees of success have been
attained and there is little doubt that such systems
will be available to agriculture in the near future.
Pheromones are extremely non-persistent (that is why
only controlled release systems represent a viable
application method), fairly target specific and
generally do not affect nontarget members of the biota.
Whether the mass use of trapping devices is a feasible
alternative to insecticides remains to be seen.
Unfortunately pheromones are only presently available
for a few insect species.

Controlled release antimorphogenetic materials are
also being investigated. Mosquitos have been
successfully controlled by this method and chitin
inhibitors are under evaluation (12, 13).

Aldicarb and dimethoate have been incorporated in
polyamide and polyvinyl chloride matrices and released
in the soil (14). The insecticidal properties were
enhanced from the standpoint of extending lifetime.
One controlled release aquatic herbicide that
displayed considerable merit in field tests has been
shown to inhibit plant growth when applied to soil(15).

Controlled release fertilizers are not new to the market place; however, the present commercially available materials are expensive for general agricultural usage and do not provide sufficiently long term nutrient release to overcome the pricing handicap (16, 17).

Although some progress has been made towards the reconciliation of a quality environment with agricultural needs through the use of controlled release systems, it is obvious that we have just begun to scratch the surface.

The merit of controlled release arises from several factors. A non-persistent material, such as methyl parathion, can be rendered persistent at the site of application so that release occurs over an extended period of time while the environmentally favored low persistence at the site of action remains. Long term continuous release provides greater efficiency from the standpoint of less frequent application, but also allows the presence of the agent over an extended interval rather than the peak-valley availability seen with conventional applications.

Agricultural chemicals, of necessity, are applied in amounts far in excess of needs. For instance it is doubtful that fertilizer take up by the growing crops ever exceeds 15% of the total amount applied. The rest is lost through downward leaching beyond the reach of the root systems or run-off with ground waters. A considerable quantity reaches major waterways, lakes, and estuaries with detrimental results on fish, shellfish and other elements of the aquatic biota. By their nature controlled release fertilizers, save with actual flooding, are not removed via run waters and downward percolation losses are decreased.

Insecticides are applied in amounts ranging to millions of times that required if each target were individually given a lethal dosage. Trapping devices overcome this in part by providing motivation for the target to seek the toxicant - and thus one need not permeate the entire area with a poisonous substance. Conventionally large amounts of toxicant are applied on day 1 so that ample amounts remain to destroy pest life on day "X" - the latter amount perhaps a millionth of the former. Controlled release mechanisms applied to many such usages will permit dramatic reduction in the quantity of chemical used through extension of the time that the agent is available to target contact.

Certain natural factors play a crucial role in the efficiency of Controlled Release. The so called "Chronicity" phenomenon, demonstrated and confirmed in

the instance of snail and water weed control, has
indicated that target populations can be managed
through exposure to ultralow toxicant concentrations
if the duration of such exposure is extended (3, 18,
19). That is; a given aquatic weed can be destroyed
by exposure to 0.001 ppm/day for 20 or so days - or
conventionally by a 2 ppm treatment dosage in one day.
Obviously the slow release method results in far less
environmental impact.

The past thrust of controlled release endeavor
has been in the antifouling and public health areas.
Agricultural work underway at this time has dealt
essentially with the use of noncontaminants such as
pheromones and insect growth regulators. It takes no
gift of prophacy to foretell that controlled release
methodology will, of necessity arising from environmental and energy considerations, be rapidly expanded
into the areas of plant nutrients; and weed, fungus,
insect and nematode control. The matrix element or
carrier will likely be a man-made polymer or natural
rubber. Theoretical effort has been underway for some
time and one can mathematically demonstrate efficacy
of controlled release systems (20, 21). Such systems
have been developed, and in some cases commercialized,
based upon several methods of release; vapor diffusion
from a plastic enclosed reservoir (6), vapor diffusion
from a solid nonporous matrix (22), microencapsulation
(23), diffusion-dissolution phenomena based upon
solution equilibrium of a toxicant in an elastomer
(3, 24, 25), leaching phenomena based upon incorporation of a nonsoluble agent in an elastomer or a
plastic (26, 27), and the addition of a control agent
as a pendent substituent to a polymeric backbone with
concommitant loss in the application environment via
hydrolysis or other degrading processes (28).

Examination of the patent and scientific literature discloses that controlled release techniques are
available. Certainly almost all control agents will
lend themselves to the extant technology. Thus it is
only a matter of time, economics, and necessity, before
those engaged in the controlled release area commit
themselves to extending their knowledge into the
challenging and wide open field of agricultural pest
control.

Literature Cited

1.   Shaw, W. C. "Need for Controlled Release
     Technology in the Use of Agricultural Chemicals."
     Keynote Address. Proc. Controlled Release

2. Cardarelli, N. F. "Controlled Release Pesticides:
    The State of the Art. Proc. Controlled Release
    Pesticide Symp." Wright State University, Dayton,
    Ohio. (Plenary Lecture), 1, Sept. 8-10, 1975.
3. Cardarelli, N. F. <u>Controlled Release Pesticide
    Formulations</u>. CRC Press, Cleveland, Ohio, 204
    pages, 1976.
4. Abrams, J. and Hinkes, T. M. Acceptibility and
    Performance of Encapsulated Warfarin. Pest
    Control, (1974), <u>42</u>, 14.
5. McLaughlin, J. R. et.al. "Evaluation of Some
    Formulations for Dispensing Insect Pheromones in
    Field and Orchard Crops." Proc. Controlled
    Release Pesticide Symp. Wright State Univ.,
    Dayton, Ohio, 209, Sept. 8-10, 1975.
6. Ashare, E. et.al. "Controlled Release from
    Hallow Fibers." Ibid 42.
7. Beroza, M. et.al. Field Trials with Disparlure
    in Massachusetts to Suppress Mating of the Gypsy
    Moth. Environ. Entomol. (1974), <u>4</u> (5), 705.
8. Hardee, D. D. et.al. Grandlure for Boll Weevils:
    Controlled Release with a Laminated Plastic
    Dispenser. J. Econ. Entomol. 1975, <u>68</u> (4), 477.
9. Beroza, M. et.al. Tests of a 3-Layer Laminated
    Plastic Bait Dispenser for Controlled Emission of
    Attractants from Insect Traps. Environ. Entomol.
    (1974), <u>3</u> (6), 926.
10. Harris, E. J. "Controlled Release Cue-Lure
    Formulations for Detection and Control of the
    Melon Fly." Proc. Controlled Release Pesticide
    Symp. Rept. #35, Univ. Akron, Akron, Ohio.
    Sept. 16-18, 1974.
11. Keiser, I. et.al. "Enhanced Duration of Residual
    Effectiveness Against the Mediterranean Fruit Fly
    of Guava Foliage Treated with Encapsulated
    Insecticides and Lures." Proc. Controlled Release
    Pesticide Symp. Wright State Univ., Dayton, Ohio,
    264, Sept. 8-10, 1975.
12. Rathburn, C. B. and Boike, A. H. "Laboratory and
    Small Plot Field Tests of Altosid and Dimilin for
    the Control of Mosquito Larvae." Rept. West Fla.
    Arthropod Res. Lab., Fla. Dept. Pub. Hlth.,
    Panama City, Fla., 1975.
13. Post, L. C. and Vincent, W. R. A New Insecticide
    Inhibits Chitin Synthesis. Naturwissen. (1973),
    <u>60</u>, 431.
14. Stokes, R. A. et.al. Use of Selected Plastics in
    Controlled Release Granular Formulations of
    Aldicarb and Dimethoate. J. Agric. Food Chem.
    (1973), <u>21</u>, 103.

15. Danielson, L. L. and Campbell, T. A. "Evaluation of a Latex Based Herbicide Formulation." Proc. Controlled Release Pesticide Symp. Rept. 41A, Univ. Akron, Akron, Ohio, Sept. 16-18, 1974.

16. Daniel, W. H. Slow Release IBDU-Promising New Tests. Weeds, Trees and Turf (1975), 14 (1), 14.

17. Allen, S. E. and Mays, D. A. Sulfur-Coated Fertilizers for Controlled Release: Agronomic Evaluation. J. Agr. Food Chem. (1971), 19 (5), 809.

18. Quinn, S. A. and Cardarelli, N. F. "Aquatic Herbicides Chronicity Study" Ann. Rept. U.S. Army Corps. Engineers, Wash., D.C. DACW 73-72-C-0031, AD903208, July 30, 1972.

19. Cardarelli, N. F. "Hypothesis Concerning Chronic Intoxication of Aquatic Weeds." Proc. Controlled Release Pesticide Symposium, Wright State Univ., Dayton, Ohio, 349, Sept. 8-10, 1975.

20. Baker, R. W. et.al. "Membrane-Controlled Delivery Systems." Proc. Controlled Release Pesticide Symp. Rept. #40, Univ. Akron, Akron, Ohio, Sept. 16-18, 1974.

21. Chandrasekaran, et.al. "A Mathematical Analysis for Controlled Delivery of Agrichemicals," Ibid. Rept. 11.

22. Anon. Controlled Release Insecticides. Soap/ Cosmetic/Chemicals Specialties, March (1975), pp. 1-4.

23. Ivy, E. E. PENCAP M: An Improved Methyl Parathion Formulation. J. Econ. Entomol. (1972), 65, 473.

24. Janes, G. A. "Polymeric Formulations for the Control of Fouling on Pleasure Craft." Proc. Controlled Release Pesticide Symp., Wright State Univ., Dayton, Ohio, 292, Sept. 8-10, 1975.

25. Shiff, C. J. "Field Tests of Controlled Release Molluscicides in Rhodesia." Ibid. pp. 177.

26. Janes, G. A. "Controlled Release Copper Herbicides." Ibid. pp. 325.

27. Evans, E. S. et.al. Larvicidal Effectiveness of a Controlled-Release Formulation of Chlorpyrifos in a Woodland Pool Habitat. Mosq. News (1975) 35 (3), 343.

28. Harris, F. W. et.al. "Polymers Containing Pendent Herbicide Substituents." Proc. Controlled Release Pesticide Symp., Wright State Univ., Dayton, Ohio, 334, Sept. 8-10, 1975.

Development of Field Evaluation of Controlled Release Molluscicides: A Progress Report

KATHERINE E. WALKER

Engineering and Science Division, Community and Technical College, University of Akron, Akron, Ohio 44325

Introduction

One vital aspect of public health programs in most tropical nations lies in the control of parasitic diseases. The major snail-borne disease, Schistosomiasis or Bilharzia, may have as many as 300 million human victims with several million deaths annually attributed directly or indirectly to it. Although death is the ultimate tragedy, all those afflicted suffer a loss in physical prowess and often in mental ability. Since the victim is usually an agricultural worker the disease manifests itself as a loss in agricultural output and the national economy is depressed accordingly.

A free swimming larva, the cercaria, develops from asexual reproduction in the snail. Released into fresh water it must find a human and penetrate the dermis. The cercaria can not obtain sustenance nor reproduce so its "infective life" seldom exceeds twelve hours.

The successful penetrant travels via the circulatory system to the mesentaries around the liver, spleen and bladder. Here development inot the adult worm takes place. Paired male and female worms produce massive numbers of eggs continuously. The ova must reach the external environment, and this is achieved via human excretion.

An ovum in water hatches into a free swimming, non-reproductive, non-feeding larval form, the miracidium. If the miracidium finds a snail of an appropriate species it penetrates and undergoes changes that lead to the asexual reproduction of cercaria, thus completing the cycle.

An infected snail may release several thousand cercariae per day, but this usually represents only a few per cubic foot of water. Of the thousands of eggs produced by the worms in the human body only a certain percentage reach the appropriate external environment, with further attrition during hatching and snail location. However, a great number of the eggs never leave the human body. They remain entrapped in capillaries and various

organs. Tissue damage and a general debility can only lead to
secondary infections and overall lowered resistance.

Control Methodology

The conventional approach to Schistosomiasis control lies in
the use of chemical agents, molluscicides, to interrupt the parasite transmission cycle by destruction of the snail intermediate
host. Medical therapy is useless if contact with infested water
is not prevented and immunization is not yet possible. The major
molluscicides used are copper sulfate, niclosamide, trifenmorph
and several pentachlorophenols. These are applied to snail
habitats as wettable powders, granules, solutions or emulsions.
Unfortunately it is literally impossible to locate and treat all
snail habitats in a given locale, and even in treated waters a
small, but relevant, number of target snails will successfully
undertake avoidance behavior. Repopulation is rapid from even
quite isolated focii and periodic retreatment becomes essential.
Economic resources are, in general, grossly inadequate in the
endemic nations to permit undertaking of the massive molluscicid-
ing program required and the necessary reapplication of the chemical every few months.
        It is generally acknowledged that the worldwide struggle
against Schistosomiasis using conventional approaches is failing
(1).
        In concept the use of controlled release molluscicides would
allow the extension of the between treatment interval to years,
provide more effective control at less cost and substantially
decrease the amount of control agent utilized thus lessening impact on the non-target biota. Controlled release also makes
attack of the miracidium, cercaria, and ova practical.

Development of Controlled Release Materials

The precursor of controlled release molluscicides is the
organotin containing antifouling elastomeric formulations developed in 1964 (2,3). The resulting 6% active chloroprene sheet
rubber material has been commercialized and applied to ship hulls,
buoys and other marine objects (4,5). The initial field applications on bouys in 1966 remain biologically effective to date(6).
That is , a chemical agent, bis(tri-n-butyltin) oxide "TBTO, has
been continuously released in levels commensurate with the pre-
vention of fouling for over 9 years! Inthis and other controlled
release applications a cost benefit of 7 to 1 or greater is realized and a reduction of 10 to 1, or greater, in terms of environmental contamination(7,8).
        The very long term sustained release materials are based upon
solution equilibrium properties common to elastomeric matrices.
An agent highly soluble in the elastomer is placed in solution in
the given material--natural rubber, styrene-butadiene copolymers,

cis polybutadiene, etc., upon water immersion surface agent molecules undergo gradual dissolution into the rubber/water interface
thus disturbing solution equilibrium. Concomitantly internal
solute molecules migrate towards the depleting surface due to solution pressure--and a gradual surface release cycle is established.
The solubility of the agent in water ought to be quite small.
System kinetics may be first or second order depending upon whether diffusion or dissolution is rate controlling (1).

Controlled release antifouling materials were found toxic to
various snail species (3,9). Trialkyltins, such as TBTO and tri-
butyltin fluoride "TBTF", and niclosamide were successfully incorporated in various elastomers and through proper compounding
techniques and vulcanization conditions caused to release at a
slow continous rate when immersed in water.

Laboratory studies performed at the University of Akron
demonstrated that various controlled release antifouling elastomers would destroy snails at ultralow toxicant release concentrations (i.e. 0.01 ppm or less). In Tanzania such materials were
examined under semi field conditions--i.e. field water continuously flowing through a laboratory bioassay tank and in small
ponds confirming that mortality did ensue (10). Laboratory tests
in Puerto Rico likewise provided positive results (11). In Brazil
antifouling rubber sheet strips placed in irrigation reservoirs
and ponds provided complete snail mortality--within 45 to 60 exposure days (12). Tests in London (Tropical Pesticide Research
Headquarters) demonstrated that the biological efficacy of a given
rubber pellet was in excess of two years (13). The formulations
involved were laboratory specimens and not optimized products.

Controlled Release Molluscicides ("CRM")

In 1972 the Creative Biology Laboratory (Barberton, Ohio)
working under the auspices of the M&T Chemical Company (Rahway,
New Jersey) undertook the optimization of a TBTO/natural rubber
formulation. This effort culminated in the 6% active material now
available as BioMet-SRM. In other effort sponsored by the World
Health Organization a TBTF/natural rubber CRM was developed to
further enlarge the controlled release arsenal (14). These substances function through a diffusion-dissolution loss mechanism
dependent upon agent solubility within the elastomer (15). In a
parallel program a CRM composed of copper sulfate in an ethylene-
propylene-diene rubber base was developed and is now commercialized as INCRACIDE E-51 (International Copper Research Organization,
New York, New York) (16). This latter material functions through
a leach type mechanism using an ammonium sulfate coleachant to
maintain appropriate rubber/water interfacial pH.

Formulations present no difficulty in mixing, extruding, vul-
canizing and pelletizing. Natural rubber, ethylene-propylene ter-
polymers, polychloroprenes, and polyacrylonitriles will retain considerable quantities of the organotins in solution and bind up to

70% by weight of copper sulfate.

Field Studies

Biomet[tm] SRM was applied at rubber dosages of 50 ppm (3 ppm active) to stationary water bodies such as ponds and marshes; and several running water channels in Brazil. Seventeen small test sites were thus established (17).

Sanil populations were reduced to zero in the static systems within a few weeks and no repopulation was observed over the course of the 14 month program. Macroscopic ovservation of vascular water plants showed no discernable damage althouh some reduction in algae was apparent. Snail destruction was insufficient in the flowing water tests.

Control has also been demonstrated in lake and reservoir tests in Rhodesia (18). BioMet[tm] SRM rubber strips and pellets were applied to irrigation reservoirs of an acre or more in surface area, irrigation channels, and along lakeside contact points. CBL-9B pellets were also applied to lake environments. Organotin containing antifouling paints were coated on the concrete walls and other structures of promary irrigation canals and weirs. All tests have given positive results to date--both in static and cynamic running water systems. Treatment dosages were but a few parts per million. Snail mortality was not observed until several months after application, and then populations dropped very rapidly--approaching zero. Focal control, i.e. treating only the human-snail interaction points or areas of large snail populations rather than area control, appears on the basis of the Rhodesian experience to be the proper approach to intervention.

Organotin paints are adequate for perhaps one year and the controlled release organotin elastomers for 2 or more years--based on Rhodesian results. Analysis of pellets returned after 14 months of exposure in Brazil showed a 15% to 20% loss of the active agent--thus allowing a 2.5 year half-life prediction.

Comprehensive analysis of non-target test site biota in Rhodesia disclosed little environmental impact on vascular plants, oligochaetes, water insects, algae, daphnia and other life forms. No fish intoxication was observed (19).

Direct observation, time lapse photography, and analysis of treated water, bottom soil, subsoil etc. strongly indicates that the organotin content in treated water is very minute--in the low parts-per-billion at best--and that it concentrates in the bottom soil where browsing snails ingest it (19). This could be expected from the extreme hydrophobicity of the organotins. Tests conducted by the author showed that where snail contact with the bottom soil was permitted a LT99 of 8 days could be expected at 10 ppm rubber (0.6 ppm TBTO or 3ppm TBTT active) dosages while snails isolated from bottom soil contact under similar regimens showed an LT99 of nearly 30 days.

BioMet[tm] SRM tests conducted in a flowing water stream in

St. Lucia, B.W.I., exhibited 100% snail mortality (20). Static water evaluation in small natural ponds in the Sudan and Iran with BioMet^{tm} SRM pellets likewise demonstrated wxcellent snail control and no gross ecological disturbance (21,22). CBL-9B pellets, supplied by the Creative Biology Laboratory, have been found effective against the amphibious snail vectors of the Asiatic form of Schistosomiasis (23).

In all instances one application provided significantly longer control than would be realized with conventional treatments and drastically less environmental impact. Efficacious dosage rates have been in the practical range of 50 ppm pellet (15 or less ppm active) at all sites. Since complete release of the active agent will require no less than 2.5 years and such release is continuous through decreasing with time--an average site concentration would be about 0.016 ppm. The actual water concentration likely does not exceed 0.002 ppm--the rest being absorbed by soil, plants, etc. Being relatively little organotin dissolved in the water, there is little available to fish and other beneficial elements of the biota (18). Microenvironmental laboratory tests affirm control without gross effects on fish or aquatic vascular plant life, at least with TBTO, TBTF and copper releasing formulations (15,24).

Although INCRACIDE E-51 CRM has not been as thoroughly tested as other materials, preliminary results from St. Lucia(20), Rhodesia (25), and the Sudan (26) indicate feasibility.

Past and present University of Akron CRM evaluations indicate that release levels of 0.007 ppm/day or less of the trialkyltins and about 0.03 ppm/day of copper ion are adequate to control host snail populations under varying water quality conditions. pH, mineral content and other environmental factors influence rates of toxicant release from the elastomeric matrix, snail uptake and detoxification mechanisms. CRM dosages are presently being established based upon water quality parameters (27).

It is believed that controlled release molluscicides are proving to be an economical and feasible method of intervening in the parasite transmission cycle. The recent decision by the Rhodesian public health authorities to utilize BioMet^{tm} SRM in an area wide control program lends support to the merit of this new approach in snail control.

Literature Cited

1. Cardarelli, N.F. (1976) Controlled Release Pesticide Formulations, CRC Press, Cleveland, Ohio.
2. Cardarelli, N.F. and Caprette, S.J. (1969) Antifouling Coverings. U.S. Patent 3426473.
3. Cardarelli, N.F. and Neff, H.F. (1972) Biocidal Elasomeric Compositions. U.S. Patent 3639583.
4. Bollinger, E.H. (1974) Controlled Release Antifouling Rubber Coating. Rept. 19. Proc. Controlled Release Pesticide Symp. Univ. Of Akron, Akron, Ohio.

5. Janes, G.A. (1975) Polymeric Formulations for the Control
    of Fouling on Pleasure Craft. Proc. Controlled Release
    Pesticide Symp. Wright State University, Dayton, Ohio.
6. Senderling, R.A. (1967) Rubber World. 157 (2), Nov.
7. Cardarelli, N.F. (1975) Controlled Release Pesticides: The
    State of the Art. Plenary Lecture. Proc. Controlled Re-
    lease Pesticide Symp. Wright State University, Dayton, Ohio.
8. Cardarelli, N.F. Address in 1975 to the Federal Working
    Group on Pest Management. NAL, Beltsville, MD. (To be pub-
    lished).
9. Cardarelli, N.F. (1968) Method for Dispersing Toxicants to
    Kill Disease Spreading Water-Spawned Larva, Trematodes,
    Molluscs and Similar Organisms; and the Products Used in
    Such Methods. U.S. Patent 3417181.
10. Fenwick, A. (1969) Wld. Hlth. Org. Inform. Rep. Ser. AFR/
    BILHARZ/14.
11. Ritchie, L.S. and Malek, E.A. (1969) Wld. Hlth. Org. Inform.
    Rep. Ser. PD/MOL/69.1.
12. Paulini, E. and Souza, C.P. da. (1969) Wld. Hlth. Org.
    Inform. Rep. Ser. PD/MOL/69.9.
13. Hopf, H.S. and Goll, P.H. (1970) Wld. Hlth. Org. Inform.
    Rep. Ser. PD/MOL/70.14.
14. Quinn, S.A. and Walker, K.E. (1972) Ann. Prog. Rept. to
    Wld. Hlth. Org. Proj. B2/181/62.
15. Cardarelli, N.F. in Molluscicides in Schistosomiasis Control.
    Ed. T.C. Cheng. Academic Press. 1974.
16. Walker, K.E. and Cardarelli, N.F. (1973) Ann. Rept. to
    International Copper Research Association. INCRA Proj. 203.
17. Castleton, C. (1974) Brazilian Field Trials of MT-1E, An
    Organotin Slow-Release Formulation. Proc. Controlled Re-
    lease Pesticide Symp. Report 22. University of Akron, Akron
    Ohio.
18. Shiff, C.J. in Molluscicides in Schistosomiasis Control. Ed.
    T.C. Cheng. Academic Press. 1974.
19. Shiff, C.J. et. al. (1975) Further Trials with TBTO and
    Other Slow Release Molluscicides in Rhodesia. Proc. Con-
    trolled Release Pesticide Symp. Wright State University,
    Dayton, Ohio.
20. Upatham, E.S. (1975) Field Studies of Slow-Release TBTO
    Pellets (BioMet^{tm} SRM) Against St. Lucian Biomphalaria
    glabrata. Proc. Controlled Release Pesticide Symp. Wright
    State University, Dayton, Ohio.
21. Amin, M. (1975) Field Evaluation of the Molluscicidal Po-
    tency of TBTO in the Sudan. Prod. Controlled Release Pest-
    icide Symp. Wright State University, Dayton, Ohio.
22. Mansoori, A. (1975) Brief Summary of the Study on MT-1E
    Slow Release Molluscicide. Controlled Release Molluscicide
    Newsletter. University of Akron, Akron, Ohio.
23. Santos, A. (1975) Summary of Results of Laboratory Screen-
    ing of Compound 443A Against O. quadrasi. Controlled Re-

lease Molluscicide Newsletter, University of Akron, Akron, Ohio.

24. Cardarelli, N.F. (1975) Microenvironmental Evaluation of Slow Release Molluscicides. Proc. Controlled Release Pesticide Symp. Rept. 29. University of Akron, Akron, Ohio.

25. Shiff, C.J. and Yiannakis, C. (1975) Controlled Release Molluscide Studies. Controlled Release Molluscicide Newsletter, University of Akron, Akron, Ohio.

26. Amin. M. (1975) Evaluation of INCRACIDE E-51 Against Biomphalaria pfeifferi and Bulinus truncatus. Controlled Release Molluscicide Newsletter. University of Akron, Akron, Ohio.

27. Walker, K.E. and Cardarelli, N.F. (1975) Quart. Rept. 1 to U.S. Natl. Inst. Hlth. Grant AI11861-01A1.

18

Polymers Containing Pendent Herbicide Substituents: Preliminary Hydrolysis Studies

FRANK W. HARRIS, ANN E. AULABAUGH, ROBERT D. CASE,
MARY K. DYKES, and WILLIAM A. FELD

Department of Chemistry, Wright State University, Dayton, Ohio 45431

Controlled-release pesticide-polymer formulations that extend the control of a wide variety of target organisms have been developed (1-3). For example, herbicide-polyethylene formulations have been prepared and studied in this laboratory (4). In these systems the herbicide is physically incorporated in the plastic matrix and release occurs by diffusion. Although formulations of this type have considerable potential, a drawback to their production and use is the large amount of inert polymer carrier (70-90% w/w) that must be employed. The development of pesticide-polymer formulations that contain a high percentage of pesticide is highly desirable.

One route to such formulations has been the synthesis of polymers that contain pesticides as pendent substituents (5-18). For example, polymers have been prepared that consist of over 80% 2,4-dichlorophenoxyacetic acid (2,4-D) or 2-(2,4,5-trichlorophenoxy)propionic acid (Silvex) as pendent side chains (14-16). Theoretically the controlled release of pesticide is then achieved by the slow, sequential hydrolysis of the pesticide-polymer chemical bonds. Bioassay studies conducted in moist soil, however, indicate that homopolymers containing pesticide residues that are attached directly to a hydrophobic polymer backbone will not undergo hydrolysis (5). The objective of this research was to prepare herbicide-polymer systems that will undergo slow hydrolysis when immersed in an aquatic environment.

In our initial approach to obtaining hydrolyzable systems, the herbicides 2,4-D and Silvex were incorporated in the alcohol residues of a series of acrylic esters (14-16). In these monomers the distance between the herbicide and the vinyl group and, hence, the resulting polymer backbone was varied by varying the length of the unit connecting the herbicide to the acrylic acid. It was postulated that increasing the length of the pendent side chain would enhance the hydrolysis of the herbicide-polymer bond since the ester linkage would be removed from the hydrophobic backbone and less sterically hindered.

The monomers, i.e. 2-acryloyloxyethyl 2,4-dichlorophenoxy-

acetate (Ia), 2-acryloyloxyethyl 2-(2,4,5-trichlorophenoxy)pro-
pionate (Ib), 2-methacryloyloxyethyl 2,4-dichlorophenoxyacetate
(IIa), 2-methacryloyloxyethyl 2-(2,4,5-trichlorophenoxy)propio-
nate (IIb), 4-acryloyloxybutyl 2,4-dichlorophenoxyacetate (IIIa),
4-acryloyloxybutyl 2-(2,4,5-trichlorophenoxy)propionate (IIIb),
4-methacryloyloxybutyl 2,4-dichlorophenoxyacetate (IVa), and
4-methacryloyloxybutyl 2-(2,4,5-trichlorophenoxy)propionate (IVb),
were polymerized by bulk- and solution-free-radical techniques to
yield the corresponding polymers (V-VIII). The polymerizations
were enhanced by low initiator concentrations and mild conditions.
Polymeric materials were obtained that exhibited inherent viscosities as high as 2.03.

This communication describes an alternate approach to enhancing the hydrolysis of herbicide-polymer bonds, i.e. the copolymerization of vinyl derivatives of 2,4-D and Silvex with
vinyl monomers containing hydrophilic residues. The rate of
hydrolysis of ester linkages connecting pendent substituents to a
hydrocarbon backbone is known to be increased by the incorporation of hydrophilic groups along the backbone (4,19,20). Preliminary studies of the hydrolysis of poly(vinyl 2,4-dichloro-
phenoxyacetate), poly(2-acryloyloxyethyl 2,4-dichlorophenoxy-
acetate) (Va), poly(4-acryloyloxybutyl 2,4-dichlorophenoxy-
acetate) (VIIa), and a series of copolymers of 2-acryloyloxyethyl
2,4-dichlorophenoxyacetate have also been carried out.

Results and Discussion

Copolymerizations. The 2-acryloyloxyethyl esters of 2,4-D
(Ia) and Silvex (Ib) were copolymerized with trimethylamine
methacrylimide (IX), 1,1-dimethyl-2-hydroxypropylamine methacrylimide (X), 1,1-dimethyl-(2-hydroxy-3-butoxypropyl)amine
methacrylimide (XI), acrylic acid (XII), and methacrylic acid
(XIII) (Table 1). The copolymerizations with the aminimides were

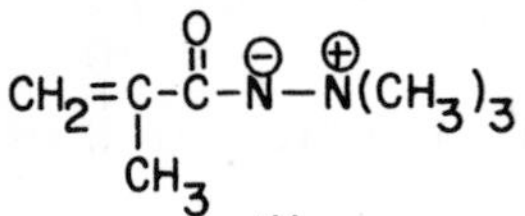

$$CH_2=C-C-N-N(CH_3)_3$$
$$\quad\ \ CH_3$$
IX

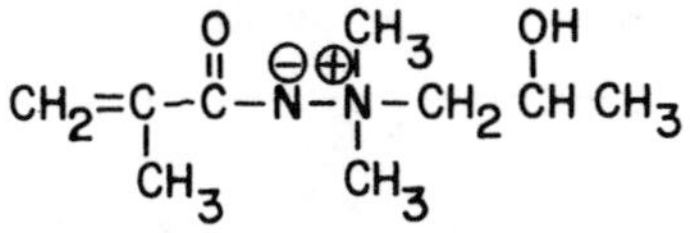

$$CH_2=C-C-N-N-CH_2\ CH\ CH_3$$
$$\quad\ \ CH_3\quad CH_3$$
X

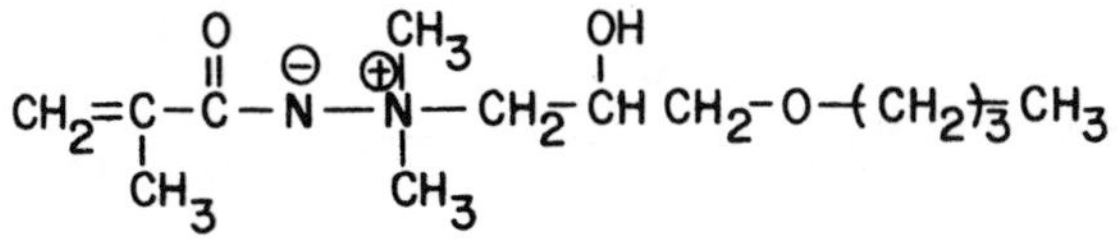

$$CH_2=C-C-N-N-CH_2 CH CH_2-O-(CH_2)_3 CH_3$$
$$\quad\ \ CH_3\quad CH_3$$
XI

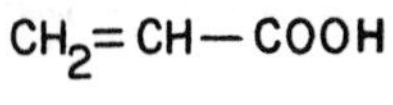

$$CH_2= CH-COOH$$
XII

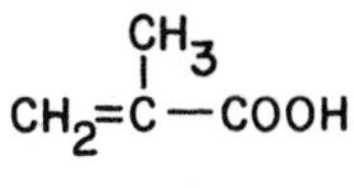

$$CH_2=C-COOH$$
$$\quad\ \ CH_3$$
XIII

carried out without solvent at 70° with azobisisobutyronitrile
(AIBN) as the initiator. The aminimides were used as comonomers
because of their extremely hydrophilic nature (21-23). The copolymerizations with acrylic acid and methacrylic acid were run in
2-butanone due to their tendency to form crosslinked gels when
polymerized by bulk techniques. In fact, the solution copolymerizations with acrylic acid also resulted in considerable
amounts of insoluble material. The presence of the appropriate

hydrophilic residues (aminimide,-OH,-CO$_2$H) in the copolymers was confirmed by infrared spectroscopy.

TABLE 1

Copolymerization Data

Copolymer	Copolymer Composition Monomer 1	Monomer 2	Mole % Monomer 1 in Feed	η [a]
XIV	Ia	IX	87[b]	0.35
XV	Ia	IX	75[b]	0.44
XVI	Ia	IX	65[b]	0.20
XVII	Ib	IX	50	0.54
XVIII	Ia	X	50	1.00
XIX	Ib	X	50	0.81
XX	Ia	XI	50	0.87
XXI	Ib	XI	50	0.78
XXII	Ib	XI	80	1.44
XXIII	Ib	XI	95	1.43
XXIV	Ia	XII	80	0.70[c]
XXV	Ia	XIII	80[b]	0.38[d]

[a]Inherent viscosity (0.50 g/dl in chlorobenzene at 30°C).
[b]Actual composition as determined by elemental analysis.
[c]Inherent viscosity (0.50 g/dl in s̲y̲m̲-tetrachloroethane at 30°C).
[d]Inherent viscosity (0.50 g/dl in 2-butanone at 30°C).

Hydrolysis Studies. The initial results of a study of the hydrolysis of poly(vinyl 2,4-dichlorophenoxyacetate), poly(2-acryloyloxyethyl 2,4-dichlorophenoxyacetate)(Va), poly(4-acryloyloxybutyl 2,4-dichlorophenoxyacetate)(VIIa), and the aminimide copolymer XIV indicate that only the copolymer is susceptable to hydrolysis (Figure 1) (18). This study is being carried out with polymer samples that were ground and sieved to a particle size of 125-400 μ, and then immersed in distilled water (pH = 7.2) at 30°C. The amount of herbicide released from each polymer is determined periodically by spectrophotometric analysis. The amounts shown in Figure 1 are the averages of three replicates. This study has now been continued for 324 days. The copolymer

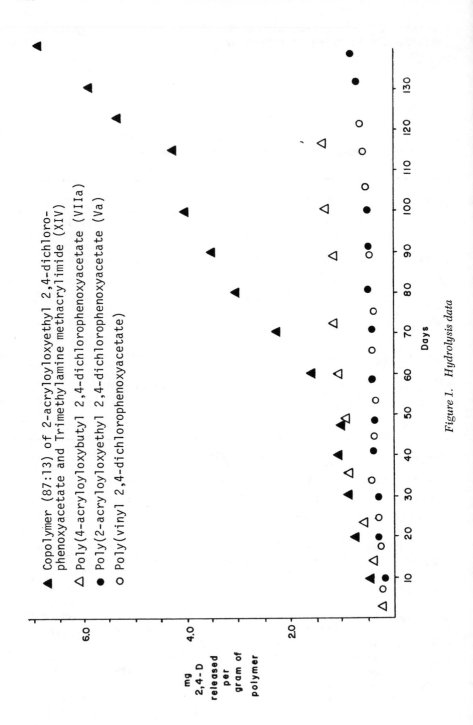

Figure 1. Hydrolysis data

samples have released an average of 23 mg of herbicide while the homopolymers have failed to hydrolyze.

An investigation of the hydrolysis of poly(vinyl 2,4-dichlorophenoxyacetate), polymer Va, copolymer XV, copolymer XVI, and copolymer XXV in a pH 8 buffer has also been initiated. The buffer was used to simulate the pH of the natural waters in the South where aquatic weed problems are the most pronounced. The data shown in Figure 2 were obtained by employing procedures described for the previous study. As can be seen from the Figure, the homopolymers are still resistant to hydrolysis at pH 8. The rate of hydrolysis of copolymer XV which contains 25% trimethylamine methacrylimide is not significantly different than that observed for copolymer XIV in the initial hydrolysis study. Copolymer XVI which contains 35% of the aminimide, however, releases herbicide considerably faster. This copolymer has released 20 mg of herbicide in 32 days. The hydrolysis data for the methacrylic acid copolymer XXV was not included in Figure 2 because the copolymer released 117 mg of herbicide in the first six days of the study. This rapid hydrolysis was accompanied by considerable swelling of the polymer particles which prevented further spectroscopic analysis of the sample solutions.

Conclusions

The homopolymers containing herbicides as pendent substituents prepared in this work will not undergo hydrolysis under slightly alkaline conditions at 30°. Increasing the length of the pendent side chains does not in itself significantly enhance the hydrolysis of the herbicide-polymer ester bonds. The incorporation of hydrophilic aminimide residues along the polymer backbone, however, results in the slow hydrolysis of the ester linkages. Increasing the percentage of aminimide in the system from 25 to 35% results in an increase in the rate of herbicide release. The rate of hydrolysis can be increased dramatically by incorporating carboxylic acid groups along the polymer backbone. These groups are very effective in catalyzing the hydrolysis of the herbicide-polymer ester bonds.

Experimental

Ultraviolet spectra were obtained with a Cary Model 14 spectrophotometer. Infrared spectra were obtained on thin films with a Perkin-Elmer Model 457 spectrophotometer. Viscosities were determined with a Cannon Number 75 viscometer. The aminimide monomers were furnished by Ashland Chemicals, Columbus, Ohio.

General Bulk Copolymerization Procedure. Herbicide monomer, comonomer, and 0.1% AIBN were thoroughly mixed and slowly heated to 70°. After heating at 70° for 3 hr, the residue was cooled, dissolved in chloroform, and precipitated in hexane. The polymer

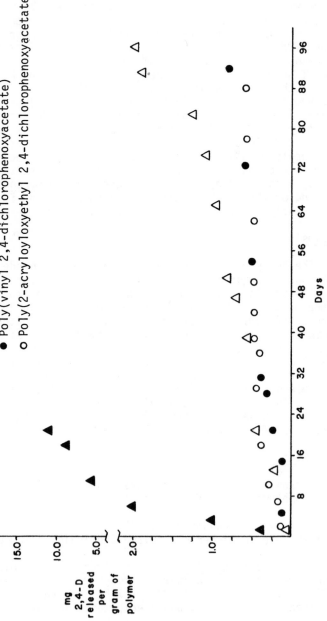

▲ Copolymer (65:35) of 2-acryloyloxyethyl 2,4-dichlorophenoxy-
   acetate and Trimethylamine methacrylimide (XVI)

△ Copolymer (75:25) of 2-acryloyloxyethyl 2,4-dichlorophenoxy-
   acetate and Trimethylamine methacrylimide (XV)

● Poly(vinyl 2,4-dichlorophenoxyacetate)

○ Poly(2-acryloyloxyethyl 2,4-dichlorophenoxyacetate (Va)

Figure 2. Hydrolysis data

was collected by filtration and dried under vacuum at 60° for 24 hr.

General Solution Copolymerization Procedure. Herbicide monomer, comonomer, 2-butanone (4 ml/g of monomers), and 0.05% AIBN were thoroughly mixed and slowly heated under nitrogen to 75°. After heating at 75° for 3 hr, the mixture was cooled, diluted with 2-butanone, and precipitated in hexane. The copolymer was collected by filtration and dried under vacuum at 60° for 3 hr.

Hydrolysis Studies. The copolymers were extracted with methanol for 18 hr to remove unreacted monomer, dried under vacuum, and then ground and sieved to a particle size of 125-400 μ. Three one-gram samples of each copolymer were placed in 500-ml erlenmeyer flasks containing 300 ml of a boric acid-sodium hydroxide buffer (pH = 8.08). The flasks were agitated in a constant temperature bath at 30±0.1°. The amount of herbicide released from each copolymer was determined periodically by spectrophotometric analysis at 198 nm.

Acknowledgement

Support of this research by the Department of the Army, U. S. Army Engineer Waterways Experiment Station under Contract DACW39-76-C-0016 (Neg.) is gratefully acknowledged. Appreciation is also expressed to AmChem Products, Inc. for furnishing the herbicides and to Ashland Chemicals Company for furnishing the aminimides used in this study.

Literature Cited

1. Cardarelli, Nate F., Ed., "Proceedings 1974 International Controlled Release Pesticide Symposium," The University of Akron, Akron, Ohio, 1974.
2. Harris, Frank W., Ed., "Proceedings 1975 International Controlled Release Pesticide Symposium," Wright State University, Dayton, Ohio, 1975.
3. Cardarelli, Nate F., "Controlled Release Pesticides," Chemical Rubber Publishing Company, Cleveland, Ohio, 1976.
4. Harris, Frank W., Norris, Steve O., and Post, Larry K., Weed Science, (1973), 21 (4), 318.
5. Neogi, A. N., "Polymer Selection for Controlled Release Pesticides," Ph.D. Thesis, University of Washington, Seattle, Washington, 1970.
6. Allan, G. G., Chopra C. S., Neogi, A. N., and Wilkins, R. M., Nature, (1971), 234, 349.
7. Jakubka, H. D. and Busch, E., N. Chem., (1973), 13 (3), 105.
8. Akagane, K. and Allan, G. G., Shikizai Kyokaishi, (1973), 46, 437; Chem. Abstr., (1974), 80, 61104k.

9. Montemarano, J. A., and Dyckman, E. J., Am. Chem. Soc., Div.
    Org. Coat. Plast., Preprints, (1974), 34 (1), 607.
10. Baltazzi, E., U. S. Patent 3,343,941 (1967); Chem. Abstr.,
    (1968), 68, 50730 n.
11. Mehltretter, C. L., Roth, W. B., Weakley, F. B., McGuire,
    T. A., and Russell, C. R., Weed Science, (1974), 22 (5),
    415.
12. Allan, G. G., Chopra, C. S., and Russell, R. M., Int. Pest
    Contr., (1972), 14 (2), 15.
13. Allan, G. G., Chopra, C. S., Friedhoff, J. F., Gara, R. I.,
    Maggi, M. W., Neogi, A. N., Roberts, S. C., and Wilkins,
    R. W., Chem. Tech., (1973), March, 171.
14. Harris, Frank W. and Post, Larry K. in "Proceedings 1974
    International Controlled Release Pesticide Symposium,"
    Cardarelli, Nate F., Ed., The University of Akron, Ohio,
    1974.
15. Harris, Frank W., and Post, Larry K., Am. Chem. Soc., Polym.
    Div., Preprints, (1975), 16 (2), 622.
16. Harris, Frank W. and Post, Larry K., J. Polym. Sci., Polym.
    Sci., Polymer Letters ed., (1975), 13, 225.
17. Feld, William A., Post, Larry K., and Harris, Frank W. in
    "Proceedings 1975 International Controlled Release Pesticide
    Symposium," p. 113, Harris, F. W., Ed., Wright State Univer-
    sity, Dayton, Ohio, 1975.
18. Harris, Frank W., Feld, William A., and Bowen, Bonnie, ibid,
    p. 334..
19. Morawetz, H. and Gaetjens, E., J. Polym. Sci., (1958), 32,
    526.
20. Davies, R. F. B., and Reynolds, G. E. J., J. Appl. Polym.
    Sci., (1968), 12, 47.
21. McKillop, W. J., Sedor, E. A., Culbertson, B. M., and
    Wowzonek S., Chem. Rev., (1973), 73, 255.
22. Culbertson, B. M., Sedor, E. A., and Slagel, R. C., Macro-
    molecules, (1968), 1, 254.
23. Culbertson, B. M., and Slagel, R. C., J. Polym. Sci.,
    Part A-1, (1968), 6, 363.

Control of Aquatic Weeds by Chronic Intoxication

GEORGE E. JANES

Creative Biology Laboratory, Inc., 3070 Cleveland-Massillon Road,
Barberton, Ohio 44203

Laboratory studies by the Creative Biology Laboratory and
others have shown that biologically active chemicals can be
released from specially compounded elastomers at relatively constant rates over long periods of time. The chemicals or "pesticides" thus released demonstrate the same biological activity as
if they were conventionally applied.

The controlled release system, however, offers advantages or
variations in approach that are not possible or at best are
impractical with conventional application. Chronic intoxication
of pest aquatic weeds with a constant low level herbicide dosage
is one example. Obviously the high cost of conventional spread-
ing or spraying herbicides precludes daily applications of ultra
low concentrations and dictates that a single acute dose be
applied.

Chronic intoxication of aquatic weeds by itself, is not an
advantage in favor of controlled release. Ultimately there must
be an economic or environmental advantage. Thus it is not sufficient to simply extend the toxicant disbursal time. There must
be an accompanying enhancement of efficacy, an extention of the
time between applications, a reduction in toxicant usage, or some
other factor altered that can be converted into a dollar savings
or environmental benefit.

With this in mind, we were quick to note during the course
of this effort that the mortality curve, in many instances, was
not proportional to the dosages used, i.e. if 0.1 ppm/day dose
killed in one week and the concentration/time (Ct) equation were
accurate, then a 0.01 ppm/day dose should give the same results
in 10 weeks. Both in laboratory and pond tests, this was not so.
The time factor was about 1.7 and not 10. Thus, it was hypothesized that whereas a Ct relationship probably held for <u>acute</u>
terminal dosages where the time period was confined to several
days, i.e. conventional treatment; the ultralow agent concentrations experienced with slow release methodology leads to a terminal <u>chronic</u> intoxication whose mechanism of action is different.
It is also suspected that the <u>slow release mechanism</u> results

in a truly <u>molecular</u> concentration in the water envelope, whereas
conventional use of granules, emulsions, etc. lead to molecular
aggregrates. The statistics of contact as well as the absorbtiv-
ity of the agent by the plant may be significantly different.

This "chronicity" phenomenon was investigated in a study
involving two basic experiments. In one the herbicide was added
daily and the toxicant was allowed to accumulate. In the other
case the herbicide was also added daily, but the test water was
changed so that the agent concentration was held fairly constant.

Watermilfoil, <u>Elodea</u>, <u>Cabomba</u>, <u>Vallisneria</u> and Southern
naiad were evaluated in one gallon jars, each with 3 liters of
water. Plants were potted, three to the jar, in 200 ml. cups.
Gro-lux lighting was used in indoor tests with intensity adjusted
for optimum growth. Other plants were tested in 5 gallon plastic
lined containers. Plants were conditioned for 4 to 8 weeks prior
to instituting a poisoning regime.

Test containers were observed daily and plant mortality sub-
jectively rated on a 100 (healthy) to 0 (mortality) scale with the
degree of thinning and browning serving as the rating criteria.

Evaluations performed during the course of this effort tend
to confirm the hypothesis that the Ct relationship does not hold
when ultralow herbicide concentrations are maintained for extended
periods of time. This is shown in the following data.

TABLE 1

EFFECTS OF FIVE TOXICANTS ON WATERMILFOIL: DOSE ACCUMULATIVE

Toxicant	Dose (ppmw)	Days to Given % Mortality		
		50%	90%	100%
Diquat	1.0	9	13	14
"	0.1	9	12	13
"	0.01	10	16	19
"	0.001	18	24	38
Fenac	1.0	14	19	21
"	0.1	22	42	43
"	0.01	24	43	48
"	0.001	never	never	never
Silvex	1.0	8	13	18
"	0.1	18	23	27
"	0.01	18	20	21
"	0.001	never	never	plants recovered
2,4-D acid	1.0	8	12	14
"	0.1	8	14	18
"	0.01	13	20	24
"	0.001	21	never	recovery

TABLE I (cont.)

EFFECTS OF FIVE TOXICANTS ON WATERMILFOIL: DOSE ACCUMULATIVE

Toxicant	Dose (ppmw)	Days to Given % Mortality		
		50%	90%	100%
2,4-D BEE	1.0	10	13	15
"	0.1	10	15	17
"	0.01	10	14	18
"	0.001	10	18	22

Water Controls average 6% mortality
Solvent Controls average 16% mortality

TABLE II

EFFECTS OF FIVE TOXICANTS ON WATERMILFOIL: DOSE CONSTANT

Toxicant	Dose (ppmw)	Days to Given % Mortality		
		50%	90%	100%
Diquat	1.0	8	10	11
"	0.1	9	14	19
"	0.01	9	13	16
"	0.001	23	27	32
Fenac	1.0	19	never	recovery
"	0.1	never	never	recovery
"	0.01	23	never	recovery
"	0.001	35	never	recovery
Silvex	1.0	8	11	15
"	0.1	20	never	never
"	0.01	21	never	never
"	0.001	never	never	never
2,4-D acid	1.0	12	18	20
"	0.1	20	never	never
"	0.01	never	never	never
"	0.001	never	never	never
2,4-D BEE	1.0	7	10	13
"	0.1	6	13	19
"	0.01	13	22	24
"	0.001	20	38	never

Water Controls 31% mortality
Solvents Controls 35% mortality

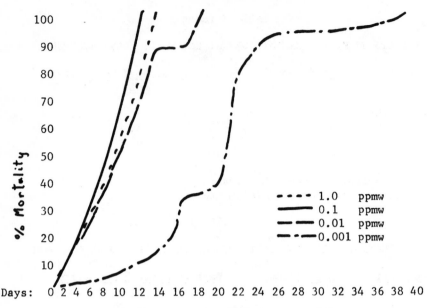

Figure 1.   Diquat vs. watermilfoil: dose accumulative

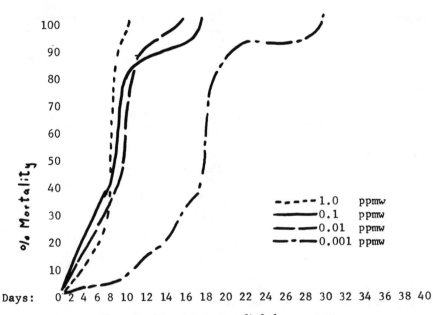

Figure 2.   Diquat vs. watermilfoil: dose constant

The preceding data represents an average reading of four test aquaria, or a total of 12 plants, for each toxicant at each concentration. Control data is an average of 12 jars or 36 plants each.

The data on 2,4-D BEE and Diquat is shown in graph form in Figures 1 through 4 to better illustrate the minimal time penalties incurred to achieve control at ultra-low toxicant concentrations.

A controlled release formulation of copper sulfate monohydrate (1) with a measured release rate of only a fraction of one percent of total available toxicant per day was evaluated against <u>Vallisneria</u>, <u>Cabomba</u>, duckweed, watermilfoil and algae to see if the "chronicity" phenomenon" was reflected in the results.

Planting, preparation and rating was the same as in the previous experiments. Toxicant pellets were added at 10 ppm, 50 ppm and 100 ppm by rubber weight with respective copper ion contents of 1.75 ppm, 8.75 ppm and 17.5 ppm. Jars were also treated with a 0.03 ppm copper ion solution to approximate the actual release from a 100 ppm pellet. Table III shows the data for the <u>Cabomba</u> exposure and the information is charted in Figure 5. The "chronicity phenomenon" is pronounced here in that a difference of only 5 days is noted for a 100% kill between the lowest and highest rates. (2)

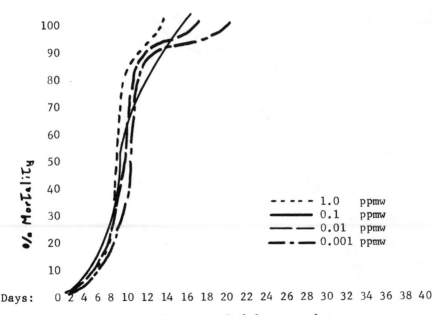

Days: 0 2 4 6 8 10 12 14 16 18 20 22 24 26 28 30 32 34 36 38 40

Figure 3.   BEE vs. watermilfoil: dose accumulative

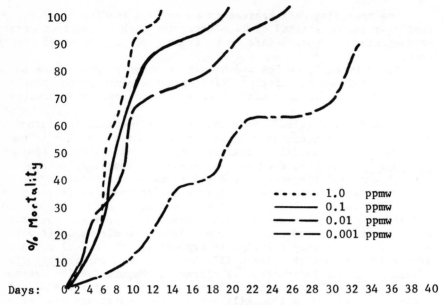

Figure 4.   2,4-D BEE vs. watermilfoil: dose constant

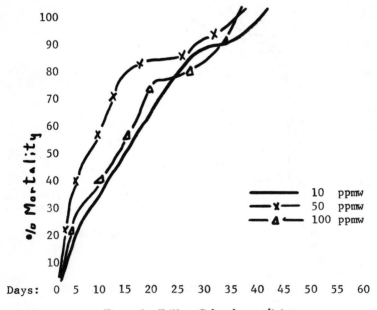

Figure 5.   E-51 vs. Cabomba caroliniana

TABLE III

E-51 vs. Cabomba caroliniana
Mortality at a given time (day)*

Day	Control	Cu++ 0.03 ppm/day	10 ppm	50 ppm	100 ppm
5	3%	10%	23%	37%	26%
10	10%	30	33	60	40
15	24	35	50	82	60
20	30	40	66	85	78
25	30	45	80	85	78
30	30	65	90	92	90
35	40	65	93	100	100
40	30	90	100	--	--
45	25	100	--	--	--
50	25	--	--	--	--

* average of replicates

The presence or absence of the "chronicity phenomenon" as noted in these studies to date is summerized in Table IV.

TABLE IV

Presence (+) or Absence (-)
of the "Chronicity Phenomenon"

Herbicide	Vallisneria	Cabomba	Milfoil	Elodea	Southern Naiad
2,4-D BEE	+	+	+	+	UNK
Diquat	+	+	+	+	+
Silvex	+	-	+	+	UNK
Fenac	+	+	+	-	+
2,4-D Acid	-	+	-	+	UNK
Endothall	-	+	-	-	+
Fenuron	-	+	UNK	+	UNK
Copper	+	+	+	+	UNK

Conclusions

The studies indicate that chronic intoxication of aquatic plants occurs and that very low doses of herbicides will destroy pest weeds given a long enough period of time. Furthermore, there is in many instances a beneficial chronic effect which minimizes the time penalty. This "chronicity phenomenon" indicates that control with slow release materials could significantly reduce environmental contamination as well as lowering costs and minimizing field hazards in handling toxicants.

Acknowledgements

Support of research on the "Chronicity Phenomenon" and controlled release aquatic herbicides by the Army, Office of the Chief of Engineers, is gratefully acknowledged.

Literature Cited

1.Walker, K.E., Cardarelli, N.F. "Development of Slow Release Copper as a Molluscicide" INCRA Ann. Rep. Proj. 203(Jul 1, 1974).
2.Janes, G.A., Bille, S.M. "Chronicity Phenomenon and Controlled Release Copper", WSSA 16th Meeting (Feb. 2-5, 1976)

Organometallic Polymers: Development of Controlled Release Antifoulants

VINCENT J. CASTELLI and WILLIAM L. YEAGER

David W. Taylor Naval Ship R&D Center, Annapolis, Md. 21402

The savings associated with the use of long-lived antifoulant coatings are quite real, especially for the Navy. Estimates of the rates of fouling for ships vary, as do the effects of these fouling rates on hull drag and the attendant increases in fuel consumption. For Navy ships, it is estimated that the increase in fuel consumption averages 8 - 10% per year from day one out of drydock. These increases are cumulative, and there is evidence that the rate increases even faster following the period of incipient antifouling coating failure. Since the current drydocking schedule for most Navy ships is five years, it is our estimate that on the average 20 - 25% of the fuel consumption per year is attributable exclusively to the fouling of the hull. Since the Navy's annual fuel bill at post energy crisis costs exceeds $700 million, this wasted fuel is costing the Navy about $150 million per year. Savings as low as 1% of these huge costs would permit extensive return-on-investment on the cost of the development of long life antifouling coatings.

The need to control the activities of plant and animal pests is well accepted. However, environmental concerns have necessitated that prudence be exercised especially when the more toxic pesticides are used. Many of these toxicants have been shown to be resistant to degradation and to possess activity toward plants and animals other than the original target specie(s). It was this concern that alerted the Navy to the problems present with its current antifouling paint systems. Antifouling paints, by their very nature, are designed to leach out a pesticide to prevent the attachment and growth of fouling organisms. The initial leaching is far in excess of the amounts required to control fouling, but since the rate of solution of the pesticide decays exponentially, large amounts of chemical are wasted in the initial phases, only to leave the coating depleted of toxin in a short period of time. Therefore, the coating is susceptable to fouling. This waste is further compounded because once these toxic substances leave the coating film, they are free to interfere with the life processes of all susceptible organisms.

THE "WHYS" OF CONTROLLED RELEASE

1. DECREASE PESTICIDE DOSE

2. LIMIT SPHERE OF ACTION

3. SAVE MONEY AND ENVIRONMENT

Figure 1

CONTROLLED RELEASE BY CHEMICAL ATTACHMENT

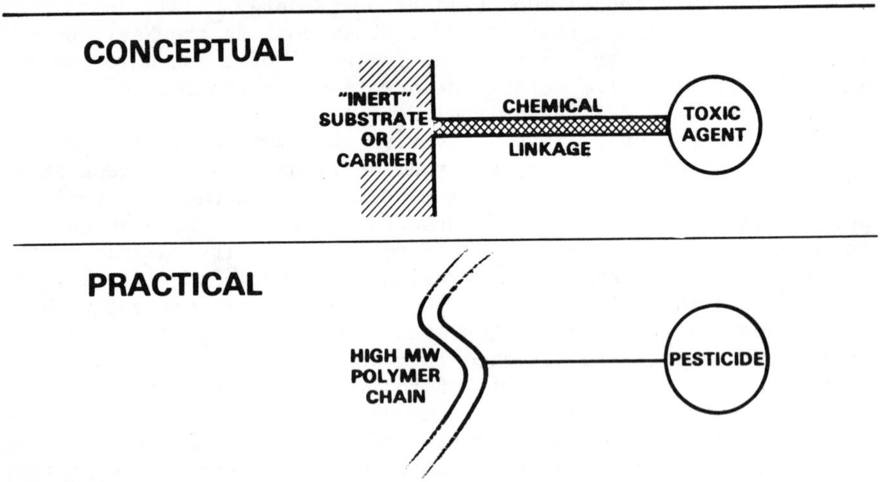

CONCEPTUAL

"INERT" SUBSTRATE OR CARRIER — CHEMICAL LINKAGE — TOXIC AGENT

PRACTICAL

HIGH MW POLYMER CHAIN — PESTICIDE

Figure 2

The idea therefore, at that time, was to produce a "non-toxic" toxicant whose effects would only be apparent on those surfaces treated with it. The quandry this posed was resolved with the idea of producing a surface which provided toxic dosages "on demand," at the instant a fouling organism started to settle. This postulated material was termed a "contact toxin," and was our first exposure to the concept of controlled release. The rationale for the controlled release approach is summarized in Figure 1.

The basic controlled release idea using chemical bonding is indicated conceptually in Figure 2. One practical rendition is also described in the same figure. This particular approach was utilized by Dyckman, et al (1972, 1974, 1975) to formulate polymeric resins whose pesticide portion was primarily organometallic toxicants, and were name organometallic polymers (OMPs). As may have been predicted, the performance of any compound of this nature will be influenced primarily by the factors described in Figure 3. These three factors all have profound effects on the ability of the system to perform effectively, but the relative contribution of each subsystem has yet to be determined. However, the characteristics of the individual pieces of the system have been well studied.

Perhaps the most intensely studied subsystem has been the pesticides, since it is ultimately their task to provide the required control. Some of the more common marine pesticides are given in Figure 4. These include the metallic materials such as copper, one of man's first antifoulants, and copper alloys, such as the various copper-nickel alloys so favored for submerged marine applications. Also included are the inorganic compounds, such as copper oxide, which presently handles over 75% of current demand for antifoulant coatings, arsenic salts, which are no longer used to any extent in marine antifouling coatings due to gross occupational hazards associated with their manufacture and application and mercuric salts, which though they have displayed fine fouling resistance suffer from the same problems as do the arsenic salts. More recent additions to the field of marine pesticides are the organic antifoulants particularly the poly-chlorinated phenols, which provide excellent control of marine plants, but possess negligible effect on most fouling animals, and the aryl and alkyl nitriles, whose benefits and drawbacks are just beginning to be explored. The newest class of antifoulants to be investigated are the organometallic pesticides, such as the trialkyl and triaryl tin compounds, which have demonstrated relatively wide spectrum activity against most species of fouling plants and animals, triaryl lead compounds, whose effectiveness has been shown to extend over a wide range of fouling organisms, and various organomercurials and organoarsenicals whose effectiveness is little disputed but which suffer from even more trouble-some manufacture and application hazards than their inorganic cousins.

FACTORS INFLUENCING
EFFECTIVE ACTION

① **PESTICIDE**

② **POLYMER TYPE**

③ **LINKAGE BETWEEN PESTICIDE**
   AND POLYMER

Figure 3

COMMON MARINE PESTICIDES

METALLIC —   Cu
                    Cu ALLOYS

INORGANIC —   CuO
                    ARSENICAL SALTS
                    MERCURIAL SALTS

ORGANIC —   POLYCHLOROPHENOLS
                    ARYL AND ALKYL NITRILES

ORGANOMETALLIC —   TRIALKYL AND TRIARYL TINS
                    TRIARYL LEADS
                    VARIOUS ORGANOMERCURIALS
                    VARIOUS ORGANOARSENICALS

Figure 4

In choosing a pesticide from the above list suitable for a controlled release formulation, certain factors need to be considered. One factor is that antifouling control should be obtained at relatively low dosage level to permit slow degradation of the controlled release formulation with attendant long service life. The Navy, for example, is presently seeking hull coatings capable of remaining fouling free for five years. Another consideration is the ability of the pesticide to provide suitable binding sites for chemical attachment. In the case of metallic and inorganic compounds, these are obviously not suitable when bonded ionicly, because of problems in maintaining effective counter-ion concentration at the surface in a medium such as sea-water. If these compounds were bonded covalently however, the effect would be the production of organometallic compounds, which might be effective agents. But by far, organic and organometallic antifoulants provide the greatest opportunity when attached through convalent chemical bonds. This is especially true for toxic compounds possessing certain types of pendants such as hydroxyl, amino and carboxylic groups, just to name a few.

The second subsystem affecting the performance of the controlled release pesticide is the "inert" polymer backbone. It is the carrier for the pesticide, and its properties determine the possible applications for the materials. Examples of polymer types, properties, and potential areas of usage are provided in Figure 5. Most present applications of plastics in the marine environment can be accomodated by the polymers listed, and for these not covered suitable modifications can be developed.

These modifications will be determined by the last element of our system, the type of chemical bond. Though, in theory, any chemical bond which can provide an adequate joint between the polymer and the pesticide is suitable, certain bond types are preferred. This preference is generally related to the ease of synthesis of the required monomers, and therefore have been limited. Those linkages which have been investigated at this Laboratory appear in Figure 6. The most encouraging results to date has been in cases where the bonding has been through an ester linkage. Field results in which the polymers have been various vinyl monomers with carboxylic groups esterfied to organometallic tin species have shown four years of 100% resistance to all forms of fouling in continuing tests. Field results of polymer systems in which the bonding has been through ether linkages is less encouraging with test samples lasting less than eighteen months. The third system in which the linkage has been through a carbon-carbon bond, has been the most disappointing with test panels not even lasting six months. With the above empirical data as a guide, emphasis at our Laboratory has been placed on refining the polymer-pesticide systems which use the ester linkage. Also work is underway investigating high performance polymeric systems - epoxies for the formulation of fouling resistant glass reinforced laminates and polyurethanes for high

POLYMER TYPES AND APPLICATION

TYPICAL POLYMERS	DESIREABLE PROPERTIES	USAGE
ACRYLICS	CLARITY	VIEWPORTS
VINYL, URETHANES	FORMS FILM	COATINGS
EPOXIES, POLYESTERS	COMPATIBILITY WITH REINFORCEMENT, STRENGTH	STRUCTURES
POLYBUTADIENES	FLEXIBILITY, WATER RESISTANCE	CABLE INSULATION, PLIANT MEMBRANES

Figure 5

INTERCONNECTING LINKAGES

$$\text{TYPES} - \quad \textcircled{1} \quad R - \overset{\overset{\textstyle O}{\|}}{C} - O\,R'$$

$$\textcircled{2} \quad R - O - R'$$

$$\textcircled{3} \quad R - R'$$

R = "INERT" CARBON BACKBONE

R' = BIOCIDE

Figure 6

performance coating applications.

With the empirical data available to date on the types of controlled release polymers described, it is beneficial to examine the possible theories which might describe the actual mode of action. The more plausible theories are outlined in Figure 7. Realistically, the true mechanism is probably a combination of some that are given.

The first postulates that the molecular weight of the majority of the polymer is low enough to permit solution of the intact toxic substituted polymer. This toxic polymer would then be free to diffuse away from the surface and then might be ingested by some potential fouling organism in which the toxic groups would be cleaved from the backbone and, disrupt the normal activities of the organism. Considering the observed long antifouling service life of some of the polymer systems of relatively high molecular weight (over 50,000 in some cases), this explanation is not entirely feasible.

The next pathway assumes that the controlled release system functions in the manner originally envisioned. Specifically, this postulates that the basic mode of bond cleavage occurs only when an organism makes intimate contact with the surface, as in attachment. It is then thought that the body fluids of the animal in some way catalyze the hydrolysis of the ester linkage and produce a local high concentration of the antifoulant which then is able to eliminate the fouling organism. After this has occurred innumerable times on the same polymer chain, the hydrophilicity of

POSSIBLE MODES OF ACTION

---

1. INTACT TOXIC POLYMER SOLVOLYSIS

2. SURFACE BIOTIC BOND CLEAVAGE (CONTACT TOXIN)

3. SURFACE ABIOTIC BOND CLEAVAGE

4. BULK ABIOTIC BOND CLEAVAGE

5. PESTICIDE DETOXIFICATION AND SUB-SEQUENT BOND CLEAVAGE

Figure 7

the chain is increased to the point where solution of the stripped
polymer chain is possible, and in so doing, a fresh, completely
toxic surface is exposed. In this model, the increase in the
hydrophilicity of the stripped polymer chain is assumed to be
sufficient to permit solvolysis, and precludes the existence
of large numbers of hydrophobic chain members, as well as limits
the chain to essentially two-dimensional structure devoid of
cross-linking. There is no evidence which discounts this theory
of the "contact toxin," in fact, bouyed by the long resistance to
fouling exhibited by many of the test panels, may indeed be
wholly or partially responsible for their apparent success.

The third pathway assumes that the fouling resistance of
these polymers is the result of a normal degree of weathering to
which all materials exposed in the marine environment are
subjected. The chemical forces which are responsible for this
degradation are also responsible for the slow hydrolysis of the
linkage anchoring the pesticide. This would provide a slow but
nearly constant outflow of pesticide from the surface which would
be in excess of the lethal concentration for the fouling organisms.
This model also assumes that after a sufficient number of
hydrolyses of the toxic pendant groups occurs the hydrophilicity
is sufficient to permit solvolysis. Also assumed is an absence
of large numbers of hydrophobic chain members as well as a limit
of the chain to essentially two-dimensional structure, devoid of
cross-linking. The available evidence does not discount this
model, and may in fact be used to support it. Since the
phenomenon of weathering is known to be essentially a slow
process, it is possible for a material to display the observed
antifouling action, and may be partially or wholly responsible
for the performance indicated.

Another model postulates that these polymeric materials can
be envisioned as tight sponges in which the "holes" are filled
by chemically bound toxicant. The toxicant bond to the polymer
is cleaved through some hydrolysis mechanism and slowly diffuses
from the boundary layer in contact with the surface into the sea-
water environment. This exposes new pendant toxicants which are
then cleaved, and then diffused, etc. All during this time
period, the stripped polymer chains remain intact on the surface.
After sufficient time has elapsed, the stripped polymer network
appears as a sponge of sorts in which the necessary agents which
affect hydrolysis are diffusing into the matrix, and the
hydrolyzed pesticide is diffusing out of the network. This model
differs in one important aspect from the currently recognized
model of conventional antifouling paints in that the rate of
toxicant outflow from the controlled release polymer is governed
by the chemical hydrolysis of the polymer-pesticide bond, not
simply the dissolution of the toxicant. This theory also is
supported by evidence from the field which indicates that even
the most highly cross-lined organometallic polymer resins are
effective antifoulants after four years of marine exposure in a

continuing series of tests.

The last model proposed is more "blue sky" than any of the preceding in that it postulates that it is the toxic surface it-self which prevents fouling by giving the fouling organisms a "bad taste" when they attempt to settle on the surface, and effectively preventing all fouling. The degradation of the surface would be concentrated primarily on the pesticide and would detoxify the agent before it ever left the surface. In effect, this would be an antifoulant which would only be toxic on the surface to which it was applied, and have only the most minor of environmental impacts, since the leachate from the surface would be of low inherent toxicity. This model cannot be elimina-ted from the data available at present, but should possibly be taken as a goal to strive for, rather than celebrating it as one achieved.

Literature Cited

1. Dyckman, E.J., J.A. Montemarano and D.E. Gilbert, "Biologically Active Polymeric Coating Materials," NSRDC Rept #4526, Apr 1975
2. Dyckman, E.J. and J.A. Montemarano, "Antifouling Organo-metallic Polymers: Environmentally Compatible Materials," NSRDC Rept $4186, Feb 1974
3. Dyckman, E.J., J.A. Montemarano, D.M. Andersen and A.M. Miller, "Non-Polluting Antifouling Organometallic Polymers," NSRDC Rept #3581, Nov 1972
4. Montemarano, J.A. and E.J. Dyckman, "Antislime Organometallic Polymer of Optical Quality," NSRDC Rept #3597, Sep 1972

21

Function of Low Polymer Fractions in Releases from Polymer Materials

MAX KRONSTEIN

Manhattan College, New York, N.Y. 10471

The paper is concerned with the releases from polymeric materials, when immersed in organic sweller solvents or in water. These releases are a function of the lower polymer fraction within such polymeric materials. They refer to such compounds which have been formed by the development of a high polymer fraction within an initial low polymer fluid which represents the monomer form or its minor modifications in this development and remains still present within the polymer material even when other fractions have already progressed to a higher polymer form. Such formations are here being referred to as "heterophase polymeric materials". These polymer formations with their fluid fraction are of particular interest because they relate to formations which occur in nature as well as in synthetic materials. Hereby the starting material is molecularly dispersible or "soluble", and the developing polymer matter is no longer molecularly dispersible or no longer "soluble" and is capable of increasing its volume in contact with the liquid sweller substance. Even though both have the appearance of a uniform material they consist of more than one phase each of which participates in the development of the characteristics of the product.

The question arises how far the lower polymer sweller fraction remains stable over extended periods of time when no exposure to specific energy applications takes place. That is, whether heterophase polymer materials will, on aging, remain in the state of mixed fractions or if under such conditions the low polymer fraction will continue to progress in polymerization and will so change the ratio between the fractions. The paper shows that, indeed, heterophase polymer materials – synthetic as well as natural ones – can maintain their condition over very long periods of time and that even afterwards it is still possible to separate their fluid sweller fraction under the same methods as established previously, and subsequently the so-isolated fluid fraction can chemically be reacted into higher polymeric forms in the same manner as in reacting their initial low polymer form. These facts are being studied experimentally in laboratory tests in the

248

first section of the paper. In a second experimental section,
various factors of this presentation are then tested also by
studying the behavior of the modified elastomeric polymers and
their released fractions under extended outdoor underwater exposure and, in particular, the resulting behavior of such selected
materials against the attack of fouling organisms.

Section I. Laboratory Investigations

The laboratory investigations concern: (a) the release of a
sweller fraction from a natural crepe rubber, (b) the varying
forms of releases from a polyether urethane compound when different forms of organo metal components have been introduced, (c)
the heterophase polymer character of selected natural resins,
and (e) of heterophase polymeric residues of the petroleum distillation.

The Release of the Sweller Fraction from Natural Crepe Rubber. In preceding papers the heterophase character of a synthetic polyisoprene, the introduction of organo metal acetates, and
the release of the soluble fraction without and with the attached
organo metal groupings have been studied (1)(2). The present
study is concerned with investigations on a natural No. IX Thick
Pale Crepe rubber. Such material is obtained by the coagulation
of the Hevea Plantation rubber latex with subsequent washing and
drying of the coagulum. Hereby the rubber globules of the latex
stage fuse into one crude rubber which has a homogeneous appearance (3). In view of this fused condition the presence of the
tridimensional insoluble fraction and of the fluid lower polymer
fraction is less readily detectable. However after the crude rubber is immersed in benzene (benzol) and allowed to swell to a
stage where it is dispersed in the solvent, the high polymer fraction can be precipitated by the addition of a poorer sweller
fluid. The precipitate can then be separated and studied. Viewed
under the electron microscope such particles are tridimensional
in appearance, but they are noncrystalline and therefore the electron diffraction pattern shows no indication of the "spot" formations typical for all crystalline materials. (Figure 1)

Studies of the presence and the release of the fluid fraction
are influenced by the fused state of the produced crepe rubber.
A specimen of fused rubber rotated in distilled water for 3 days
shows in the infrared spectrum of its ether-extracted matter,
the presence of the released rubber around 2950 cm^{-1}; the expected band around 1750 cm^{-1} is very little developed. But when
the crepe rubber has been loosened by swelling in benzol and
after driving off the sweller the resulting gel under water immersion releases an increased ratio of the lower polymer fraction and
gives an increased band at around 1750 cm^{-1}. When an organo
metal grouping is being introduced, using tributyllead acetate
(10% of the rubber solids in the dispersion), the underwater release from the new gel material shows in its ether extracted

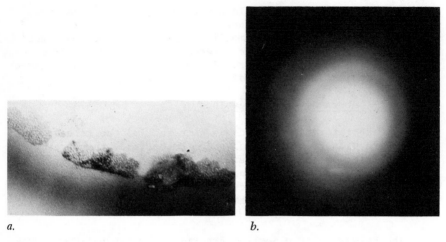

a.   b.

*Figure 1. Natural crepe rubber: (a) precipitated phase (125,000×); (b) its electron dif-
fraction pattern*

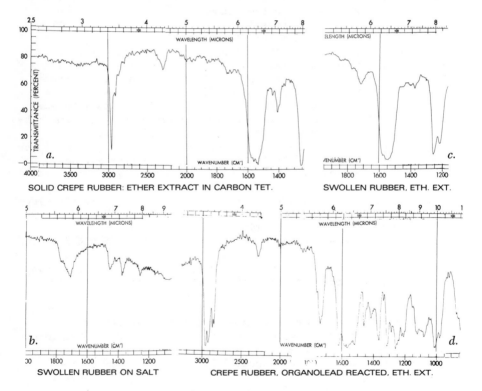

Figure 2. Infrared spectra of released fractions of natural crepe rubber

matter the 1750 cm^{-1} band where the lower polymer fraction has reacted strongly with the new groupings besides the same bands as
had been observed on organo lead modifications of elastomers (4).
The infrared spectra are made with the P-E Model 621 grating spectrophotometer. The released lead content in the exposure water
is determined using the dithizone test of ASTM C-555-64 T.
(Figure 2)

Comparative studies have been made of a synthetic elastomeric
polymer material with introduced triphenyllead acetate groupings:
studying once the released matter from an immersion in water and
again from immersion of the applied polymer in an organic solvent
which is, in particular, a solvent for the low polymer fractions.
The spectra of two recovered releases (in water and in hexane)
show that the low polymeric fraction has been released together
with the incorporated organolead grouping. The release in hexane
is hereby considerably higher in the ratio of release than in
water. (Figure 3)

The Influence of the Introduced Organometal Component on a
Polyurethane Resin. In the preceding studies the organo metal
grouping is introduced into the lower polymer fraction of the
heterophase polymers in the form of organo metal acylates such as
triphenyllead acetate, dibutyltin diacetate, and others. The resulting released matter combines the organic spectrum as well as
the organo metal grouping of the developing polymer. On the other
hand the author has shown that many thermoplastic polymer resins
as well as elastomeric polymers increase rapidly into highly developed tridimensional formations when reacted with tetra alkyl
titanates (5)(6). It is therefore of interest to explore whether
or not such gel formation with alkyl titanates also will release,
under water, corresponding lower polymeric and organo metal group-
carrying fractions which can be identified in their infrared spectra. For this investigation a fluid polyether urethane was selected. The resin as obtained has a low ratio of tridimensional
to liquid fraction. When dispersed 1:1 in benzol, the addition of
petroleum ether or of acetone causes a limited precipitation; and
when this is left on a glass slide over night, no gelation of the
precipitate is visible. But when this resin is exposed to the infrared light of the GE R-40 250 watt lamp at 50°C. the ratio of
tri-dimensional matter increases considerably and can be precipitated from a benzol dispersion. Such a precipitate fuses on the
slide into a coherent film. This demonstrates the available re-
activity in the initial product. Gelation products were prepared
with organo metal acylates as well as with tetra alkyl titanates.
Both were immersed in water and their releases were studied under
the infrared spectrophotometer. The released matter from the
gelation product with tributyllead acetate shows in the IR spectrum the typical bands of the urethane groupings as well as of the
organo lead matter, but the gelation product with a tetraethyl-
hexyl titanate does not show the corresponding bands. This form
of gelation is therefore of a different nature due to the
specific nature of the titanate itself. (Figure 4 and 5)

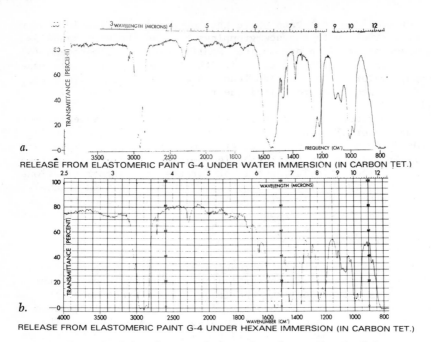

Figure 3.   Infrared spectra of releases from elastomeric paint G-4

Recovering the Lower Polymer Fraction from Aged Polymer Formations: An Aged Highly Polymerized Polystyrene. Without the introduction of any of these organo metal groups into the heterophase polymers, the low polymer fraction itself remains unchanged
and is therefore being released into organic sweller solvents as
well as into water in its own form. On the other hand, experiences in the large scale production of polystyrene and polystyrene
-butadiene rubbers have shown that the styrene vapors on sudden
cooling can be obtained in highly insolubilized polymer forms,
which because of their appearance have been referred to as popcorn
styrene.   In 1948 the author has shown that gelled or solid drying
oil polymers (that is, insoluble polymers of unsaturated glycer-

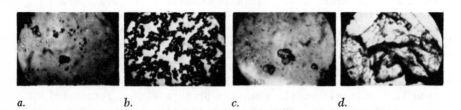

a.   b.   c.   d.

Figure 4.   Fluid polyurethane (450×): (a) fresh precipitate; (b) same, after exposure to
ir; (c) on glass slide 24 hr; (d) ir-exposed precipitate, left on slide 24 hr

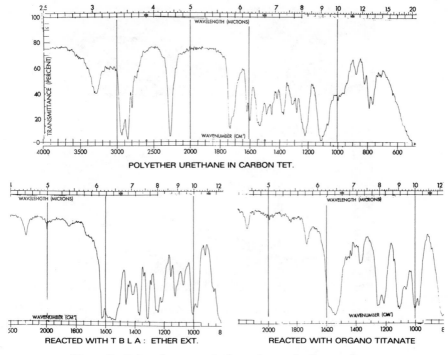

POLYETHER URETHANE IN CARBON TET.

REACTED WITH T B L A : ETHER EXT.

REACTED WITH ORGANO TITANATE

Figure 5.   Infrared spectra of releases from polyether urethane

ine fatty acid ester-oils) can be redispersed by heating them with
metal soaps whereafter they may be "diluted" with volatile solvents.   Film forming dispersions had so been obtained and such resulting films contain the dispersed high polymer units imbedded
solidly within the films.   When strips of such films are immersed
in freshly distilled monostyrene there occurs at around 50°C. a
formation of film-shaped infusible polystyrene, following in its
pattern that of the immersed polymer film.   Such a formation which
had been prepared in 1948, that is about 27 years ago (7), has now
been studied in order to determine how far this early formation
of insoluble polystyrene still contains a lower polymer fraction
or if during the long storage in the laboratory the polymerization
has progressed and has insolubilized this initially soluble fraction.   On breaking off parts of the old polystyrene sample, pow-
dering it, and dispersing it in carbon tetrachloride the recovered
monostyrene was found within the IR spectrum of this dispersion;
and in swelling the old polystyrene in benzol the low polymer
fraction was released into the sweller, isolated, and identified
from there. (Figure 6 and 7)

<u>Heterophase Condition of a Polymer Tung Oil Gel after 25</u>
<u>Years in the Soil</u>.   The behavior of a low polymer sweller fraction
has been studied under more severe storage conditions in the case

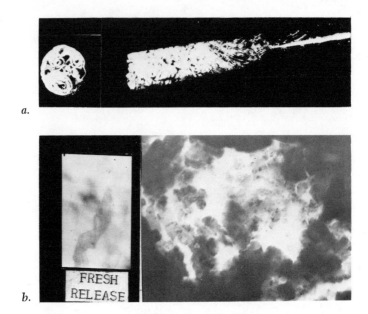

Figure 6. Grown polystyrene of 1949: (a) whole sample, and in cross-section; (b) electron micrograph (100,000×), with inset (450×)

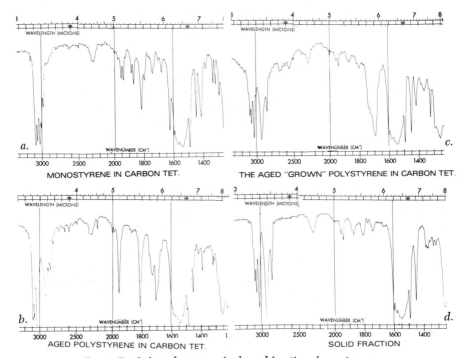

Figure 7. Infrared spectra of released fractions from styrene

of a polymer Chinawood oil, which was recovered after having been
spilled during production into the earth a long time ago. The
Chinawood-, or tung, oil is the most readily polymerizing drying
oil, since it is an alpha-elaeostearic acid triglyceride having
three conjugated double bonds in each of its three acid groups.
On heating, it turns readily into an insoluble gel. However in
this coherent gel form it shows, when dispersed in a solvent upon
precipitation under an electron microscope, the solid high polymer
units surrounded by a fluid fraction and it is possible to study
the progress of the formation of its solid phase progressingly
under varying heating conditions. For the present studies on the
stability of its fluid fraction a special gelled form has been
used. About forty years ago when the author was in charge of a
varnish factory in Europe considerable amounts of Chinawood oil
were prepolymerized into a heat bodied oil, heating it in venti-
lated kettels under carbon dioxide gradually to a viscosity somewhat higher than the Z-2 viscosity of heat-bodied linseed oil. It
was then transferred to 500 gallon storage tanks which had been
placed on shelves above the bare ground under a wooden roof. When
the crew took out some of the pretreated oil regularly, they evi-
dently spilled some oil which sank into the ground. But when 25
years later the factory was enlarged and the soil excavated con-
glomerates of solid polymerized oil were recovered, and some of it
was sent to the author's lab. On removing the earth and washing
the product with solvent to remove some residual stickiness, the
solvent was again removed. The obtained material represents a
solidified reddish conglomerate instead of the fluid bodied oil
form which sank into the ground. When now the recovered conglom-
erates were broken into fine particles and pressed between salt
crystals, their IR spectrum shows only minor differences from that
of a freshly prepared oil gel. And when swollen in benzol for 3
weeks, it is possible to recover from the sweller solvent a freed
fluid oil which has a spectrum very similar to that of fluid tung
oil. This establishes that despite the extended exposure the
fluid fraction of the polymerized material is still present.
(Figures 8, 9 and 10)

Application of the Test Methods to Heterophase Natural Polymers. Extending the study further into the preservation of heterophase polymeric conditions over extended periods of time, a natural fossil polymer resin has been studied, the Congo copal gum.
This fossil plant-derived resin is obtained in diggings from
swampy ground in the spring flood area of the Congo River in central Africa. For the present studies the underground harvested
gum was used in a clear, transparent grade known as Grade No. 1.
Despite the large amounts of gum used around the world the knowledge of its chemical nature is limited to the facts that it is insoluble in common varnish solvents and that it can be made soluble
by a partial breaking down of the polymer gum. Certain long chain
acids have been identified from this resin, but its polymeric and

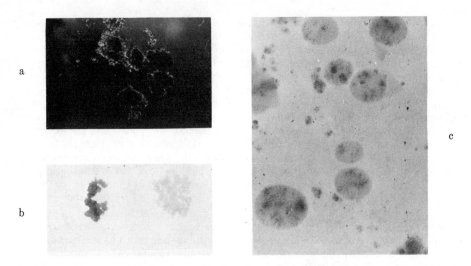

Figure 8.   Aged Chinawood oil (tung oil) gel: (a) solids viewed against light (5×); (b) after 25 years in the soil; (c) precipitated fresh gel (100,000×)

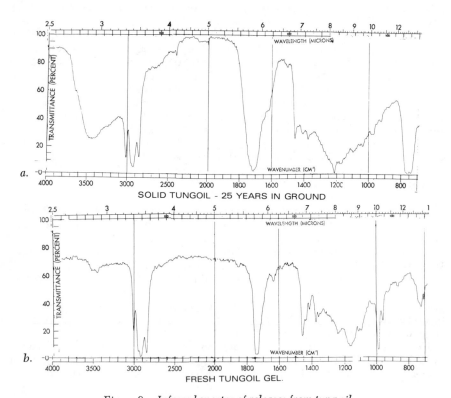

Figure 9.   Infrared spectra of releases from tung oil

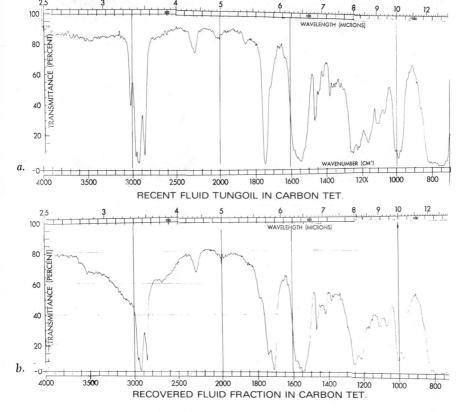

Figure 10.   Infrared spectra of releases from tung oil

in particular its heterophase nature has not been investigated. When, now, the powdered fossil gum was entered into benzol as a sweller fluid and exposed there for 3 days at a temperature of 38°C, the lower polymeric fraction enters the solvent, and can from there be isolated as an oil. This then can further be poly-merized with di-t-butyl peroxide whereby it turns into a trans-parent resin. Infrared spectra indicate, in the isolated fluid oil, strong characteristic bands around 1800 cm^{-1} which are not defined in the powdered Congo copal gum; the spectra of the perox-ide treated fluid fraction are nearly the same as of the gum. On stirring the powdered fossil gum in water for 1 month, the ether extract indicates released matter with a strong band at 3000 cm^{-1} and between 1750 and 1600 cm^{-1}. (Figures 11, 12, 13 and 14)

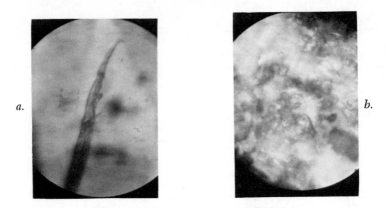

*Figure 11.   Congo copal gum (450×): (a) swollen in benzol; (b) oily
fluid further polymerized*

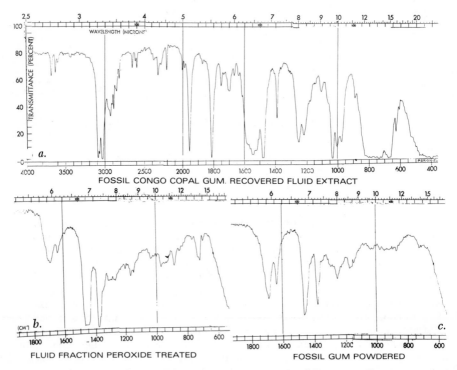

Figure 12.   Infrared spectra of releases from fossil Congo copal gum

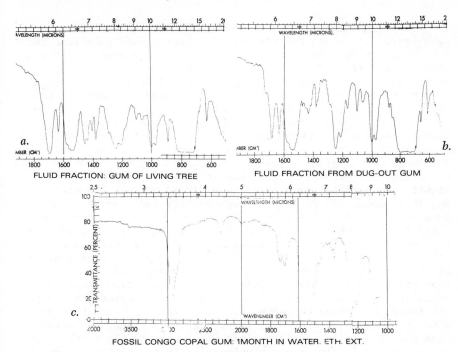

Figure 13.   Infrared spectra of the separated fluid fraction

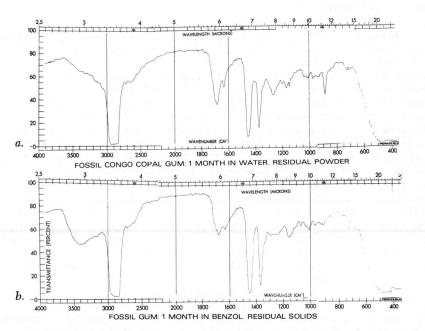

Figure 14.   Infrared spectra of fossil gum after fluid fraction has been removed

A polymerizing resin derived from an insect secretion
(shellac): In nature the formation of heterophase polymeric resins is not limited to plant exudations. Another resin which was
studied is derived from the secretion of an insect, the *laccifer
laca*, and is hardening on trees and shrubs in India where the insect protects its larvae by the resinous covering. When it has
been scraped off, the natives obtain a thermoplastic resin from it
which, in warm state, they form into sheets, whereafter the
hardened sheets are broken into the well known flakes of shellac.
(The material used in the tests is a Lemon No. 1 Orange Flake
Shellac). It is alcohol-soluble and its output from India amounts
to millions of pounds a year. But it is known that this thermoplastic and soluble resin turns on extended storage and on heating it at about 150°C. into a tough rubbery and insoluble gel.
This indicates that its earlier form has contained an unsaturated
fluid fraction which is capable of undergoing further polymerization under limited heat application. Since it is capable of
allowing an entry of an organometal acrylate grouping, a mixture
of shellac with 10% tributyllead acetate was included in the gelation tests. The straight shellac gel and the gelled shellac-
organolead product were immersed in water and rotated for 5 days.
Afterwards the released matter was recovered from both by ethyl
ether extracts and studied by IR spectroscopy. That the organolead modified gelled shellac gives off lead into the water at a
gradual rate of release was studied also by the dithizone test.
All these tests confirm the heterophase polymer character of the
products. (Figure 15)

Release Studies on the Heterophase Polymer Residues of Petroleum Asphalts. Finally, the release of a low polymeric matter
under water immersion was studied also on petroleum asphalts. The
author has pointed out in an earlier presentation already that
these petroleum asphalts represent colloidal substances of heterophase polymeric nature. Hereby the tri-dimensional insoluble
fraction has been referred to by an earlier author as the "as-
phaltenes" fraction and the still soluble fraction of these asphalts has been referred to as "maltenes" (8). In the present
work such a petroleum asphalt has been used in its initial state,
and in a second form the polymeric fraction has been increased by
reacting the asphalt with dicumyl peroxide. Even though this
treatment increases the softening point from 41.5°C to 53°C and
lowers the penetration index (0°C) from 166 to 66.5, upon water
immersion the released fractions from both have the same infrared
spectrum. It indicates that the peroxide treatment has increased
the ratio of higher polymer fraction without essentially changing
the residual low polymer and the released fraction. (Figure 16)

SectionII. Underwater Outdoor Exposures

The aforementioned laboratory experiments established general
principles of the release of low polymer fractions from heterophase polymer coatings. They were studied further under seawater

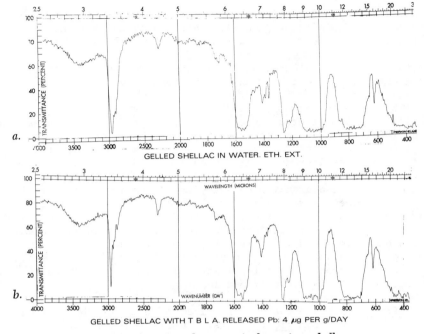

a.   GELLED SHELLAC IN WATER. ETH. EXT.

b.   GELLED SHELLAC WITH T B L A. RELEASED Pb: 4 μg PER g/DAY

Figure 15.   Infrared spectra of releases from shellac

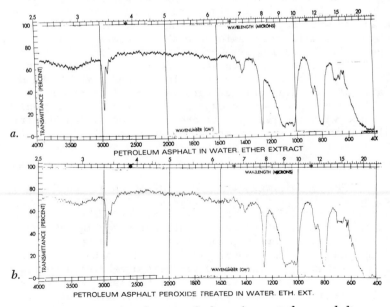

a.   PETROLEUM ASPHALT IN WATER. ETHER EXTRACT

b.   PETROLEUM ASPHALT PEROXIDE TREATED IN WATER. ETH. EXT.

Figure 16.   Infrared spectra of releases from petroleum asphalt

exposure of applied coatings. By using in particular an organolead toxicant such as triphenyllead acetate (TPLA) for these
tests, the underwater released fractions were tested for their resistance to the growth of algae and of barnacles in highly fouling
waters in the coastal area of Connecticut throughout the fouling
season of 1975. The following observations were made:

The Influence of organolead toxicant in antifouling paints.
The introduction of organometallic toxicant groupings, such as
using TPLA, provided in elastomeric polymer vehicles and in a
vinyl copolymer paint - without wood rosin - satisfactory fouling
resistance. The introduction of metallic lead powder as a toxicant in a vinyl copolymer antifouling paint was ineffective.
Without the organo-grouping no entry of the lead was possible into
the lower molecular fraction of the vehicle-polymer. Replacing a
considerable part of the vinyl copolymer - following present paint
practices - by wood rosin increased the rate of released contamination nine times. Nevertheless the exposed panels showed, at
least on the shaded side of the exposure site, a higher rate of
algal growth than on the all-polymer vehicle paint, despite its
low release rate. (Figure 17 and 18)

Effect of the Amount of Organolead Toxicant on the Fouling
Resistance of Elastomeric Coatings. In the same Connecticut
coastal area, early in 1974, the underwater section of a ship was
painted with an elastomeric paint G-4 containing TPLA as the only
toxicant. This paint contained 10% of the solids in the form of
TPLA and no growth of marine fouling was observed throughout the
spring and summer fouling seasons. During the 1975 fouling season, one-fourth of the shipbottom (toward the bow) was exposed
for a season with the 1974 G-4 coating. The remaining three-
fourths of the hull was repainted with elastomeric coatings containing 2.5%, 5% and 10% TPLA, respectively. At the end of the
1975 fouling season, the ship was inspected. No growth was de-
tected on any of these four areas. In another test at the Miami
test site of the Naval Ship Research and Development Center,
epoxy fiberglass panels were exposed in duplicate groups which
were coated with the test paint: one group containing 10% triphenyllead acetate, another group having 2.5% TPLA. After 11
months exposure the panels are reported to have 100% fouling resistance.

Introduction of Organolead Toxicant in Water-Based Elastomeric Paints. Porous concrete blocks, coated with new water-
based elastomeric paints containing TPLA, were free of blistering,
were nonporous, and showed no sign of marine fouling at the end of
the 1975 fouling season in Connecticut coastal waters. Corresponding coatings with dibutyl tin diacetate as toxicant showed
after this exposure period - due to their accelerated toxicant release rates - increasing development of fouling. When the same
water-based paints had been applied on the concrete blocks,

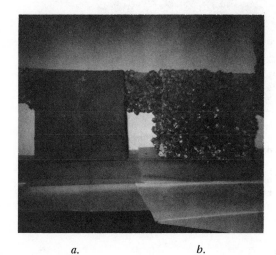

a.   *b.*

Figure 17.   Underwater exposures of vinyl copolymer paints: (a) with organolead; (b) with metallic lead

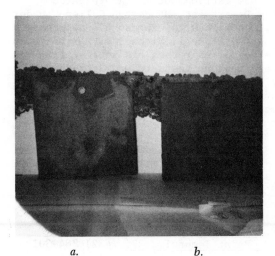

a.   *b.*

Figure 18.   Underwater exposures of vinyl copolymer paints: (a) with organolead with rosin; (b) with organolead without rosin

a.   *b.*   *c.*   *d.*

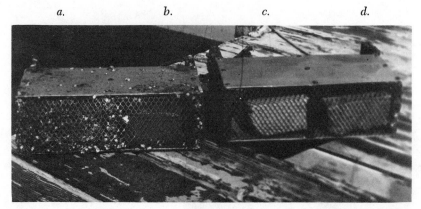

Figure 19. Water-based elastomeric antifouling coatings on concrete (in exposure boxes) after exposure season 1975: (a,b) formulation with organotin without and with top coat; (b,c) formulation with organolead, without and with top coat

followed by a top coat, using either the same TPLA paints as used on the ship tests or using the same paint formulation but containing a triphenyltin acetate as toxicant, both of these topcoated blocks were free of fouling   (Figure 19).

Acknowledgements

The work discussed here was carried out in the research laboratories of the Chemistry Department, Manhattan College, under the direction of the author, who wishes to express his appreciation to his assistants James P. O'Connell, Michael A. Marchiarullo and Mary Beth Siegrist. The author expresses his appreciation for cooperation in the underwater exposure tests to Dr. Schrade F. Radtke and Dr. Dodd S. Carr of the International Lead Zinc Research Organization, Inc. and to Dr. Eugene C. Fischer of the U.S. Naval Research and Development Center in Annapolis, Maryland for the exposures in Miami test site.

Literature Cited

(1) Kronstein, M., Chem. Abstr. 77, 153992Q (1972).
(2) Kronstein, M., ACS, ORPL Preprints, 35, (2)(1975).
(3) Van Rossem, A., ACS Monograph Series No. 74, p 11, Reinhold
              Publishing Corp., New York (1937).
(4) Kronstein, M., ACS, ORPL Preprints, 35, (2) p. 70 (1975).
(5) Kronstein, M., et al., J. Paint Technol., 37, (482) 284-301
              (1965).
(6) Kronstein, M., et al., J. Paint Technol., 38, (492) 37-42
              (1966).
(7) Kronstein, M., Chem. Abstr. 44, 5608h.
(8) Pfeiffer, J. Ph., "The Properties of Asphaltic Bitumen,"
              Elsevier, New York (1950).

Use of Pheromones in Insect Control Programs: Slow Release Formulations

B. A. BIERL, E. D. DeVILBISS, and J. R. PLIMMER

Agric. Environ. Qual. Inst., USDA, Beltsville, Md. 20705

Among the newer strategies for insect pest management are techniques that make use of naturally occurring compounds that affect the behavior of insects. These compounds are extremely specific in their action and have minimal impact on non-target species. They must be protected during the period required for activity because they are usually readily degradable by oxidants or sunlight. For this purpose, synthetic or natural polymers may be used as permeable coatings to protect labile materials and permit their controlled release. The U.S. Department of Agriculture supports a number of pest control programs involving the use of insect attractants. Such compounds are ideally suited for incorporation in controlled-release formulations. We have examined a number of these formulations and studied some properties that affect the practical application of polymeric formulations for release of attractants, including the emission rate and its dependence on temperature and other parameters. It is to be anticipated that more sophisticated theoretical treatment can ultimately provide a direction for improved technology.

During the past decade, increased knowledge of the chemical basis of sensory communication among insects has contributed to the science of pest management. Mating behavior, aggregation attraction to sites for feeding or oviposition, and other forms of insect behavior are mediated by chemicals known as "pheromones". Such chemicals are used for communication among members of the same species. In particular, some lepidopteran species are equipped with well-developed antennae which can detect pheromones at extremely low concentrations. Often a specific blend of two or three chemicals is used by a particular insect species. However, in the case of the gypsy moth, <u>Lymantria dispar</u> (L.), evidence to date indicates that a single compound, identified as cis-7,8-epoxy-2-methyloctadecane, disparlure, is the sex pheromone emitted by the virgin female to attract the male (<u>1</u>).

The last decade has witnessed considerable advancement in our knowledge of the chemistry of natural pheromones, largely because instrumental techniques have improved to the extent that microgram quantities of material can be used for structural studies. The minute amounts of pheromones that are secreted by the insect may be obtained by extraction or by collection of volatiles emitted by caged insects. Sex attractant pheromones are emitted by insects of one sex to attract the other and stimulate mating. The value of virgin female moths as baits for trapping was recognized during the eighteenth century. The use of synthetic chemicals as attractants for trapping insects is a well-established practice and the identification of pheromones has supplemented and extended the value of this technique.

Insect traps containing chemical baits are used for surveying or monitoring insect infestations. In some cases, grids of traps may be adequate to achieve some degree of population control by mass trapping. Damage to ornamental or economic plants may thus be reduced. Trapping for survey purposes is important if insecticide applications are to be used effectively. Reductions in cost and in chemical contamination of the environment can be achieved if insecticides are applied on a local basis only when the need exists.

The use of attractant traps for proper timing of insecticidal spray applications has achieved considerable savings in the cost of insecticides used to control fruit flies (2). Other benefits may be cited. For example, regular applications of orchard sprays to control the codling moth, Laspeyresia pomonella (L.), have affected the balance of population of other insects with the result that some of these have now become major pests. Traps baited with the sex attractant pheromone, trans,trans-8,10-dodecadien-1-ol (codlelure) (3,4) have been used to improve timing of pesticide applications and to reduce their frequency. Thus, savings in costs have also been accompanied by benefits in pest management practices (5,6,7).

A promising technique for control of some insect species is the use of pheromones for reduction of mating. Permeation of the infested area with sex attractant pheromones or related compounds may lead to disorientation of the male and a reduction in frequency of mating. Effective reduction of mating should result in a decline of the pest population. Experimental evaluation of this technique has demonstrated its ability to reduce mating of the gypsy moth, the pink bollworm, Pectinophora gossypiella (Saunders), and other insect pests. In one experiment (8), the sex pheromone of the pink bollworm, gossyplure, was evaporated into the air from evaporators spaced at 40 m. intervals in all cotton fields in the Coachella Valley of California. The amount of larval boll infestation was comparable to that provided by conventional insecticide applications and there was about a month delay in the onset of larval infestations in the bolls, as compared to previous years.

Mating reduction of the gypsy moth has been successfully achieved using formulations of the sex pheromone, disparlure (9, 10). Disparlure is a stable liquid of relatively low volatility

that can be evaporated slowly into the air from a wick or reservoir. However, consistently successful application of a
control technique based on air permeation must depend on formulations of 'delivery systems' that can be used under a variety of
environmental conditions.

Demonstration of the value of a particular chemical in pest
control is of great scientific interest, but practical application is necessary to prove its worth. The use of pheromones has
great promise since they are species-specific and will not ad-
versely affect predators or beneficial insects. Environmentally,
they present a few problems since they are effective at application rates of few grams per acre (2 to 16 grams per acre in
the case of disparlure). Chemicals that are readily degradable
in the environment and that can be used at such extremely low
rates of application offer valuable alternatives to conventional
pest control chemicals. Therefore, research efforts to demonstrate the use and practical application of pheromones as alternative techniques of pest control are being undertaken in many
parts of the U.S. Success depends in part on the use of the
correct pheromone or blend, combined with a reliable technique
for release into the environment.

Our research on formulation of insect pheromones had the
following two major objectives. The first was to achieve optimum
rates of release from a dispenser that could be used in a survey
trap. The second was to provide a formulation that would permeate the forest atmosphere with the desired concentration of
pheromone throughout the mating period of the insect.

The principal topic of the discussion to follow is the gypsy
moth and its attractant pheromone, disparlure. The gypsy moth
is a serious pest of forest, shade, and orchard trees in the
northeastern U. S. and in Europe. Larvae emerge in early May
from eggs laid in the previous year. Leaves are consumed by the
larvae and the resulting defoliation kills many trees. The
larvae pupate and emerge as adult moths in early summer; a
flight period of six to eight weeks follows. The male is a strong
flier but in North America, at least, the female does not normally
fly. The female emits the pheromone to attract the male for
mating. For effective use of disparlure in traps, the rate of
emission of disparlure from the source must be similar to that
from the female moth and should remain at that level throughout
the mating period. Several types of dispensers have been used. [1]
The one in current use (the Hercon Ⓡ dispenser, manufactured by
the Hercon Div. of Health-Chem Corp., New York, N.Y., 10010)
has proved effective for the controlled emission of disparlure
and a number of other insect pheromones (11). It consists of a
plastic laminate fabricated in three layers; two outer plastic

---

[1]/ Mention of a proprietary product does not imply endorse-
ment by the USDA.

layers cover an inner layer impregnated with disparlure. The
rate of emission of lure is controlled by its concentration and
by the thickness of the outer layers (Table I).

Table I. Emission Rate of Hercon Dispenser

% Lure	mils	Per Dispensers mg lure	µg/hr *	Season Used
2.4	7	3.4	0.10	–
2.0	12	4.8	0.09	–
2.0	21	7.4	0.08	1974
5.0	7	7.0	0.24	–
6.0	13	14.4	0.22	–
3.9	6	6.2	0.22	1975

* Emission rate at room temperature

By using a simple technique for trapping and measurement of released pheromone (12), we have shown that the emission rate of
disparlure from a Hercon® dispenser under controlled conditions
is relatively constant (13, 14). The emission rate of disparlure
from the dispensers used in 1974 field tests was very low
(0.1 µg/hr) in proportion to the amount of material originally
present. Although the rate of emission remained constant over
extremely long periods, the loss of disparlure was low. Approximately 90% of the lure remained in dispensers that had hung in
traps for the entire season.
     Current studies of emission rates have taken into account
not only concentration and thickness of outer layers of the dispenser but also factors such as temperature and air movement.
     The dispensers used in 1975 field tests, manufactured in
1975, again contained 6 mg disparlure but the thickness of the
laminate was only 6 mils. From such a dispenser, the rate of
emission was 0.24 µg/hr at 80°F in a constant flow of dry air
at 100 ml/min (Table II).

Table II. Temperature Dependence of 1975 Hercon Dispensers

Temp	µg/hr *
80° F	0.24
90° F	0.45
100° F	0.83

Rate of Increase: 1.8 µg/hr per 10° F

* Emission rate for dispenser containing 6.2 mg of
   lure

The rate approximately doubled with each increment of 10°F., and
at 100°F, the rate was 0.83 µg/hr. Under our experimental condi-

tions, the increase in emission rate with flow rate was linear.

Emission rates for efficient trapping cannot be arrived at by precise laboratory measurement. Biological and atmospheric variations will be responsible for wide fluctuations in the concentration of the natural pheromone. Overall constancy of emission rate from the dispenser must be maintained throughout the flight period, but emission must also be maintained at an adequate rate over the range of environmental conditions encountered in the field. Hercon Ⓡ dispensers appear to satisfy these conditions. Thus, current dispenser technology appears adequate but there are other subtle factors which may enter into the consideration of insect trapping efficiency.

Mating disruption techniques that rely on permeation of the forest environment by pheromones are subject to similar limitations. The technical problem is that of providing a uniform concentration of pheromone in the forest atmosphere throughout the flight period of the gypsy moth. Conventional formulations, such as those used for pesticides would require application at frequent intervals. Since this is impractical, a controlled-release formulation is essential. The effects of environmental conditions on such formulations would be expected to be even more important than those observed with the Hercon Ⓡ dispensers. It is important that an effective level of pheromone be maintained in the forest atmosphere during the entire flight period of the moth.

One of the most promising methods of controlled release of insect pheromones is microencapsulation. Although various methods of encapsulation are available, our own research has been primarily directed toward the study of the behavior of gelatin-walled microcapsules containing a 2% solution of disparlure in xylene/amyl acetate. The capsules range from 25 to 250 microns in size and are formulated by the National Cash Register Corp., Dayton, Ohio. The formulation was applied as an aerial spray at the rate of 2 to 16 grams disparlure per acre. To improve the performance of the microencapsulated material during application and in the field, thickeners and stickers were added. Such additives will affect rates of emission and our laboratory studies were aimed at accumulating comparative data on formulations of varying composition. Ultimately we hope to correlate laboratory data with field behavior so that the performance of candidate formulations may be predicted from the laboratory results.

During the 1975 field season, microencapsulated disparlure was applied by air over large acreages in Pennsylvania, Massachusetts, New Jersey, and Maryland; by taking field samples, we had an opportunity to observe the behavior of microcapsules under practical conditions. Subsequently, these observations were supplemented by laboratory measurements. However, our ultimate goal is to study the distribution of disparlure under forest conditions. Experiments to measure disparlure concentrations in air have been successful on experimental plots and further experiments along these lines will be continued during the 1976 field season.

Emission rates of the microcapsules produced in 1975 were determined for 250 mg of capsules containing 4.2 mg of disparlure. The capsules were mixed with 2 other ingredients of the formulation, hydroxyethyl cellulose and Rhoplex B-15, and were then allowed to dry overnight on a microscope slide. Dry air was continuously passed over the capsules for 672 hours (28 days) at 80°F. Over this period there was no reduction in emission rate, although some fluctuations were observed. The average rate of emission was approximately 2 µg per hour and at this rate, the lure content would be reduced to 50 percent of its original value after 43 days. The experiment did not take into account factors such as humidity, temperature variations, sun, etc.

In another experiment, microscope slides coated with capsules were maintained indoors at room temperature; outdoors, inverted, covered; outdoors, inverted, uncovered; and outdoors, totally exposed to the effects of sunlight, air, etc. Under these conditions, the time required for the disparlure content of the capsules to fall to half of its initial value was 123 days, 34 days, 15 days and 10 days respectively (Table III).

Table III. Aging Effects of Microencapsulated Disparlure

Location	Exposed to			$t_{1/2}$ *
	Rain	Sun	Wind	(days)
Indoors	No	No	No	123
Outdoors	No	No	Yes	34
Outdoors	No	Yes	Yes	15
Outdoors	Yes	Yes	Yes	10

* Based on residual lure contents

Many capsules, especially those of larger diameter, appeared to lose their spherical shape; this collapse of the capsule wall seemed to be related to high humidity. The effects of humidity and temperature on the 1975 NCR capsules were determined in the laboratory. Increasing temperature had a greater effect on the emission rate of disparlure from microcapsules than it did with the Hercon ® dispensers; the rate from capsules was 0.59 µg/hr at 100°F (Table IV).

Table IV.   NCR Microencapsulated Disparlure

Temp.	μg/hr *
80°F	0.59
90°F	1.6
100°F	4.2

Rate of Increase: 2.7 μg/hr per 10°F

*   Emission rate for 4.2 mg of lure encapsulated in
    250 mg of wet capsules

The rate had therefore increased by a factor of 2.7 per 10°F
compared with a factor of 1.8 for the Hercon℞ dispensers. If
the air passing over the capsules was saturated with moisture
there was also an increase in emission rate; the effect of
passing humidified air over capsules for one week was to increase the rate of emission by 13-26%. However after 20 days of
aging there was a 30 to 40% reduction of emission rate in moist
air compared with that in dry air.
    The rate of emission of disparlure from Hercon℞ dispensers
or NCR microcapsules was affected by environmental parameters in
a predictable manner. Although minor modifications of the formulations affected the rate of emission, the observed changes were
not comparable in magnitude to those resulting from temperature
variations or fluctuations in other environmental parameters.

Literature Cited

1. Bierl, B. A., Beroza, M., and Collier, C. W.   Science (1970)
        170, 87-9.
2. Chambers, D. L., Cunningham, R. T., Lichty, R. W., and
        Thrailkill, R. B.   BioScience (1974) 24, 150-2.
3. Roelofs, W., Comeau, A., Hill, A., and Milicevic, C.   Science
        (1971) 174, 297-9.
4. Beroza, M., Bierl, B. A., and Moffitt, H. R.   Science (1974)
        183, 89-90.
5. Batiste, W. C.   Environ. Entomol. (1972) 1, 213-8.
6. Batiste, W. C., Berlowitz, A., Olson, W. H., DeTar, J. E., and
        Loos, J. L.   Environ. Entomol. (1973) 2, 387-91.
7. Madsen, H. F., and Vakenti, J. M.   Environ. Entomol. (1973)
        2, 677-9.
8. Shorey, H. H., Gaston, L. K., and Kaae, R. S., in "Pest
        Management with Insect Sex Attractants and Other Be-
        havior-Controlling Chemicals", M. Beroza, ed.   ACS
        Symposium Series, Number 23.   American Chemical Society,
        Washington, D.C.   1976.   pp. 67-74.
9. Beroza, M., Hood, C. S., Trefrey, D., Leonard, D. E., Knipling,
        E. F., Klassen, W., and Stevens, L. J.   J. Econ. Entomol.

(1974) <u>67</u>, 659-64.
10. Cameron, E. A., Schwalbe, C. P., Beroza, M., and Knipling,
     E. F. Science (1974) <u>183</u>, 972-3.
11. Beroza, M., Paszek, E. C., Mitchell, E. R., Bierl, B. A.,
     McLaughlin, J. R. and Chambers, D. L. Environ. Entomol.
     (1974) <u>3</u>, 926-8.
12. Beroza, M., Bierl, B. A., James, P, and DeVilbiss, D. J.
     Econ. Entomol. (1975) <u>68</u>, 369-72.
13. Beroza, M., Paszek, E. C., DeVilbiss, D., Bierl, B. A., and
     Tardif, J. G. R. Environ. Entomol. (1975) <u>4</u>, 712-4.
14. Bierl, B. A., and DeVilbiss, D., Proceedings of the Inter-
     national Controlled Release Pesticide Symposium, Dayton,
     Ohio; September, 1975. pp. 230-46.

Controlled Release from Hollow Fibers

E. ASHARE, T. W. BROOKS, and D. W. SWENSON

CONREL, An Albany International Co., 735 Providence Highway,
Norwood, Mass. 02062

In recent years controlled release of active materials has
emerged as a distinct technology in answer to a great many end-
use needs in medicine, agriculture, forestry and the home. The
subject has gained enough prominence to deserve a book (1) and
two international symposia (2). A growing number of commercial
products are based on controlled release formulations including
such familiar items as time release oral medications, fragrance
dispensing wicks and gels, and impregnated plastic pesticide
strips or animal collars. Modern controlled release devices
and systems such as impregnated plastic or rubber matrices, membrane envelopes, laminated poromerics and microcapsules testify
to the growing level of sophistication being demanded of this
technology to satisfy increasingly complex end-use requirements.

A novel controlled release device for vaporizable materials
has been developed, consisting of hollow fibers which function
both as a reservoir and as a means of control over dissemination
of vapors from the open end of the fibers. There is great flexibility in the use of this system in that it is capable of dispensing any vaporizable material at a release rate which is dependent on the inside diameter and number of fibers and for an
effective life dependent on fiber length. This system shows
promise for use with insect pheromones, insecticides, animal
repellents, and fragrances.

Mass Transport Theory

The mechanism for dispensing of volatile materials from
capillary channels consists of three steps:
  a. evaporation at the liquid-vapor interface;
  b. diffusion from the liquid-vapor interface to the open
      end of the hollow fiber;
  c. convection away from the open end.
Generally, the diffusion step will be the rate-controlling
factor. The rate of diffusion can be predicted by use of the
transport equations.

The molar flux (Fig. 1), N_a is given by ($\underline{3}$, p. 522):

$$N_a = - \frac{cD}{1-x_a} \frac{dx_a}{dz} \tag{1}$$

where x_a is the mole fraction of the volatile material, c its molar density, and D the diffusion coefficient.

A mass balance, $dN_a/dz=0$, combined with Eq. (1) and assuming ideal gas behavior gives:

$$-\ln (1-x_a) = C_1 z + C_2 \tag{2}$$

where C_1 and C_2 are constants which must be determined by the boundary conditions.

$$\text{B.C. 1} \quad \text{at } z=0, \; x_a = 0 \tag{3}$$

$$\text{B.C. 2} \quad \text{at } z=1, \; x_a = P_a^{vap}/P \tag{4}$$

The first boundary condition indicates that there is zero concentration at the open end of the fiber, i.e., convection is sufficient to remove the volatile material away from the fiber. The second boundry condition implies vapor-liquid equilibrium at the liquid-vapor interface, and P_a^{vap} is the vapor pressure of the volatile material.

Applying these boundary conditions gives:

$$(1-x_a) = (1-P_a^{vap}/P)^{z/\ell} \tag{5}$$

The liquid-vapor interface is continuously moving away from the fiber open end and the rate of this movement can be related to the molar flux, N_a.

$$-N_a = \frac{\rho}{M} \frac{d\ell}{dt} \tag{6}$$

where ρ is the liquid density, M the molecular weight, and ℓ is the distance between the fiber open end and the liquid-vapor interface.

Combining Eqs. (1), (5) and (6) gives:

$$\frac{d\ell}{dt} = - \frac{cMD}{\rho\ell} \ln (1 - \frac{P_a^{vap}}{P}) \tag{7}$$

This then leads to

$$\frac{d\ell}{dt} = \left[\frac{-McD}{2\rho} \ln (1 - \frac{P_a^{vap}}{P}) \right]^{1/2} t^{-1/2} \tag{8}$$

For most materials and temperatures considered $P_a{}^{vap} \ll P$. A Maclaurin expansion of the ln term gives:

$$\ln \left(1 - \frac{P_a{}^{vap}}{P}\right) \approx -P_a{}^{vap}/P$$

so that

$$\frac{d\ell}{dt} = \left[\frac{McD}{2\rho} \frac{P_a{}^{vap}}{P}\right]^{1/2} t^{-1/2} \qquad (9)$$

Thus, the change in meniscus level with time, $d\ell/dt$, which is related to the dispensing rate, is predicted to be inversely proportional to the half power of time. Note that this relationship makes use of a pseudo-steady state; i.e., a steady state is assumed at each instant even though the meniscus is continuously moving. The validity of this relationship was checked by measuring the movement of the meniscus for carbon tetrachloride. The results are shown in Figure 2 where the solid line represents Eq. 9 and points are measured values for release rate. The agreement is quite good considering that the diffusion coefficient, D, was calculated by using an empirical equation (3, Eq. 16.3-1). The slope of the experimental curve is -1/2 as predicted by Eq. 9.

The vapor pressure used in Eq. 9 is not the true equilibrium vapor pressure of the material but a reduced value due to the curved meniscus in the capillary. This reduction is a function of the radius of curvature of the meniscus(4) and as a result is dependent on the diameter of the hollow fiber. The curvature is also a function of surface tension and is therefore dependent on the nature of the material from which the hollow fiber is made. (In practice, a hollow fiber dispenser is best designed by making laboratory measurements using a hollow fiber of the size and material which will be used in the final product.)

The rate of release is dependent on temperature since the material properties, $P_a{}^{vap}$, D and c are temperature dependent. The major contribution to this dependence is the vapor pressure and is given by the Clausius-Clapeyron equation.

$$\frac{d \ln P^{vap}}{dT} = \frac{\Delta H^{vap}}{RT^2} \qquad (10)$$

A 30°F temperature change (e.g., from 70°F to 100°F) will result in a vapor pressure increase for pheromone-type materials of about 200%, while the diffusivity, D, increases by only about 10% and the molar gas density, c, decreases by about 5%. Thus, from Eq. 9 it is noted that the dispensing rate will about double for a 30°F temperature rise.

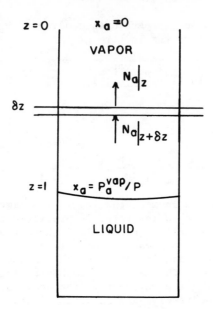

Figure 1. Diffusion through a stagnant gas layer

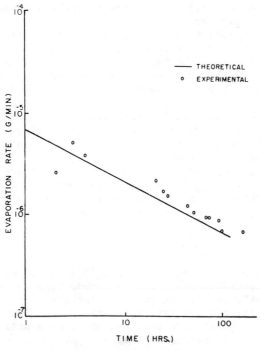

Figure 2. Release curve for carbon tetra-chloride

Evaporation Studies

The rate of release of volatile materials is determined in the laboratory by following the meniscus movement in the hollow fiber via a cathetometer. These menisci readings can be made to ±0.002 cm with the equipment used. This is equivalent to about ±1 μg for a fiber with 8 mil inside diameter. This type of release rate measurement has been shown to give approximately the same result as by cold trapping the effluent vapors and analyzing by gas chromatography (5).

Figure 3 is a typical plot of amount dispensed as a function of time for several different materials at 70°F. The slope of each curve is the dispensing rate. Note that there is an initial high slope (or dispensing rate) which corresponds to the time in which the meniscus is near the open end. As the meniscus recedes down the fiber with time, the change in dispensing rate becomes less pronounced. A relatively steady dispensing rate occurs after only a very short time and is usually the value to which the system is designed.

Fiber material selection is dictated largely by the compatibility between fiber and active material. It is essential that active material be nonreactive with the fiber and that the fiber walls are impermeable to the active material. These requirements are necessary for reasons of shelf life, and in the case of biologically active materials such as pheromones, for preservation of activity.

Field Tests

Hollow fiber dispensers have been designed for use with insect pheromones for field evaluations. The evaluations include survey, mass trapping, and disruption approaches for pheromone application. The use of pheromones of about 20 insects are being investigated.

For insect survey or monitoring, sex pheromones are employed to determine the presence of an insect infestation, from which it is determined if and when an insecticide should be used. For this method of use, it is desired to have a delivery system with a relatively constant release rate throughout a season. Hollow fiber dispensers were extensively evaluated in 1975 for use as a survey tool with sex pheromones of many lepidoptera insects. These tests indicated that the hollow fiber concept shows promise as a survey tool. The initial investigation brought out a distinct advantage for the hollow fiber concept, namely, the release rate can be easily varied by changing the number of fibers, thus making it simpler to determine the optimum rate of release for a pheromone system for survey purposes. This has been done for pink bollworm (6) and gypsy moth (7).

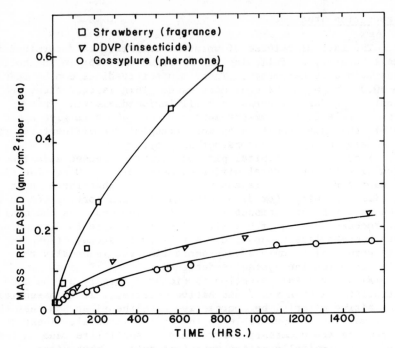

Figure 3.   Vapor release curves for various materials

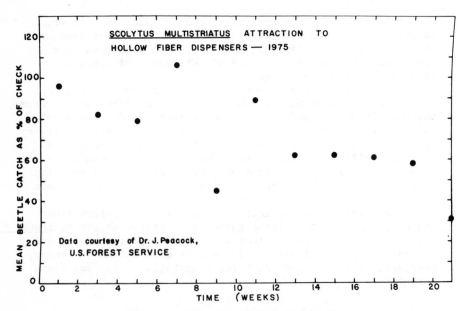

Figure 4.   Mass trapping of elm bark beetle

Hollow fiber pheromone dispensers have also been used for mass trapping, i.e., a procedure of using pheromones to attract and trap a large percentage of an insect population to minimize the pest damage. To date, the largest evaluation of these dispensers is mass trapping of the elm bark beetle, the vector for Dutch elm disease. This field work was done by the U. S. Forest Service, Delaware, Ohio. The versatility of the hollow fiber dispenser is illustrated by this study. The elm bark beetle pheromone is a mixture of three components and the desired dose rate is obtained by supplying each component in separate fibers, the number of fibers of each being dependent on the relative delivery rate of each component. Employing separate fibers for each component eliminates any problem of a distillation effect, that is, the changing concentration of a vapor mixture due to the different evaporation rates of each component of the mixture.

Dispensers were field tested in traps set out in Australia in early 1975 when U.S. beetle populations were dormant. The results are presented in Table I (8). The hollow fiber dispensers consistently out-captured beetles when compared to a polyethylene vial type of dispenser which is frequently employed by experimenters. Further, as the season progressed the hollow fiber dispensers improved in performance relative to the plastic vials. Since no data were collected after the fifth week, no comment can be made on total performance. The data as indicated by beetle catch do suggest that the hollow fiber dispensers adhered more closely to release design specifications than did the plastic vials. This demonstrates the potential hollow fibers offer in designing dispensers for multicomponent pheromones.

Data are presented in Figure 4 for elm bark beetle mass trapping studies carried out in Detroit, Michigan and Ft. Collins, Colorado in the summer of 1975 (8). The data are presented as beetle catch with a hollow fiber dispenser compared to beetle catch with a standard. The standard used was a freshly activated hollow fiber dispenser replaced every two weeks. As the theoretical analysis and release rate data presented above indicate, the rate of release drops with time, and it is therefore expected that the beetle catch with an aged dispenser will be less than the catch with a freshly activated dispenser, as is shown in Figure 4.

In the mating disruption technique, an area is permeated with a quantity of sex pheromone, sufficient to interfere with the insect's olfactory sexual communication system. The result is no mating, and therefore a reduction in the population of the next generation. This is extremely useful for lepidoptera, since it is in the larval stage when the insect does its damage.

Hollow fibers have recently been used for a mating disruption experiment for grape berry moth (9), a very serious pest in Eastern U.S. grape growing regions. The results of these experiments are presented in Table II. Dispensers were placed

Table I

Elm Bark Beetle Trapping Results
with Hollow Fiber Pheromone Dispensers

Trap No.	Trap Installed On Tree Species	Dispens- er Type[b]	Beetle Catch on Dates (1975)			
			2/6	2/12	2/26	3/17
1	Eucalyptus saligna	PV	31	175	13	54
3[a]	Archontophoenix cunninghamiana	--	0	0	0	0
4	"	HF	15	37	15	143
5	Nothofagus sol- anderi	PV	6	15	5	7
7	Ulmus procera	HF	3	35	53	112
8	"	PV	17	99	35	193
9[a]	Prunus spp.	--	0	0	0	0
11	Ulmus procera	HF	18	144	8	220
12[a]	Quercus spp.	--	0	0	0	0
13	Eucalyptus calo- phylla	PV	4	5	1	9
14	Ulmus procera	HF	16	302	130	200
16	Cedrus deodara	PV	23	75	4	7
17	Ulmus procera	HF	210	786	209	990
19	Pinus radiata	PV	33	70	16	32
21[a]	Pinus ponderosa	--	0	0	0	0
22	Ulmus procera	HF	54	235	34	160
23[a]	"	--	0	0	0	0
	Total Catches		430	1978	497	2127
	% of Total with HF Dispensers		73	78	90	86

[a]Control trees, traps installed without baits
[b]PV = polyethylene vials
HF = hollow fiber dispenser

in the test plot, one per vine and 605 per acre. Both in the treated and untreated plots pheromone baited survey traps were used to determine the presence of males. If the male could find its way to the trap, it was presumed it would be able to find the female. If the male could not find the trap, it was presumed that disruption was effective, i.e., the male could not find the female for mating purposes.

The data in Table II indicate that orientation to pheromone baited survey traps was disrupted for a 2-1/2 month period, after which time the experiment was terminated. Disruption of E. argutanus was also observed for the same period of time. The latter insect is a local species of no economic consequence. The record of its disruption serves only as additional evidence that the technique is working. The grape berry moths in this test were lab-reared insects while E. argutanus were from the local wild population.

Table II

Grape Berry Moth Orientation Disruption Tests
with Hollow Fiber Pheromone Dispensers - 1975[a]

Number of Males Captured in 6 Traps

		Treated Plot		Untreated Check Plot	
Date		GBM	E. Argutanus[b]	GBM	E. Argutanus
Jul	15	0	0	2	2
	20	0	0	19	45
	25	0	0	14	65
	30	0	0	7	39
Aug	6	2	2	28	199
	16	0	0	9	49
	26	0	1	11	26
Sept	5	0	0	15	8
	15	0	0	7	0
	25	0	0	11	0
Totals		2	3	123	433

---

[a]These data were obtained by Dr. E. F. Taschenberg, Vineyard
Laboratory New York State Agricultural Experiment Station,
Fredonia, New York.
[b]E. argutanus is a non-pest insect attracted by (Z)-9-dodecenyl
acetate, the sex pheromone of the grape berry moth.

This is the first time, to our knowledge, that orientation
disruption of a pest insect was achieved for a two and one-half
month period with a single pheromone treatment. This fact,
coupled with the very modest rate of pheromone application of
about 1 gm per acre per season, clearly indicates that mating
disruption with pheromones could be an economically feasible
approach to insect control in agriculture. These tests showed
only disruption to a survey trap. Tests planned for the 1976
season will be designed to ascertain whether disruption of the
grape berry moth also protects the crop against insect-caused
damage, the ultimate measure of economic value for any treatment
method.

Acknowledgements

The technical assistance of JoanEllen Hoar and Roger Kitterman in preparing formulations and obtaining field test data is gratefully acknowledged. We wish also to acknowledge the invaluable contributions of E. F. Taschenberg and W. Roelofs of the New York State Agricultural Experiment Station who conducted the grape berry moth experiment, and J. W. Peacock and R. A. Cuthbert of the U.S. Department of Agriculture Northeast Forest Experiment Station who arranged for the elm bark beetle tests.

Literature Cited

1. Tanquary, A.C., and Lacey, R.E., (eds.), "Controlled Release of Biologically Active Agents," Plenum Press, New York (1974c).
2. Cardarelli, N. F. (ed.), "Proceedings of the 1974 Controlled Release Pesticide Symposium," University of Akron, Akron, Ohio, September 16-18, 1974; Harris, F. W., (ed.), "Proceedings of the 1975 Controlled Release Pesticide Symposium," Wright State University, Dayton, Ohio, September 8-10, 1975.
3. Bird, R. B., Stewart, W. E., and Lightfoot, E. N., "Transport Phenomena," John Wiley & Sons, New York, (1960c).
4. Pippard, A. B., "The Elements of Classical Thermodynamics," Cambridge University Press, London (1961c).
5. Gore, W. E., private communication, February 17, 1975.
6. Kitterman, R. W., private communications.
7. Forrester, T., private communications.
8. J. W. Peacock and R. A. Cuthbert, private communications.
9. E. F. Taschenberg and W. Roelofs, private communications.

Controlled Release of Pheromones Through Multi-Layered Polymeric Dispensers

AGIS F. KYDONIEUS and INJA K. SMITH

Hercon Division, Health-Chem Corp., 1107 Broadway, New York, N.Y. 10010

MORTON BEROZA

M. Beroza & Assoc., 821 Malta Lane, Silver Spring, Md. 20901

The purpose of this article is to discuss and review the experiences with the new 3-layer HERCON® polymeric dispenser for controlled release of such volatile organic chemicals as the insect sex pheromones and related potent behavior-controlling chemicals. The dispenser is manufactured by The Hercon Division of Health-Chem Corporation, New York, N.Y., 10010, and its first use in dispensing pheromones was reported in December 1974. (1) During the 1974 and 1975 seasons, millions of these dispensers containing sex pheromones were sold. This paper will report and examine the results that have become available and comment on the future potential of the product.

First, some background material is in order. In the mid-fifties we began to hear of insects becoming resistant to insecticides and of pesticide residues appearing in our food. Later we heard of wildlife being affected, beneficial insects being destroyed along with the injurious ones, and that our air, soil, and water were becoming polluted with pesticides. Spurred by these ominous reports scientists began to cast about seriously in search of alternatives to the use of insecticides for insect control. One of the alternatives involved the use of insect attractants. At first, it was more fruitful to test a great variety of chemicals to find an attractant than to try to isolate and identify an attractive chemical from an insect. About half dozen attractants were found this way by the USDA, and they were put to good use. For example, traps each baited with synthetic lures for 3 of the world's worst insect pests, the Mediterranean fruit fly, oriental fruit fly, and the melon fly, were deployed about ports of entry to the U.S. since the early 1960s to detect an accidental importation of any of these subtropical pests. Infestations of all of these species were found, and they were eradicated quickly with the traps showing where and when to apply the appropriate counter measures. USDA has stated that the traps have saved them millions of dollars in potential eradication costs, but they saved the agricultural community and the public far greater in increased prices of food that would have resulted if we had to live with these insects.

With the great value of insect attractants established, the possibility of similar use of the attractants that the insects themselves manufacture, e.g., their sex attractants or pheromones, became most appealing. We have already heard from Dr. Bierl and her co-workers (2) about pheromones and their biological function, particularly their role in aiding the insect reproductive process. They also noted potential uses; i.e., how pheromones are useful in monitoring the whereabouts of injurious insect species, in timing control measures such as insecticide sprays to achieve optimum effects, and how pheromones may be useful in direct control, i.e., by mass trapping or by sowing pheromone-emitting particles among insect populations to prevent the sexes from finding each other and mating.

For a long time, the isolation, identification, and synthesis of these materials--mainly the sex attractants--were hampered by the minute amounts of these potent substances present in insects. Fortunately, by the late 1960s, this situation was largely reversed by the introduction of remarkable improvements in spectrometric, chromatographic, instrumental, and specialized techniques, which greatly facilitated the isolation and identification of minute amounts of the pheromones. Progress has been so rapid in the past five years that pheromones or chemicals believed to be pheromones are now known for hundreds of insect species, (3), and many of these species are of great economic importance.

What is needed now is the Technology to use the pheromones effectively.

As a partial answer to this need, the HERCON® dispensing system was developed. In its simplest form, the Hercon dispenser is a three-layer plastic laminate with the pheromone reservoir in the inner layer. (See Figure 1). A pressure sensitive adhesive can also be incorporated for ease of application. When the dispenser is exposed (as in a trap), the pheromone gradually diffuses out through the outer layers and is thereby released much as an insect releases its pheromone to lure a mate. Great flexibility in regulating the emission rate of the pheromone from the dispenser is readily achieved by adjusting the area of the dispenser (readily cut to size with scissors), the thickness of the outer layers, and the amount of pheromone per dispenser. Since most pheromones are potent, very little pheromone

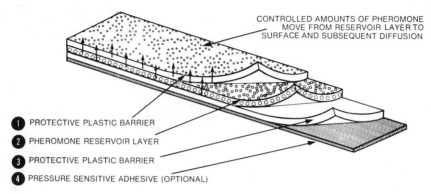

CONTROLLED AMOUNTS OF PHEROMONE
MOVE FROM RESERVOIR LAYER TO
SURFACE AND SUBSEQUENT DIFFUSION

1 PROTECTIVE PLASTIC BARRIER
2 PHEROMONE RESERVOIR LAYER
3 PROTECTIVE PLASTIC BARRIER
4 PRESSURE SENSITIVE ADHESIVE (OPTIONAL)

Figure 1

is needed and a dispenser may contain enough pheromone to last an entire season. A major point is that the pheromone is released at a near-constant rate. As a further feature, the position of the pheromone in the plastic laminate protects it from degradation by light or air. The importance of this protection should not be underestimated. Some pheromones, e.g., aldehydes, are rather unstable and have to be protected. Also, the degradation products of some sex attractants are inhibitors which quickly nullify attraction. For example, the sex lure of the cabbage looper (Tricoplusia ni [Hubner]) and the oriental fruit moth (Grapholitha molesta [Busck]) are acetates, and their corresponding alcohols (formed by deacetylation) are highly inhibitory (4)(5); as little as a few percent conversion of these acetates to their alcohols (hydrolysis) severly diminishes trap captures.

The USDA gypsy moth (Lymantria dispar [L]) survey program was the first to use the HERCON® dispenser in their traps (6). In 1974, and again in 1975, at least 100,000 of the traps were strategically placed in the Eastern half of the U.S. to monitor the whereabouts of the gypsy moth. The rate of emission of disparlure, the gypsy moth sex attractant, from the dispensers has been shown to be ample and fairly constant (6), and the dispensers are effective for an entire season. Compare Figure 2 and Figure 3 which give the emission rates of the Hercon dispenser and the previously used cotton wick dispenser.

Mass-trapping with a new, inexpensive, highly efficient trap baited with the new dispenser has shown potential for direct control of the gypsy moth in light infestations (7). Further improvements of this trap are being made by the Animal and Plant Health Inspection Service of the USDA. Earlier demonstrations that mass-

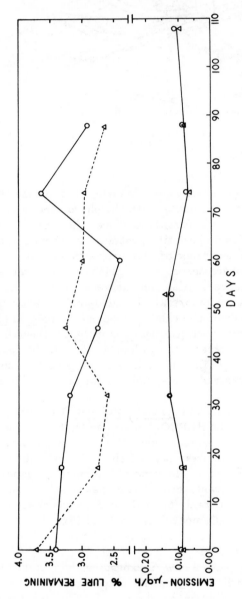

Figure 2. Rate of emission of HERCON laminated plastic dispensers of disparlure (lower graph) and percentage lure found in these laminates (upper graph) after aging at room temperature. Points for laminates with sealed ends designated by circles; points for laminates with open ends designated by triangles.

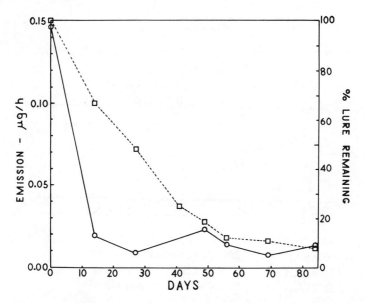

Figure 3. Rate of emission of cotton wicks, each initially containing 300 μg disparlure and 2 mg trioctanoin (solid line, ordinate on left), and percentage lure remaining (dashed line, ordinate on right, lure initially = 100%) after aging up to 84 days at room temperature

trapping can prevent a buildup of low-level populations have been reported.

The HERCON dispenser has also been used successfully by the USDA (8) with grandlure, the boll weevil (<u>Anthonomus grandis</u> Boheman) sex pheromone, a 4-component mixture of chemicals (9), two of which are aldehydes. As one part of an integrated control program designed to determine the feasibility of eradicating the boll weevil (the worst pest of cotton), the dispenser is used to lure weevils into traps. Of 4 types of dispensers recently tested by scientists of the Boll Weevil Research Laboratory, the HERCON dispenser performed best (10). After 12 weeks in the field, it caught 177% as many weevils as the next best type of dispenser, which was the standard 3 mg lure on a filter in a vial that had to be changed weekly throughout the test. (See Table I). The HERCON grandlure dispenser has now been designated as the standard in the Belt-wide tests being conducted against the boll weevil. The release rate of grandlure is also constant with time as shown in Figure 4.

<u>TABLE I</u>

MEXICO GRANDLURE FORMULATION TEST (1975)
BOLL WEEVIL CATCHES

Week	HERCON®	USDA STANDARD (changed weekly)
2	71	17
4	138	50
6	115	75
8	40	41
10	17	27
12	7	9
TOTAL	388	219

H
HERCON	177% Catches of Standard
PRODUCT A	29% Catches of Standard
PRODUCT B	25% Catches of Standard
PRODUCT C	91% Catches of Standard

Source: T.B. Davich, Boll Weevil Research Lab, USDA.

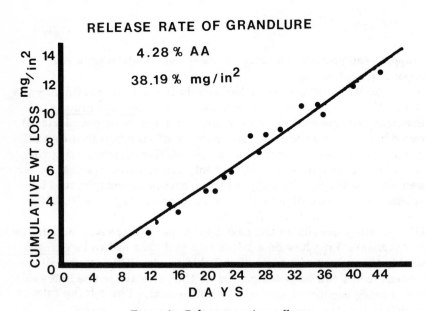

RELEASE RATE OF GRANDLURE

4.28 % AA

38.19 % mg/in^2

Figure 4.   Release rate of grandlure

The HERCON dispenser has also been adopted for use in the USDA pink bollworm (Pectinophora gossypiella [Saunders]) survey program. This insect is the second most injurious pest of cotton in this country. Dispensers, 1 sq cm in size and containing about 1.5mg of the lure, a 1:1 mixture of (Z, Z)- and (Z, E)-7, 11-hexadecadien-1-ol acetates, have been highly effective in capturing pink bollworms in the field tests in different parts of the country.

A recent report by McLaughlin, Mitchell and Tumlinson (12) stated that HERCON dispensers provide an "excellent means for baiting pheromone traps" for the peachtree borer (Synanthedon exitiosa [Say]), the lesser peachtree borer (Synanthedon pictipes [G.Y.R.]), the soybean looper, (Pseudoplusia includens [Walker]), and the cabbage looper. They state further that the HERCON system is excellent for baiting traps because the dispensers "can be stored and handled with relative ease, and the rate of release of active compound is readily adjusted."

The smaller European elm bark beetle, Scolytus multistriatus (Marsham), has been responsible for the decline of the American elm tree (Ulmus americana L.) in this country. After the ingredients of the sex pheromone of this beetle were reported by Pearce et al. to be 4-methyl-3-heptanol, cubebene, and a chemical called multistriatin (13), formulations of HERCON dispensers containing these ingredients were tested by Dr. John Peacock and R.A. Cuthbert of the USDA Forest Service (14), and some were found highly attractive to the beetle. A production run of the best dispensers was tested over a prolonged period by comparing captures of traps baited with it versus captures made by traps with the same dispenser but freshly baited every two weeks. For 11 weeks, captures with the aged and freshly baited dispensers were not too different, which indicates that the rate of release of lure from fresh and aged dispensers was not too different; if a 70% level of captures by aged versus fresh dispensers is considered acceptable, the HERCON dispenser gave a total of 13 weeks of acceptable performance (5/22 - 8/20/75) without rebaiting (See Table II). These results indicate that only one rebaiting would be needed to retain trap effectiveness for the 150-180-day season of the beetle.

HERCON dispensers have been prepared with virelure, the sex attractant of the tobacco budworm (Heliothis virescens (F.)), which consists of a mixture of (Z)-11-hexadecenal and (Z)-9-tetradecenal. Our latest information indicates that the HERCON dispensers with virelure are catching well compared to other commercial formulations It outcatches several live females in a trap and remains effective for at least a month (15). Favorable results have also been reported in tests of the 3-layer laminate against other insect species, e.g., fall armyworm (Spodoptera frugiperda [J.E. Smith]), Douglas-fir

TABLE II

Catches of Elm Bark Beetle
at traps baited with HERCON® dispensers
May 22 - August 20, 1975

Mean beetle catches for 20 traps

	WEEKS						
	I	3	5	7	9	11	13
HERCON	391	368	476	162	95	515	567
CHECK[a]	342	283	477	128	294	518	820
% of Check	114	130	100	127	33[b]	100	69

[a] Fresh dispenser every two weeks
[b] Probably anomalous due to high value for check

Source: Drs. John Peacock and Roy Cuthbert
N/E Forest Expt. Station, USDA, Delaware.

tussock moth (Orgyia pseudotsugata [McDunnough]), eastern spruce
budworm (Choristoneura fumiferana [Clemans]); but again the data
have not been released by the investigators doing the testing.

The 3-layer laminates also have potential for dispensing
chemicals other than pheromones. For example, in an experiment
with trimedlure, a synthetic lure for the Mediterranean fruit fly,
(Ceratitis capitata [Wiedemann]), HERCON laminates attracted
more than 2 1/2 times as many flies as the bait dispenser in current
use, and this throughout a 2-month period. Furthermore, the
HERCON dispenser achieved these results with less than 1/4 of the
amount of lure used in the current bait dispenser.

Before we leave the subject of trapping, it is well to note
that the design of an optimum trapping system, whether for
detection or control, requires consideration of many parameters.
In addition to emission rate of lure, lure stability and quantity, and
duration of effectiveness -- which are related to the lure dispenser,
consideration must also be given to trap design and color, trap
height, trap placement, trapping means (e.g., use of adhesive or
insecticide), position of bait dispenser in trap, effect of host crop,
effective distance of attraction, time of insect response, cost of
trap, and ratio of ingredients if the lure is multi-component. More
attention to the determination of these parameters for the many
different species of insects is needed.

A device now under investigation by the Herculite Protective
Fabrics Corporation comprises a long-lasting combination of the
HERCON pheromone dispenser with a similar laminate that releases

insecticide at a controlled rate. The objective of the device is to attract the target insect to an insecticide-containing plastic sheet that will dispatch the insect on contact.

Permeation of the atmosphere with sex pheromone to disorient insects trying to find mates has already been mentioned. This technique has proven successful in experiments with the gypsy moth (up to 98% suppression in mating) (7) (16), oriental fruit moth (17), codling moth (Laspeyresia pomonella [L]) (18), pink bolloworm moth (19), and many other insect pests (12). In most of these applications, micorencapsulated solutions of the pheromone were dispensed from aircraft or ground equipment. In some cases, metal planchets were used to evaporate the chemical into the atmosphere.

USDA workers Mitchell and Tumlinson have come up with a simple means of accomplishing this disruption of pheromonal communication between the sexes. Thus, in a preliminary experiment, they demonstrated such disruption with the boll weevil in a cotton field by using HERCON dispensers as evaporators of the boll weevil pheromone (20). The 1-inch-square dispensers were arrayed in a checkerboard pattern in a test plot with a pheromone baited trap at its center. The general idea of the test is that the boll weevils in the cotton field would have difficulty finding the trap if the pheromone emitted by the dispensers disoriented the weevils, and, in fact, this is what happened. Over a 20-day period, trap captures of weevils in the plot with the dispensers were suppressed 83% compared to trap captures in a similar plot without the dispensers. Similar suppression in captures was also obtained with dispensers containing two of the four grandlure components.

In another similar experiment, C.R. Gentry and coworkers disoriented the peachtree borer and the lesser peachtree borer (20). Laminated HERCON strips (1-inch-square) containing the pheromone of the peachtree borer, (Z, Z,)-3, 13-octadecadien-1-ol acetate (21), were hung on trees in two 2-acre peach orchards; another orchard was left untreated as a check. Traps baited with the pheromone of each insect were placed in each orchard to monitor the ability of the borers to find the traps. In comparison with the check, captures of the lesser peachtree borer in the plots with the dispensers were suppressed 100% for 9 weeks; then results became erratic. Fresh HERCON strips restored almost complete suppression of captures for another 10 weeks. (See Table III). Similar results were recorded for the peachtree borer, but because the population of this insect was extremely low, the significance of these results are questionable.

TABLE III
Effect of air-permeation trials on captures
of lesser peachtree borer males
in pheromone traps [a]

Week	Treated Orchard I[b]		Orchard 2		Untreated Orchard 3
1	1	(86)	0	(100)	7
2	0	(100)	2	(93)	27
3	2	(92)	0	(100)	24
4	1	(93)	0	(100)	15
5	0	(100)	0	(100)	2
6	1	(90)	0	(100)	10
7	0	(100)	1	(92)	12
8	0	(100)	0	(100)	4
9	0	–	0	–	0
10	0	(100)	2	(83)	12

[a] Each orchard had 5 traps baited with 100 mg of pure E Z.
[b] Value in parenthesis is percent reduction compared to the untreated orchard.

A preliminary report on the foregoing was made by McLaughlin et al (12) who also noted that HERCON formulations of (Z)-7-dodecen-1-ol acetate were tested in soybean fields as disruptants of soybean looper communication. "Several formulations were quite effective with excellent longevity", according to these workers.

If ground application of the pheromone formulation for air permeation is contemplated, use of the HERCON 3-layer dispensers as evaporators of the pheromone, e.g., by fastening them to foliage or other objects throughout the crop area, appears to offer a means that is simpler, more controllable, more dependable, and less expensive than any other means now available.

In another variation of the air-permeation technique, sheets of the 3-layer laminate containing pheromone were reduced to a confetti or granules, which were then distributed over the crops to be protected. Although data are lacking on the results of such tests, we have been told that such material tested against the pink bollworm was effective for about 3 weeks. For application from aircraft or ground equipment, the pheromone granules or confetti will probably have to be dispensed with a sticker so the particles will adhere to the foliage upon impact and then slowly emit their lure to the atmosphere over a prolonged period and not be washed off by rain or removed by wind. Use of the HERCON granules may have advantages over other slow-release methods in terms of efficacy or cost or both.

Mitchell has recently proposed the development of integrated pest management systems that use the atmospheric permeation technique with several chemicals to disrupt the mating of some or all of the offending coexisting species in a given vicinity (22). In seeking appropriate systems for Heliothis species, he has successfully disrupted insect communication with HERCON 3-layer laminates that volatilized (Z)-11-hexadecenal and (Z)-9-tetradecenal into the atmosphere at a controlled rate. These unsaturated aldehydes are sensitive compounds. However, in most cases, the addition of an anti-oxidant has not improved performance of HERCON pheromone dispensers. In his article (22), Mitchell outlines how the laminated plastic strips would be used in simultaneous release of several chemicals.

Summarizing Contents

With pheromones of economically important insects species rapidly becoming available (see recent listing of pheromones) (3) (23), the HERCON dispensing system appears to have excellent potential for use in trapping, air permeating, and in lure-insecticide combinations. The flexibility of the system makes it easy to adjust the rate of emission of the behavior chemical to values approaching optimum and greatly facilitates their use as dispensers in traps or as evaporators of pheromone in the air-permeation technique. Ease of handling and storage, protection of a broad variety of chemicals from degradation by light and air, and excellent weathering qualities are other unique features of the HERCON multi-layered polymeric dispenser.

Literature Cited

(1) Beroza, M., Paszek, E.C., Mitchell, E.R., Bierl, B.A., McLaughlin, J.R., and Chambers, D.L. Environ. Entomol. (1974) 3, 926-8.

(2) Bierl, B.A., DeVilbiss, E.D., and Plimmer. The Use of Pheromones in Insect Control: Slow Release Formulations. This Symposium.

(3) Mayer, M.S., and McLaughlin, J.R., "An Annotated Compendium of Insect Sex Pheromones", Fla. Agric. Exptl. Station, No. 6, Univ. Fla., Gainesville, August 1975.

(4) Tumlinson, J.H., Mitchell, E.R., Browner, S.M., Mayer, M.S., Green, N., Hines, R., and Lindquist, D.A. Environ. Entomol. (1972), 1, 354-8.

(5) Beroza, M., Gentry, C.R., Blythe, J.L., and Muschik, G.M., J. Econ. Entomol. (1973) 66, 1307 - 11.

(6) Beroza, M., Paszek, E.C., DeVilbiss, D., Bierl, B.A., and Tordif, J.G.R., Environ. Entomol. (1975) 4, 712-4.

(7) Beroza, M., Hood, G.S., Trefrey, D., Leonard, D.E., Knipling, F.F., and Klassen, W., Environ. Entomol. (1975) 4, 705-11.

(8) Hardee, D.D., McKibben, G.H., and Huddleston, P.M., J. Econ. Entomol. (1975) 68, 477-9.

(9) Tumlinson, J.H., Hardee, D.D., Gueldner, R.C., Thompson, A.C., Hedin, P.A., and Minyard, J.P. Science (1969) 166, 1010-2.

(10) Private Communication.

(11) Hummel, H.E., Gaston, L.K., Shorey, H.H., Kaae, R.S., Byrne, K.S., Silverstein, R.M., Science (1973) 181, 873-5.

(12) McLaughlin, J.R., Mitchell, E.R., and Tumlinson, J.H., Proc. 1975 International Controlled Release Pesticide Symposium, Sept. 8-10, 1975, Wright State Univ., Dayton, Ohio, P. 209-15.

(13) Pearce, G.T., Gore, W.E., Silverstein, R.M., Peacock, J.W., Cuthbert, R.A., Lanier, G.N. and Simeone, J.B., J. Chem. Ecol. (1975) 1, 115-124.

(14) Peacock, J.W., and Cuthbert, R.A., Proc. 1975 Intn'l Controlled Release Pesticide Symposium, Sept. 8-10, 1975, Wright State Univ., Dayton, Ohio, P. 216.

(15) Private Communication, E.R. Mitchell, USDA.

(16) Schwalbe, C.P., Cameron, E.A., Hall, D.J., Richerson, J.V., Beroza, M., and Stevens, L.J., Environ. Entomol. (1974) 3, 589-92.

(17) Gentry, C.R., Beroza, M. Blythe, J.L., and Bierl, B.A., Environ. Entomol. (1975) 4, 822-4.

(18) Anonymous. Agric. Res. (Wash., D.C.) (1974), May 15.

(19) McLaughlin, J.R., Shorey, H.H., Gaston, L.K., Kaae, R.S., and Stewart, F.D., Environ. Entomol. (1972), 1, 645-50.

(20) Mitchell, E.R., and Tumlinson, J.H., USDA, Gainesville Fla., Private Communication.

(21) Tumlinson, J.H., Yonce, C.E., Doolittle, R.E., Heath, R.R., Gentry, C.R., and Mitchell, E.R., Science (1974) 185, 614-6.

(22) Mitchell, E.R., Bioscience (1975) 25, 493-9.

(23) Inscoe, M.N., and Beroza, M. ACS Symposium Series. In Press.

Application of a New Controlled Release Concept in Household Products

A. F. KYDONIEUS, A. R. QUISUMBING, and S. HYMAN

Health-Chem Corp., 1107 Broadway, New York, N.Y. 10010

As the public became more increasingly aware of contamination of our environment, they joined efforts with environmentalists to force federal and state governments to pass legislation regulating the use of harmful pesticides or industrial pollutants that may ultimately endanger man and his surroundings. This has resulted in many legal control measures emphasizing the need for effective, safe pesticides.

In the area of pesticides, proposed regulations dealt not only with the active ingredients but were also extended to propellant gases used in various aerosol products. Arguments - pro and con - on the effect of these gases upon the atmosphere's ozone layer are a constant subject of debate.

The rampant use of chemicals, among other things, has often resulted in the development of pesticide-resistant strains of pests. In addition to hazards arising from pesticide residues, increased outbreaks of secondary pests have also resulted from the accidental destruction of natural predators (1).

In spite of limitations of the use of pesticide chemicals, however, there is little other than these chemicals that man can use to avoid damage and to obtain the desired immediate reduction of pest populations. And since man has the right to protect himself, his crops and possessions from pest attack, it appears that pesticides will continue to be used as an important part of pest management programs.

There is a need to judge the use of each chemical independently. It will be a gross mistake to replace chemical control with sophisticated but untested or ineffective pest management techniques. An effort must be exerted to find a new revolutionary approach for applying the existing tools for pest control. Traditional methodology must be modified to utilize pesticides in a manner that will be both effective and safe to user and off-target organisms.

Spraying, fogging and dusting methods have been reviewed to insure that problems from drift and residues do not arise. Proper application procedures, amounts, persistence and placements of

pesticides are continuously underscored by government and industry
to help make our environment a safe and clean place to live in.
Recently, researchers became interested in mixing the active ingredients with unconventional materials, e.g., lacquer, resins and
plastics, to lengthen the pesticide's residual activity.

Health-Chem Corporation's patented HERCON® controlled release
process utilizes a multi-layered polymeric dispensing system. The
basic characteristics of this HERCON technology have been described elsewhere (2). Utilizing its unique controlled release
concept, Health-Chem is introducing household products designed
not only for insect control, but also as room air fresheners or
deodorizers. This paper describes these household products.
These include I. ROACH KILLERS, II. FLY STRIPS, and III. AIR
FRESHENERS.

Health-Chem has been involved in controlled release technology for 15 years. Through its Herculite Protective Fabrics, a
New York-based subsidiary, Health-Chem introduced the Staph-Chek®
line of fabrics which featured a controlled release anti-bacterial
agent. Some Staph-Chek mattress coverings were found to be effective in controlling Staphylococcus and Klebsiella bacteria even
after six years usage (3).

I. Roach Killers. HERCON INSECTAPE® Insecticidal Strips
is the household product marketed for control of cockroaches or
"waterbugs". These multi-layered plastic strips kill the insects
on contact as they walk across its surface. The insecticide on
the surface is replenished continuously from a specially designed
storage layer sealed in the strip (Figure 1).

The use of INSECTAPE allows the homeowner more control over
insecticide placement than many other formulations or application
techniques. Additionally, the strips are installed in out-of-
sight locations, away from likely contact with children, pets or
clothing.

After extensive laboratory and field testing in 12 states,
the INSECTAPE was registered for general use roach control by the
U.S. Environmental Protection Agency (EPA). The currently registered INSECTAPE dispensers use either propoxur (®BAYGON) or
diazinon insecticides. Submissions for registration of insecticidal strips which will dispense chlorpyrifos (DURSBAN®) insecticide were submitted to EPA in late 1975.

The three insecticides used in INSECTAPE formulations have
been proven to be effective pesticides for roach control. There
are distinct advantages of having these different chemicals as
active ingredients in INSECTAPE. An important benefit is that a
choice of insecticide will help counter the development of roach
resistance to a specific kind of insecticide.

The INSECTAPE product will be available in three different
product versions depending upon the strips' length of effectiveness. The household consumer INSECTAPE is designed to be effective for six months. Exclusive sales rights were granted to the

Johnson Wax organization for sale of the six-month product in
supermarkets and other retail outlets in the United States. This
product will be marketed under their RAID® ROACH-TAPE® label.

For professional and institutional use, an INSECTAPE product
which will be effective for 12 months has been developed. The
12-month efficacy is beneficial to pest control operators involved
in roach control in residences, institutions and industry.

Another long-life INSECTAPE which will deliver the pesticide
for up to five years is also being tested. This latter delivery
system is designed to protect vending machines, refrigerators,
washers and dryers, and telephone equipment from future roach
infestations. These strips are intended to be installed in fact-
ories where the above equipment are manufactured.

When the INSECTAPE was first produced, the challenge was to
prove that HERCON dispensers of chemical roach killers were at
least as effective as, or more effective than, the standard spray
treatments. Tests on residual activity of INSECTAPE insecticidal
strips were shown to be equal to or superior to those of conventional means ($\underline{4}$, $\underline{5}$, $\underline{6}$).

Table I summarizes the comparisons between conventional spray
treatments and INSECTAPE only treatments. Efficacy is expressed
in terms of percentage reduction of the original roach infestation
($\underline{6}$). The following equation was used:

$$\text{ROACH INFESTATION REDUCTION} = \frac{\text{PRE-COUNT} - \text{FOLLOW-UP COUNT}}{\text{PRE-COUNT}}$$

where pre-count is the number of roaches counted when INSECTAPE
strips were initially applied, and follow-up count is the number
of live roaches found during a subsequent visit (or follow-up).

To obtain roach counts in test sites, the 3-minute sub-lethal
flush method was used. A pressurized spray of non-residual pyre-
thrin and piperonyl butoxide was directed into suspected harbor-
ages and counts taken when the roaches emerged.

The percent infestation reduction reflects the decrease in
number of live roaches, and also indicates percent mortality due
to the control measures.

Table I shows that control by INSECTAPE strips containing
either propoxur, diazinon or chlorpyrifos were similar to each
other, but were superior to control due to spray applications.
Reduction of roach infestation, as a result of INSECTAPE applications, remained high even five months after strip installation.
Roach control due to residual sprays, on the other hand, though
appreciably high two to three months after spraying, eventually
decreased. The latter may be due to a gradual loss of the sprayed
chemical's efficacy in time. After three to five months, percent
infestation reduction obtained by the use of INSECTAPE strips with

Table I. Summary of tests comparing efficacy of RESIDUAL SPRAY TREATMENT ONLY, and HERCON INSECTAPE ONLY, containing either propoxur (BAYGON), diazinon, or chlorpyrifos (DURSBAN).

| Variables | SPRAY ONLY | HERCON INSECTAPE | | |
| | | BAYGON | DIAZINON | DURSBAN |
		Insecticidal Strips Only		
No. of sites tested	19	38	27	28
No. of roaches/site	47.74	30.92	36.33	12.18
AVE. % INFESTATION REDUCTION				
After 1 - 1.5 months	43.31	85.78	71.10	78.70
After 2 - 3 months	65.28	92.07	92.59	88.42
After 3 - 5 months	34.37	86.69	90.18	92.91

propoxur, diazinon or chlorpyrifos were 86.69%, 90.18% and 92.91%, respectively; percent reduction due to sprays was only 34.37%.

Laboratory studies with German roaches, Blattella germanica (L.), also showed that length of time of contact required for 100% knockdown and kill was shorter with the INSECTAPE than with a sprayed surface (7). Moore reported that a two-second roach contact with the strip knocked down 93% of a roach sample within two hours, and killed all roaches within three days. Increasing the contact time to four minutes shortened the killing time to two days. In a similar test, Moore (8) discovered that a 30-second contact with a plate sprayed with BAYGON insecticide did not result in any knockdown even after seven hours.

It was also interesting to note that when sprayed plates were assayed, the rate of application of propoxur was found to be 667.6 mg/sq.ft. (8). Significantly, INSECTAPE has a smaller concentration of propoxur on the strip's surface. Infra-red spectrophotometric analyses of an INSECTAPE strip containing propoxur showed that the amount of active ingredient on the surface was only 270 mg/sq.ft. Determinations of concentration of the pesticide, and the reduction in cockroach infestations indicate that an effective roach killer need not carry large amounts of the active ingredient.

Moore (7) also indicated that there was minimal fumigant action by the HERCON insecticidal strips. The absence of a fumigant action is desirable since possibility of contamination of non-target surroundings is minimized. This characteristic will also be useful in treating areas where spray drift may be hazardous and the use of dusts may be unsightly or messy. Such areas include pet shops or shelves where a fish aquarium or a hamster cage may be found.

To expand the INSECTAPE's uses as registered currently with EPA, Health-Chem is analyzing data from tests conducted to prove that these roach killers will also control other household pests, including ants, silverfish and spiders.

II. Fly Strips. Another controlled release product designed for households is an insecticide dispenser for use in controlling flies. The fly strips, now undergoing extensive field tests, are designed also for use in dairy and cattle barns, and livestock sheds. Also multi-layered, the HERCON Fly Strip has both outside surfaces active.

To improve the effectiveness of this HERCON fly control product, a separate strip containing a fly attractant will be attached to the insecticide dispenser. The fly attractant has been shown to stimulate flies to come in contact with the insecticide-containing surface, thus resulting in a greater percentage of fly kill.

The fly strip's active ingredient is resmethrin (SBP 1382), a relatively non-volatile, solid synthetic pyrethroid. With its low mammalian toxicity, resmethrin is desirable for use in the house where safety of humans and pets is always an important consideration. A non-volatile insecticide is preferred to minimize contamination of the immediate surroundings.

Since resmethrin kills by contact, there is no release of undesirable toxic vapors. Also, unlike the standard fly strips which release volatile DDVP or dichlorvos insecticide, the HERCON product may be used continuously in nurseries and kitchens. Since the insecticide is non-volatile, air movement will not be a serious factor in decreasing the HERCON fly strip's efficacy.

The specific non-toxic attractant was chosen after screening dozens of materials known to be attractive to flies. Test data have shown that efficacy of aged strips was "revitalized" when the attractant strip was added. In one test, the addition of a fly attractant dispenser to a 4½ months old fly strip resulted in fly mortality not different from control obtained with new fly strips.

Studies on the release rate of resmethrin indicate that after 40 days, only 1.5 mg/sq.in. out of the original 16.21 mg/sq.in. active ingredient were lost (Figure 2). Extrapolating from this rate, the fly strip is expected to kill flies for at least nine months.

Figure 3, on the other hand, shows the release rate of the fly attractant. With the HERCON controlled release system, only 16% of the attractant present in the strip was lost after 50 days, thus making this dispenser effective for at least eight months.

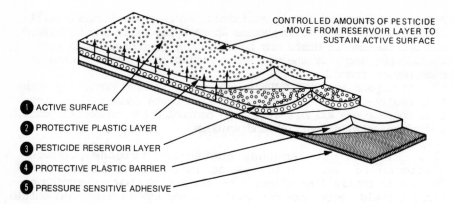

CONTROLLED AMOUNTS OF PESTICIDE
MOVE FROM RESERVOIR LAYER TO
SUSTAIN ACTIVE SURFACE

1 ACTIVE SURFACE
2 PROTECTIVE PLASTIC LAYER
3 PESTICIDE RESERVOIR LAYER
4 PROTECTIVE PLASTIC BARRIER
5 PRESSURE SENSITIVE ADHESIVE

*Figure 1.   Schematic of HERCON® INSECTAPE®, a multi-layered polymeric dispenser
of an insecticide for cockroach control*

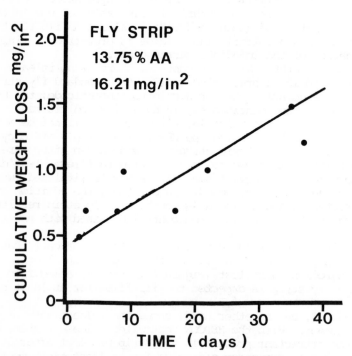

*Figure 2.   Release rate of active ingredient Resmethrin (SBP 1382)
from HERCON fly strip*

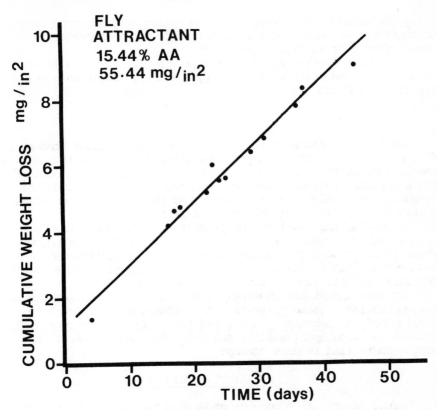

Figure 3. Release rate of non-toxic fly attractant from HERCON dispenser fly strip

III. Air Fresheners. In addition to research on pest control, Health-Chem is currently developing the SCENTSTRIP™which utilizes the HERCON concept instead of the conventional aerosol or gel systems. In this household product, the inner reservoir of the multi-layered unit contains a fragrance or perfume.

The introduction of air freshener strip dispensers into the household market hopefully will contribute to the further reduction of dependence on aerosol products.

Over 30 different kinds of fragrances, scents and perfumes have already been tested in the laboratory for possible use as room fresheners or deodorizers. Because of varying compositions of the fragrances, release rates from the SCENTSTRIPs have been recorded regularly to determine the best construction of a dispenser for each product.

In laboratory tests, linear release rates of fragrances from standard solid fresheners (wherein the fragrance is carried in a gel which shrinks and evaporates in time) have been duplicated

using the SCENTSTRIPs. Complete evaporation of fragrances from
conventional gel dispensers were observed, on the average, to
occur after four to five weeks.

Tests are continuing to develop a SCENTSTRIP with a linear
release rate and which will last significantly longer than conventional products.

CONCLUSION

We believe that with the HERCON controlled release concept of
dispensing active agents, a positive effort is exerted to minimize
the contamination of our environment - by reducing the amount of
toxic material released into our ecosystem, and by reducing the
frequency of pesticide applications. At the same time, we still
obtain the high level of control that is always desired.

Potential applications for products utilizing the HERCON
process are numerous, stretching into every field of entomology
where there is need for toxicants, repellents and attractants -
and beyond, into fields or industries involving fragrances, deodorizers, paints, floor coverings and pet care.

To date almost 100 chemical agents have been incorporated in
our controlled release polymers. As a consequence, there is a
growing body of laboratory and field test data which increasingly
attests the wide applicability and practical importance of this
unique controlled release concept.

LITERATURE CITED

1. Smith, Ray F. In "Concepts of Pest Management". R. L. Rabb
    and F. E. Guthrie (editors). North Carolina State University,
    Raleigh. 1970.
2. Kydonieus, A. F., I. K. Smith, and S. Hyman. Proc. 1975 In-
    ternational Controlled Release Pesticides Symposium, Sept. 8 -
    10:60-75. Wright State University, Ohio. 1975.
3. Anonymous. Chemical Week, August 21:43. 1974.
4. Anonymous. Pest Control, December: 13-14, 38. 1974.
5. Anonymous. Pest Control Technology, November: 28, 30-31.
    1974.
6. Quisumbing, A. R., D. J. Lawatsch, and A. F. Kydonieus. Proc.
    1975 International Controlled Release Pesticides Symposium,
    Sept. 8 - 10:247-257. Wright State University, Ohio. 1975.
7. Moore, Richard C. Efficacy of HERCON Roach-Tapes for German
    Cockroaches. Paper presented at Annual Meeting, Entom. Soc.
    Amer., Nov. 30 - Dec. 4. New Orleans, La. 1975.
8. Moore, Richard C. Personal communication.

Controlled Release from Ultramicroporous Cellulose Triacetate

A. S. OBERMAYER and L. D. NICHOLS

Moleculon Research Corp., 139 Main St., Cambridge, Mass. 02142

A broad range of controlled release investigations have been carried out recently based on the unique properties of an ultra-microporous, open-celled form of cellulose triacetate which has the trade name POROPLASTIC® when in film or membrane form and SUSTRELLE™ when in microbead or powder form for controlled release.

Since this product as formed normally contains between 70% and 98% liquid, it is often referred to as "a solid composed mostly of liquid" or as a "molecular sponge." It is made by a coagulation process which results in a crystalline, non-crosslinked polymer matrix.

For some applications, the properties of Poroplastic are comparable to a typical membrane, sometimes it is considered similar to a hydrogel, and sometimes it responds more like a porous polymer or plastisol. Sustrelle powder is usually compared to a microencapsulated product or an absorbent. However, none of these other materials have the same unique combination of properties.

Experiments which have been performed on Poroplastic film and Sustrelle powder have, thus far, shown no difference in properties that could not be accounted for solely by the difference in surface area-to-volume ratio between film and powder. In almost all cases, initial laboratory investigations are best carried out with the product in film form, because (1) film samples have well-defined dimensions and internal loading capacities; (2) they can easily be handled and weighed; (3) phase changes and shrinkage can be visually observed in the transparent film; (4) excess surface liquid can readily be removed by blotting; and (5) experience gained with film can be roughly translated into subsequent experiments with powder. Any liquid (as long as it is not a solvent for cellulose triacetate) can be impregnated into Sustrelle or Poroplastic by a simple diffusional exchange process of miscible liquids. The most common liquid impregnants are aqueous solutions, alcohols, alcoholic solutions, essential oils, aliphatic or aromatic hydrocarbons, silicone oils, esters, ketones, and liquid monomers. Table I provides a comparison of mechanical properties as a function of content for water and mineral oil filled material.

TABLE I

PROPERTIES OF POROPLASTIC FILM

Property	Aqueous MA-70	Aqueous MA-92	Oil MA-70	Oil MA-92
Composition —				
Resin %	30	8	30	8
Water %	70	92	—	—
Mineral Oil %	—	—	70	92
Apparent Pore Size, Angstroms	14	60	14	60
Specific Gravity	1.09	1.02	1.01	0.91
Tensile Strength, psi	1,300	175	2,300	400
Elongation at Break, %	44	20	41	32
Tensile Strength after Drying, psi	2,600	550	—	—
Elastic Modulus, psi	21,000	200	41,000	3,400
Elongation at Elastic Limit, %	2.4	4.0	2.4	3.1

Hydraulic flux data indicates that Poroplastic film acts as a homogeneous membrane whose flux varies linearly with pressure and inversely with film thickness. The characteristic pore size of either film or powder can be varied by control of the liquid content of the product. Measurements of characteristic pore diameter have been made by determining the ability of film to act as a filter and retain molecules of well-defined dimensions. Table II and Figure I demonstrate the variation in characteristic pore dimensions with the water content of the film.

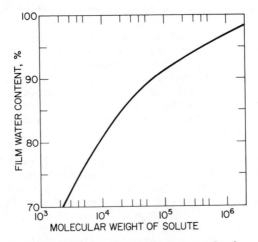

Figure 1. Effect of water content on molecular weight cutoff (90% retention, 0.004-in. film)

TABLE II

RETENTION CHARACTERISTICS OF POROPLASTIC FILM

Solute	Molecular Weight	% Retention at 30 psi on 4 mil Films			
		MA-70	MA-85	MA-92	MA-97.5
Phenyl-Alanine	165	0	0	0	0
Sucrose	342	0	0	0	0
Vitamin B-12	1,355	70	0	0	0
Inulin	5,200	—	10	0	0
Cytochrome C	12,400	>99	87	7	0
Beta Lactoglobulin	35,000	>99	—	—	0
Hemoglobin	64,000	>99	97	—	0
Albumin (Bovine)	67,000	>99	95	25	0
Gamma Globulin	153,000	>99	>99	>98	0
Apoferritin	480,000	>99	>99	>99	42
Blue Dextran 2000	2,000,000	>99	>99	>99	93
Apparent Pore Diameter in Angstroms		14	25	60	>200
Apparent Pore Diameter in Microns		0.0014	0.0025	0.006	>0.02
Water Content by Weight		70%	85%	92%	97.5%

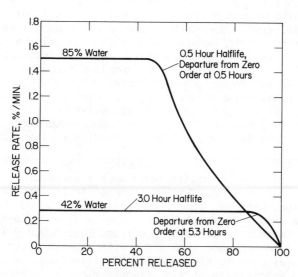

Figure 2.   Release of precipitated zinc fluorescein from MA-85 (85% water) poroplastic film and from a similar sample dried to 42% water

In contradistinction to most gels, Poroplastic and Sustrelle shrink irreversibly when liquid is removed from them, for example, by evaporation. This result occurs because it is not crosslinked and, therefore, is no more stable in its swollen state than after it has been dried. When an internal liquid such as water is partially or wholly removed, shrinkage appears to occur initially with the collapse of the smallest pores and eventually also includes the larger pores. Thus, liquids or solutions can initially be diffused into the ultramicroporous matrix. Subsequently, by a drying process the pores can be partially collapsed so as to reduce the rate of active agent diffusion to the surface of the matrix. This pore collapse process represents the most common method of fixation or reducing the rate of release of active agent.

In general, a three step process is involved in the controlled release of active agent. The steps are: (1) impregnation, (2) fixation, and (3) diffusional release. The impregnation step normally involves a series of diffusional exchanges of miscible liquids until the liquid within the polymer matrix is the active agent or a solution of the active agent to be released. The fixation step utilizes some procedure to retard the rate of diffusion of active agent to the environment. In addition to the pore collapse fixation method described above, there are a number of fixation methods based on the precipitation of active agent within the porous matrix. For example, when the porous matrix is impregnated with a saturated solution, evaporation of the solvent can cause the solute to precipitate within the porous matrix. The solvent evaporation causes partial pore collapse, and the precipitated active agent fills the remaining pore structure and prevents complete collapse. Internal precipitation of an active agent can also be accomplished by a solvent substitution method. In this case, after impregnation with a solution of the active agent, another liquid is added with which the original solvent is miscible but in which the active agent is insoluble. A third precipitation technique involves chemical reaction within the porous matrix to produce a precipitate.

Diffusional release may require a trigger mechanism for initiation. It differs from microencapsulation in that no outer shell is broken, and it differs from common adsorbents such as activated carbon in that no chemical bonding to the substrate is involved.

A specific example which demonstrates the steps involved in this process is the controlled release of fluorescein from a MA-85 Poroplastic film matrix. Sodium fluorescein is very soluble (over 20%) in water, whereas, zinc fluorescein is reported to be soluble only to the extent of about 0.16%. When a 5% aqueous solution of sodium fluorescein is allowed to diffuse into a 0.009 inch water-containing film from one side and a 0.5% aqueous solution of zinc chloride is allowed to diffuse into the film from the other side, an internal precipitate of zinc fluorescein occurs close to the middle of the Poroplastic film. The precipitate can be observed

in the transparent film by the onset of cloudiness and eventually
the film may become distended or brittle as large amounts of zinc
fluorescein precipitate are formed near the center of the film.
In order to insure that only the slightly soluble zinc fluorescein
is present within the film, a final water wash is carried out to
remove excess sodium fluorescein. A film sample so prepared was
then placed in well agitated water and the rate of release of zinc
fluorescein was measured. An almost constant or zero order release
was observed for 30 minutes representing 50% of the loaded material.
This was followed by a declining release rate giving 90% delivery
after two hours. A second piece of zinc fluorescein film prepared
as above was dried from 85% water to 42.5% water and showed a constant release rate for over 5 hours, representing more than 80% of
the contained loading. Rate data for both film samples are shown
in Figure 2.

This type of experiment has been extended to capsule forms.
Poroplastic film can be fabricated into the shape and appearance
of a typical 2-piece hard gelatin capsule. Zinc fluorescein, or
other active agents, can be placed directly within the capsule,
and the rate of release can be measured through the permeable walls
of the capsule. Since the rate determining step is diffusion
through the capsule walls and there is a large reservoir of solid
active agent to maintain a saturation level within the capsule,
constant release rates are commonly measured. Such experiments
have been carried out not only with zinc fluorescein but also with
such diverse compounds as methylene blue and potassium chloride.
Methylene blue is about 3% water soluble, and potassium chloride
is about 30% water soluble. From an experimental standpoint, the
principal complicating feature is the need for the capsule to
withstand an osmotic pressure build up, or alternatively one can
balance the ionic strength and resultant osmotic pressures on both
sides of the capsule wall. When solubilities are below 1%, these
osmotic pressures generally can be ignored. Poroplastic capsules
also offer a convenient form for carrying out laboratory experiments and releasing active agents at a constant rate. We anticipate
that many new applications for Poroplastic capsules will be found.

There are many other similar types of experiments that can be
performed with active agents that have practical utility as
pharmaceuticals, cosmetics, air fresheners, toiletries, household
products and pesticides.

INDEX

INDEX